Combination Therapies 2

Biological Response Modifiers in the
Treatment of Cancer and
Infectious Diseases

Combination Therapies 2

Biological Response Modifiers in the
Treatment of Cancer and
Infectious Diseases

Edited by
Enrico Garaci
University of Rome "Tor Vergata"
Rome, Italy

and
Allan L. Goldstein
The Institute for Advanced Studies in Immunology and Aging
Washington, D.C.

**Sponsored by The Institute for Advanced Studies in
Immunology and Aging**

Springer Science+Business Media, LLC

Library of Congress Cataloging-in-Publication Data

Combination therapies 2 : biological response modifiers in the
  treatment of cancer and infectious diseases / edited by Enrico
  Garaci and Allan L. Goldstein.
       p. cm.
    "Sponsored by the Institute for Advanced Studies in Immunology and
  Aging."
    Proceedings of the Second International Symposium on Combination
  Therapies, held May 1-3, 1992, in Acireale, Sicily, Italy.
    Includes bibliographical references and index.
    ISBN 978-1-4613-6289-0   ISBN 978-1-4615-2964-4 (eBook)
    DOI 10.1007/978-1-4615-2964-4
    1. Biological response modifiers--Congresses. 2. Cancer-
  -Chemotherapy--Congresses. 3. Communicable diseases--Chemotherapy-
  -Congresses. 4. Chemotherapy, Combined--Congresses. I. Garaci, E.
  (Enrico) II. Goldstein, Allan L.   III. Institute for Advanced
  Studies in Immunology & Aging. IV. International Symposium on
  Combination Therapies (2nd : 1992 : Acireale, Italy) V. Title:
  Combination therapies two.
    [DNLM: 1. Biological Response Modifiers--congresses. 2. Combined
  Modality Therapy--congresses. 3. Communicable Diseases--therapy-
  -congresses. 4. Drug Therapy, Combination--congresses.
  5. Immunotherapy--congresses. 6. Neoplasms--therapy--congresses.
  WB 330 C7312 1992]
  RC271.B53C662 1993
  615'.704--dc20
  DNLM/DLC
  for Library of Congress   93-36641
                                                             CIP

Proceedings of the Second International Symposium on Combination Therapies:
New and Emerging Uses for Biological Response Modifiers in the Treatment
of Cancer and Infectious Diseases, held May 1-3, 1992, in Acireale, Sicily, Italy

ISBN 978-1-4613-6289-0

© 1993 Springer Science+Business Media New York
Originally published by Plenum Press New York in 1993
Softcover reprint of the hardcover 1st edition 1993

PREFACE

The 2nd International Symposium on Combination Therapies brought together several hundred of the leading researchers, scientists and clinicians in this area to discuss new and emerging uses for biological response modifiers (BRM's) in the treatment of cancer and infectious diseases. The meeting was held during May 1-3, 1992 in Acireale, Sicily (Italy). It was hosted by Professor G. Nicoletti (U. of Catania) and organized by the Institute for Advanced Studies in Immunology and Aging (Washington, D.C.) in collaboration with the University of Rome "Tor Vergata," the University of Catania and The George Washington University Medical Center. The synergy exhibited between BRM's and conventional therapies including bone marrow and other lymphoid cell transplants is a rapidly expanding area with significant promise for the treatment of human diseases. Advances in this area of biomedicine are leading to the rapid development of new therapeutic approaches that are being applied clinically as both primary and adjuvant therapy to enhance the effectiveness of conventional treatments.

The 2nd International Symposium on Combination Therapy provided a setting for the exchange of new scientific information regarding the emerging uses for BRM's alone or in combination with conventional therapies. The 1st International Symposium on Combination Therapies was held in 1991 in Washington, D.C. The very rapid advances in this field of immunology have led the organizers and participants to conclude that it would be worthwhile to hold yearly meetings alternating between Europe and the United States in order to facilitate the rapid communication of new ideas, technologies, and advancements in this area so that developments can be translated into meaningful clinical treatments in the shortest time possible.

It is clear to the scientists and clinicians in this field that the decade of the 90's offers enormous opportunities for utilizing the myriad of immune molecules produced by the lymphoid system to augment and regulate the immune network and to influence therapy. Recent studies indicating the BRM's may synergize with conventional treatments are expanding our knowledge of their use and are providing broad and novel insights into understanding the underlying mechanisms utilized by neoplastic and infectious agents to evade destruction by the immune system. The increased ability to intervene to correct immune dysfunctions with one or more BRM's in combination with other BRM's or by conventional therapies is rapidly expanding our knowledge of the ways in which the immune system is regulated.

The scientific program, which was organized by Professor Enrico Garaci (President of the University of Rome "Tor Vergata" and President of the Medical Committee of Consiglio Nazionale delle Ricerche [C.N.R.]) and Professor G. Nicoletti (University of Catania), brought together many outstanding scientists and clinicians from the United States and Europe with diverse interests in the field of BRM's. The program included first reports of a number of experimental and clinical studies in cancer and infectious diseases as well as an interesting number of basic research projects which are helping to elucidate the ever-widening range of the action of BRM's.

The book is divided into three major sections. In the first section, entitled "Mechanism of Action and Rationale for the Use of Biological Response Modifiers, Differentiating Agents and Nucleoside Analogues in Combination," the strategy for utilizing BRM's such as IL-2, thymosin α_1, interferon, TNF and other compounds is reported along with the rationale for using these agents in combination as well as the challenges presented for the clinical lab with regard to monitoring these agents.

In the second section, entitled "Combination Chemotherapy and BMR Therapy in the Treatment of Cancer," attention is focused on the role of triazene compounds, BRM's and conventional therapies in protocols specifically designed to stop the growth of malignant tumors.

The third section of the book reviews novel approaches to the use of single agent and combination BRM therapy in the treatment of infectious diseases, AIDS and autoimmunity. In this section, results are presented for a number of interesting experimental studies in mice involving BRM and anti-cytokine therapy along with the first report (in English) from China of the results of clinical trials with a thymic hormone extract (thymopeptidin) as well as the results of promising new treatments of Hepatitis B and C with thymosin α_1 or combinations of beta interferon and inosine pranobex. This section also presents a number of papers dealing with approaches to the treatment of AIDS including potential novel combinations of antivirals and BRM's.

In a period of only one year since the last meeting, extraordinary progress in the clinical utilization of BRM's as primary therapy and as adjuncts to current treatment regimens has been made. This volume should be of significant interest to both basic and clinical scientists interested in an excellent overview of current and projected clinical applications of BRM's that are under investigation or are being considered for clinical studies. This volume should also be of major interest to other health care professionals who are interested in getting a future snapshot of many of the novel therapeutic approaches that are emerging in the treatment of cancer, AIDS and other diseases associated with immune dysfunction in one of the most rapidly changing areas of biological investigation.

Enrico Garaci

Allan L. Goldstein

CONTENTS

SECTION II - COMBINATION CHEMOTHERAPY AND BRM THERAPY IN THE TREATMENT OF CANCER

SECTION III - SINGLE AND COMBINATION THERAPY WITH BRM'S IN THE TREATMENT OF INFECTIOUS DISEASES, AIDS AND AUTOIMMUNITY

CYTOKINE SYNERGY IN IMMUNOTHERAPY

John W. Hadden, Piotr Malec, Anutosh Saha and Elba M. Hadden

Department of Internal Medicine
University of South Florida Medical College
Tampa, FL 33612

The normal function of the immune system involves a myriad of synergistic interactions among cytokines of many types (e.g. lymphokines, monokines and thymic hormones). It seems then eminently logical that efforts to modify immune function with exogenous cytokines should involve the employment of combinations. It will be the intent of this chapter to summarize our recent efforts to employ combination therapy to restore and direct the thymus-dependent T cell system.

The origins of the work go back to initial efforts to determine the relevant molecules involved in T lymphocyte development. It was initially thought that thymic hormones induced T lymphocyte differentiation[1] and promoted intrathymic development,[2] yet subsequent studies failed to show that thymic hormones induced intrathymic maturation.[3,4] It became evident that interleukin-2 (IL_2) was involved in T cell maturation as well as T cell proliferation.[3,4] Information then emerged concerning the IL_2 receptor (IL_2r) α and β and the regulation of IL_2r display by interleukin-1 (IL_1) and it was subsequently shown that the synergy between IL_1 and IL_2 which involves the regulation of high affinity IL_2r display is expressed throughout the T cell lineage from the prothymocyte on.[7,8] Developing thymocytes were shown to be responsive to interleukins including IL_1, IL_2, IL_3, IL_4, IL_6, IL_7, IL_{10} and granulocyte-macrophage colony stimulating factor (GM-CSF) (see 1 for review). It became evident that thymic epithelial cells and perhaps stromal cells also produce interleukins (e.g. IL_1, IL_6, IL_7, G-CSF and GM-CSF). These interleukins are envisioned to regulate T cell development in a complex way which involves cellular interactions and T lymphocyte cytokine production, as well. For example, T lymphocytes bind to thymic epithelial

Combination Therapies 2, Edited by A.L. Goldstein
and E. Garaci Plenum Press, New York, 1993

cells (TEC) and respond with IL_2-dependent proliferation mediated by IL_2r expression. TEC and thymocytes bind via CD-2: LFA-3 and LFA-1:ICAM-1 ligands (11,12) and the former is a secretory signal for TEC to produce IL_1 (12).[14] IL_1 induces in turn IL_6 and GM-CSF production by TEC. It also induces the secretion of zinc-thymulin complex by TEC.[15] Collectively, these interleukins can be viewed as promoting thymocyte proliferation and maturation.

The role of thymic hormones in this process of thymocyte maturation becomes unclear since the hormones seem to have little effect on the process. TEC secrete thymosin α_1 and zinc-thymulin complex, the first in a constituitive manner and the latter in a regulated way induced by IL_1, prolactin, hydrocortisone, sex steroids, thyroid hormone and zinc itself (see 9 for review and references, 15). Experiments on mature T lymphocytes indicate that thymosin α_1 and thymulin-zinc complex regulate the expansion of IL_2r^+ cells in a synergistic manner with IL_1; this process apparently involves IL_2 production and high affinity IL_2r expression.[15,16] Collectively, these thymic hormone peptide actions can be viewed as enforcing the expression of a T lymphocyte program involving IL_1, IL_2 and IL_2r in the expansion of IL_2r^+ T lymphocytes. One hypothesis which serves to integrate these various observations is that thymic hormone peptides induce pre-T lymphocytes to express this genetically determined program and that they maintain its continued expression throughout the life of the T lymphocyte in the thymus and in the periphery. It follows then, that interleukins are the moment-to-moment signals which regulate the stepwise development of T lymphocytes. It follows further that if one wants to maximize the ability to induce T lymphocyte development, a combination of cytokines and thymic hormones would be most effective.

We designed experiments[17] to test this postulate using aged, retired breeder mice (female, Balb/c, 9-12 months of age) whose thymuses had undergone a degree of involution compared to 6-8 week old mice (thymus (mg)/body weight (gm) ratio $0.92 \pm .05$ vs 2.64 ± 0.16). We administered two doses of hydrocortisone (0.5 mg) which further involute the thymus (70%) by depleting the double positive ($CD4^+$ $CD8^+$) cortical thymocytes. Spleen weight was also reduced with a 30% loss of mature T lymphocytes. To attempt to restore T lymphocytes in thymus and spleen, we administered five daily treatments from the nadir of the thymic and splenic involution and then assessed organ weight, cellularity, T cells and subset numbers and functions. Function was evaluated with proliferative responses in vitro to stimulation with rIL_1, r or natural IL_2, mixed interleukins (BC-IL), or the T cell mitogen, concanavalin A (Con A).

The treatments included:

1) natural buffy coat interleukins (BC-IL, 50 units IL_2 equivalence/mouse)
2) natural IL_2 (50 units/mouse)
3) $r-IL_1$ (4 ng/mouse)
4) combination of 2 and 3
5) thymosin fraction V (TF5, 100 ug/mouse)
6) combination of 1 and 5

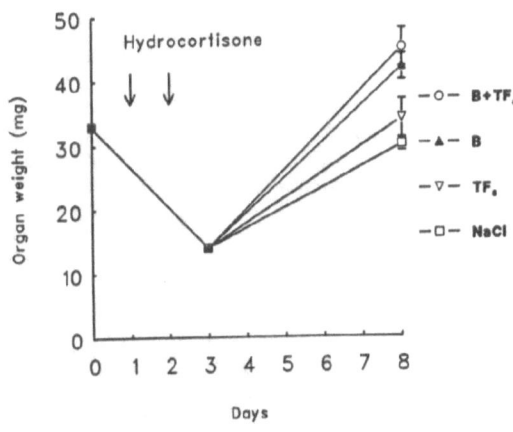

Figure 1

Balb/c female mice, 9-12 months old were given a chemical thymectomy with 2 consecutive doses of hydrocortisone. On the third day, groups of 5 mice were injected daily for 5 days with saline, TF_5, BC-IL (B), or combination of the last two. The mean weight of the thymuses at the end of each treatment are shown $\pm$ SEM (p < .01).

In vitro responses of thymocytes and splenocytes to interleukins after various in vivo treatments.

In vivo treatments for 5 days were with BC-IL, TF_5, and the combination of BC-IL with TF_5 or thymosin α_1 ($T\alpha_1$). The in vitro proliferative responses to r-IL, $r-IL_2$ and BC-IL were measured and expressed as ratios to control $\pm$ SEM (p < 0.05).

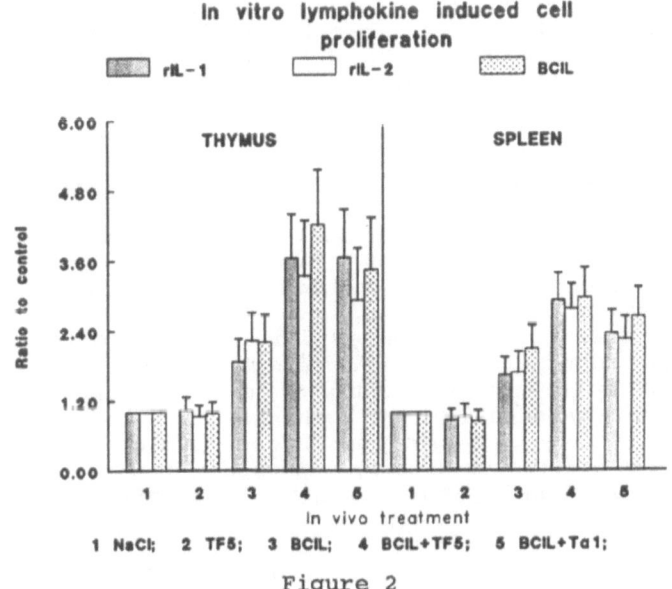

Figure 2

The results were clear cut in showing that of the treatments only BC-IL accelerated the recovery of organ weight and cellularity. Figure 1 shows the recovery of thymus weight induced by BC-IL $\pm$ thymosin fraction V. The recovery of thymocytes involved significant increases in both immature (double positive $CD4^+ CD8^+$) and mature (single positive $CD4^+$ or $CD8^+$) phenotypes. Also, BC-IL treatment greatly increased the in vitro response of thymocytes to interleukins (ILs) and Con A stimulation and of splenocytes to IL stimulation. IL_1, IL_2, their combination or thymosin fraction V had no significant effect on these parameters.

Interestingly, thymosin fraction V showed a marked synergy with BC-IL on the responses of thymocytes to ILs and Con A and of splenocytes to ILs.[17] Figure 2 shows the effect of in vivo treatment with BC-IL $\pm$ TF5 (columns 3 and 4) on in vitro responses of thymocytes and splenocytes to ILs. Column 5 shows that much of the effect of TF5 (100 ug/mouse) is reproduced by thymosin α_1 ($T\alpha_1$) (5 ug/mouse). These studies support the hypothesis that ILs and thymic hormone peptides act in concert to promote T lymphocyte development and function.

Studies by Fabris and coworker[18] point to a central role of zinc supplementation in restoring age-related thymic involution and increasing the number of zinc-thymulin secreting cells in thymus and zinc-thymulin levels in serum. Our preliminary studies (A. Saha and J.W. Hadden, unpublished) show that, in the hydrocortisone induced "chemical thymectomy" model discussed above, both oral zinc supplementation or zinc-thymulin treatment with BC-IL treatment promotes the responsiveness of thymocytes to ILs and Con A and of splenocytes to ILs in a manner similar to thymosin fraction V and α_1. These results suggest that, with BC-IL, oral zinc supplementation may achieve the same effect as thymic hormone peptide injection.

In an effort to put this hypothesis to the test in humans, we devised a cancer therapy treatment protocol involving the employment of BC-IL and oral zinc supplementation in conjunction with low-dose cyclophosphamide and indomethacin in four patients with head and neck cancer. This study was performed with Dr. James Endicott, Paulette Skipper and Dr. Paul Baekey at the University of South Florida Medical College and presented at the 3rd International Conference on Head and Neck Cancer.[19] The origins of this protocol are complex. As I have detailed, we have developed evidence that BC-IL with zinc supplementation should be immunorestorative via effects to promote T cell development. Head and neck cancer patients are known to develop significant cellular immune deficiency even when the cancer is regional and not widespread. This cellular immune deficiency involves T lymphocytopenia, depressed mitogen and mixed leukocyte culture (MLR) responses, and hypoergy or anergy.[20,21,22]

These patients also show evidence of suppressor cells of both the adherent and nonadherent type.[20] Nonadherent suppressor cells are presumably T cells and the suppressive function of these cells have been shown[23] to be abrogated for up to 21 days by a single low dose of cyclophosphamide (300 mg/m^3).[24] The use of low dose cyclophosphamide has been shown by others[24,25] to enhance immunotherapy in patients with malignant melanoma. The adherent suppressor cells are presumably monocytes and the suppressive function of these cells has been shown to be abrogated by administration of a prostaglandin synthesis inhibitor like indomethacin. The use of indomethacin to enhance tumor responses has been presented by Lala in this text. We thus incorporated low dose cyclophosphamide into the trial to abrogate suppressor cell function, that is as a "contrasuppressive" therapy.

Finally, the BC-IL was administered perilymphatically in the contralateral neck region where the lymphatic system was perhaps intact despite irradiation. The rationale for this approach derives from work which indicates that cytokines act as an adjuvant, particularly when administered to regional lymph nodes.[26,27] Pulley et al.[28] showed that intralymphatic BC-IL had a potent effect in malignant melanoma patients to expand regional nodes. Finally, and importantly, Cortesina et al.[29,30] had observed that perilymphatic low dose natural IL_2 induced partial responses in 13 of 20 head and neck cancer patients and this was associated with infiltration of tumor with eosinophils and $CD25^+$ T cells presumed to be lymphokine activated killer (LAK) cells. Others could not reproduce this with a r-IL_2[31]; we thus employed the BC-IL in low dose (200 units IL_2 equivalence) perilymphatically as 10 daily injections after the low dose cyclophosphamide in an effort to provide an adjuvant stimulus for tumor antigen resident in the region.

Three of the four patients treated had been previously treated with unilateral radical neck dissection and irradiation but had failed and had significant regional recurrences. These patients had T lymphocytopenia (mean CD3 count 600/mm^3) and two had inverted CD4/CD8 ratios (without evidence of HIV infection). Two showed depressed DTH responses to recall antigens and to intracutaneous injection of the BC-IL; the third was anergic to renal antigens as well as the BC-IL. The fourth patient was treated on diagnosis of the primary with neck metastases prior to surgery and was immunologically normal.

All of the tumors were squamous cell cancers of the head and neck and all showed evidence of tumor infiltrating lymphocytes (TIL) but no tumor necrosis prior to treatment. It is notable that these TILs are routinely unrecorded by the pathologist in such specimens. The responses of these patients are interesting. The two patients who had recurrent disease after surgery and irradiation and who responded to intradermal injection of the BC-IL with a DTH response underwent partial regression (>80%) of their tumors over two 21 day cycles. The regressions are notable in that they began at day 7 of the BC-IL treatment and continued when the BC-IL was not given (days 12-21). The responses occurred on the contralateral side and "upstream" from a lymphatic standpoint. The treatment was performed on an outpatient basis and had negligible side effects (only fatigue in one patient). These two responding patients were treated for seven 21 day cycles and maintained substantial regressions. When treatment ceased, tumor recurrence and death followed at approximately six months due to local complications (carotid blow out) without known visceral metastases. Initially, survival was predicted to be < 3 months without treatment.

The patient who was anergic to recall antigens and the BC-IL showed no tumor response, as expected. The fourth patient was treated postoperatively on the ipsilateral side and showed a partial response (50%) prior to surgical resection. Apparently complete removal of tumor was achieved.

It is notable that all three of the lymphopenic patients showed significant increases in total T (CD3) cells (Figure 3). $CD4^+$ T lymphocytes increased in all 3 patients and $CD8^+$ T lymphocytes increased in 2 of the patients. We take these increases to reflect tentative support for the thymic mobilization hypothesis although other sources (e.g. spleen and lymph node could be postulated).

The three responding patients showed evidence of increased infiltration tumor sites with both $CD4^+$ and $CD8^+$ T lymphocytes with negligible B lymphocytes. In one patient, tumor sloughing from patent neck sites with granulation tissue formation obscured tumor immunhistochemistry; however, in the other two responders, the histology was that of classic DTH with accumulation of activated macrophages and granulomatous changes in association with tumor necrosis and fragmentation. Nonspecific tumoricidal processes (e.g. NK, LAK) could not account for the nature and timing of these responses. The appearance of classic DTH and T lymphocyte mobilization in blood and in the tumor sites distinguish our findings from the previous studies.[30,31] Our findings indicate that the combination treatment employed here activated the immune system to tumor-related antigens and induced, without significant side effects, major progressive tumor responses mediated by cellular immune mechanisms.

These studies are preliminary but they allow several important insights when integrated with the prior literature. These patients with head and neck cancer had pre-existing immunity to squamous cell cancer (as evidenced by the TIL). Although they had only regional disease they developed profound immunodeficiency following surgery and irradiation. Combined immunotherapy partially reversed the immunodeficiency and elicited effective, apparently tumor specific, immunity. Since this is a first attempt yielding palliative responses, it seems likely that modification of this protocol will be necessary to effect more lasting and perhaps complete responses. A challenge exists to obviate iatrogenic immunosuppression to improve the chances of response and to more effectively restore endogenously suppressed responses as evidenced in the anergic, unresponsive patient. The immunodeficiency of these patients involves not only depressed T cell numbers but also depressed efferent limb responses i.e. the monocyte/macrophage mediated responses to intradermal BC-IL. The nature of the immunosuppressive mechanisms have not been adequately elucidated; we have found evidence in several of the head and neck patients of potently immunosuppressive serum suggesting soluble tumor derived factors as well.

It is difficult to conclude more from these initial experiments but solid hints have been obtained that suggest combination therapy (BC-IL, thymic peptides, and zinc supplemention) is useful to reverse thymic involution associated with hydrocortisone treatment in one model which mimics stress. It will be important to determine whether similar effects occur in thymic involution due to aging, polytrauma, irradiation, retrovirus infection, etc. Solid hints have also been obtained to indicate that multiagent immunotherapy offers the prospect of less toxic, more effective treatment for cancer patients. Twenty years of development in immunopharmacology is beginning to pay off in clinical progress. The future prospects seem immense.

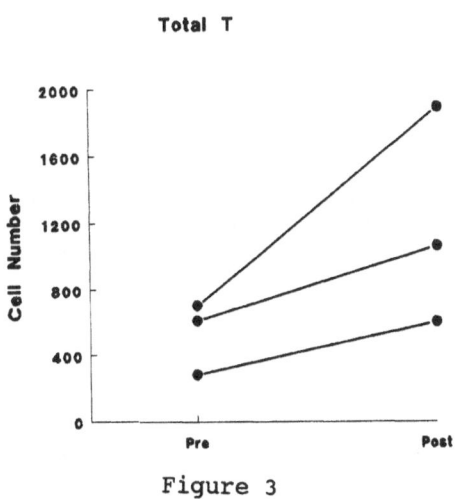

Total T

Figure 3

Effect of BC-IL treatment on total T-lymphocyte counts in blood of 3 patients pre and post BC-IL treatment.

Bibliography

1. K. Komuro and E.A. Boyse, Induction of T lymphocytes from precursor cells in vitro by a product of the thymus, J. Exp. Med. 138:479-484 (1973).

2. A.L. Goldstein, Ed., "Thymic hormones and lymphokines", Plenum Press, New York (1984).

3. S.S. Chen, J.S. Tung, S. Gillis, R.A. Good and J.W. Hadden, Changes in surface antigens of immature thymocytes under the influence of T cell growth factor and thymic factors, Proc. Natl. Acad. Sci. 80:5980-5984 (1983).

4. P. Andrews, K. Shortman, R. Scollay, E.F. Potworowski, A.M. Kruisbeek, G. Goldstein, N. Trainin and J-F. Bach, Thymus hormones do not induce proliferative ability or cytolytic function on PNA+ cortical thymocytes. Cell. Immunol. 91:455-466 (1985).

5. P.J. Conlon, C.S. Henney and S. Gillis, Cytokine-dependent thymocyte responses, J. Immunol. 128:797-804 (1982).

6. J.W. Hadden, S. Specter and E.M. Hadden, Effects of T cell growth factor (interleukin 2) and thymic hormones on prothymocytes and immature thymocytes, Lymph. Res. 5:49-54 (1986).

7. W. Falk, B. Kyewski, D. Mannel and P.H. Kramer, Growth of double negative mouse thymocytes is initiated by the combined action of interleukin I and interleukin 2, Lymph. Res. 6:75 (1987).

8. J.W. Hadden, H. Chen, Y. Wang and E.M. Hadden, Strategies of immune reconstitution: effects of lymphokines on murine T cell development in vitro and in vivo, Life Sci. AIDS Comm. 44:5-12 (1989).

9. J.W. Hadden, Thymic endocrinology, Int. J. Immunopharmacol. 14:345-352 (1992).

10. P.T. Le, L. W. Vollger, B.F. Haynes and K.H. Singer, Ligand binding to the LFA-3 cell adhesion molecule induces IL-1 production by human thymic epithelial cells, J. Immun. 144:4541-4547 (1990).

11. M. Wiranowska, T. Kaido, G. Caspritz, J. Cook and J.W. Hadden, Interleukin-2 and coculture with thymic epithelial cells synergistically induce prothymocyte differentiation and proliferation, Thymus 10:231-235 (1987).

12. S.M. Denning, J. Kurtzburg, P.T. Le, D.T. Tuck, K.H. Singer and B.F. Haynes, Human thymic epithelial cells directly induce activation of autologous immature thymocytes, Proc. Natl. Acad. Sci. 85:3125-3129 (1988).

13. A. Galy, E.M. Hadden, J-P. Touraine and J.W. Hadden, Effects of cytokines on human thymic epithelial cells in culture: IL1 induces thymic epithelial cell proliferation and change in morphology, Cell Immunol. 124:13-27 (1989).

14. A. Galy, C.A. Dinarello, T.S. Kupper and J.W. Hadden, Production of cytokines by recombinant IL1-stimulated human thymic epithelial cells in vitro, Cell Immunol. 129:161-175, (1990).

15. J.A. Coto, E.M. Hadden, M. Sauro, N. Zorn and J.W. Hadden, Interleukin 1 regulates secretion of zinc-thymulin by thymic epithelial cells and its action on T lymphocyte proliferation and nuclear protein kinase C, Proc. Natl. Acad. Sci. (1992, in press).

16. M.B. Sztein, S.R. Serrate and A.L. Goldstein, Modulation of interleukin 2 receptor expression on human lymphocytes by thymic hormones, Proc. Natl. Acad. Sci. 83:6107-6111 (1986).

17. E.M. Hadden, P. Malec, M. Sosa and J.W. Hadden, Mixed interleukins and thymosin fraction V synergistically induce T lymphocyte development in hydrocortisone-treated aged mice, Cell. Immunol. (1992, in press).

18. E. Mocchegiani and N. Fabris, "In vivo" and "in vitro" effect of zinc on thymic efficiency in old age, in: "Abstracts of 6th Int. Cong. of Int. Assoc. Biol. Gerontol.", Ancona, Italy, (1991).

19. J.W. Hadden, E.M. Hadden, P. Baekey, P. Skipper and J. N. Endicott, Adjuvant nonrecombinant interleukins and contra-suppressive agents induces immune regression in head and neck cancer, Arch. Otolaryngol. (1992, in press).

20. N.T. Berlinger, E.Y. Hilal, H.F. Oettgen and R.A. Good, Deficient cell-mediated immunity in head and neck cancer patients secondary to autologous suppressive immune cells, Laryngoscope 88:470-481 (1978).

21. G.T. Wolf, Head and neck tumor immunology, in: "Immunobiology, Histophysiology and Tumor Immunology in Otolaryngology", Proc. 2nd Int. Acad. Conf., Utrecht, The Netherlands, (1987).

22. H.J. Wanebo, T. Jones, R. Pace, R. Cantrell and P. Levine, Immune restoration with interleukin-2 in patient with squamous cell carcinoma of the head and neck, Amer. J. Surg. 158:356-360 (1989).

23. D. Berd, H.C. Maguire and M.J. Mastrangelo, Potentiation of human cell-mediated and humoral immunity by low-dose cyclophosphamide, Cancer Res. 44:5439-5443 (1984).

24. D. Berd, H.C. Maguire Jr., P. McCue and M.J. Mastrangelo, Treatment of metastatic melanoma with an autologous tumor-cell vaccine: clinical and immunologic results in 64 patients, J. Clin. Oncol. 8:1858-1867 (1990).

25. M.S. Mitchell, R.A. Kempf, W. Harel, H. Shau, W.D. Boswell, S. Lind, G. Dean, J. Moore and E.C. Bradley, Efficacy of low-dose cyclophosphamide and interleukin-2 in melanoma, in: "Advances in Immunopharmacology 4", J.W. Hadden, F. Spreafico, Y. Yamamura, K.F. Austen, P. Dukor and K. Masek, eds, Pergamon Press, Oxford (1989).

26. J.H.L. Playfair and A.W. Heath, Cytokines - The new generation of adjuvants for vaccines?, in: "Immunotherapeutic prospects of infectious diseases", K.N. Masihi and W. Lange, eds., Springer-Verlag, Berlin, (1990).

27. K. Kelly, Harvey, Sadler and D. Dumonde, Accelerated cytodifferentiation of antibody-secreting cells in Guinea pig lymph nodes stimulated by sheep erythrocytes and lymphokines, Clin. Exp. Immunol. 21:141-154 (1975).

28. M.S. Pulley, V. Nagendran, J.M. Edwards, D.C. Dumonde, Intravenous, intralesional and endolymphatic administration of lymphokines in human cancer, Lymph. Res. 5:S157-S163, (1986).

29. G. Cortesina, A. DeStefani, M. Giovarelli, M.G. Barioglio, G.P. Cavallo, C. Jemma amd G. Forni, Treatment of recurrent squamous cell carcinoma of the head and neck with low doses of interleukin-2 injected perilymphatically, Cancer 62:2482-2485, (1988).

30. G. Cortesina, A. DeStefani, E. Galeazzi, M. Bussi, C. Giordano, G.P. Cavallo, C. Jemma, S. Vai, G. Forni and G. Valente, The effect of preoperative local interleukin-2 (IL-2) injections in patients with head and neck squamous cell carcinoma, Acta. Otolaryngol. 111:428-433 (1991).

31. V. Mattijssen, P.H. DeMulder, J.H. Schornagel, J. Verweij, P. Van den Broak, A. Galazka, S. Roy and D.J. Ruiter, Clinical and immunopathological results of a phase II study of perilymphatically injected recombinant interleukin 2 in locally far advanced, nonpretreated head and neck squamous cell carcinoma, J. Immunother. 10:63-68 (1991).

MONITORING COMBINATION THERAPY TRIALS: NEW CHALLENGES

FOR THE CLINICAL LABORATORY

Jeffrey L. Rossio[1], Helen C. Rager[1], Carol S. Goundry[1], and
Walter J. Urba[2]

[1]Lymphokine Testing Laboratory, Clinical Immunology Services
[2]Clinical Services Program
PRI/DynCorp, NCI-Frederick Cancer Research & Development Center
Frederick, Maryland 21702, USA

INTRODUCTION

Cytokines are, with few exceptions, normally undetectable in serum. This is primarily due to their role as local mediators of immunological signals among cells participating in immune or inflammatory reactions. However, therapeutic administration of cytokines often results in measurable serum cytokine levels which may be clinically informative. In addition, clinical and animal model data show that injection of one cytokine often leads to the induction of appearance of significant amounts of other cytokines. For example, the administration of IL-1 leads to measurable serum IL-6 and G-CSF; IL-2 administration induces interferon-gamma production. Clinical side effects may be due to the presence of such induced cytokine(s); these side effects may or may not be related to the intended therapeutic role(s) of the agents. Thus, knowledge of the spectrum of cytokines present may guide clinical cytokine use (Oppenheim, et al., 1992; Rossio et al., 1992). It is now possible to measure a large number of cytokines by immunoassay (ELISA or RIA) to a sensitivity of 50 picograms/ml or less. Levels of some cytokine receptors (e.g., IL-2, TNF) can also be measured in serum and other body fluids. The decisions as to which cytokines or receptors to monitor during clinical trials, and when to look for them, depends partly on empirical observations, and partly on an understanding of the immunological interactions involved (Clemens, et al., 1987; Coligan, et al., 1991; Dawson, 1991). The addition of secondary therapeutic agents, which may be immunosuppressive or stimulatory, further complicates the picture.

ACTIVITIES OF CYTOKINES

Because many cytokines have been described, and new cytokines are continually being discovered, it is useful to classify these substances according to their primary in vivo biological effects. Figure 1 shows one such classification.

Combination Therapies 2, Edited by A.L. Goldstein
and E. Garaci   Plenum Press, New York, 1993

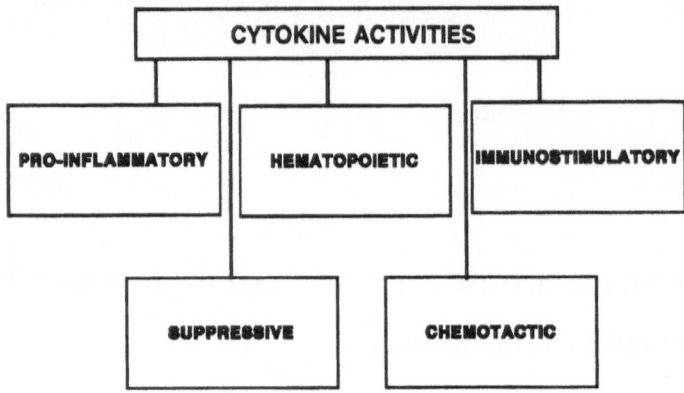

Figure 1. Classification of Cytokine Activities.

Most cytokines have many activities, involving numerous target tissues or cell types. Because of this, some cytokines may appear in more than one of the arbitrary categories set up in Figure 1. A preliminary sorting of cytokines by the above scheme is shown in Table 1 (Aggarwal, et al, 1991; Thomson, 1991; Wagstaff, 1990).

THE PRO-INFLAMMATORY CYTOKINES

One of the clinically most interesting aspects of cytokine monitoring is based on the observation that certain cytokines appear to be associated with ongoing inflammatory conditions, and are inferred to have a role in the initiation and propagation of inflammatory responses (Dinarello, 1990). IL-1, IL-6 and TNF are measurable in the serum of patients with a number of inflammatory conditions. IL-1 was first described as an inflammatory mediator in bacterial infections, and has been implicated in fever production, induction of acute phase protein, effects on vascular endothelium, and as a lymphocyte activator. TNF has been shown to have a similar spectrum of effects, including a primary role in the induction of toxic shock. IL-6 is currently being promoted as an early indicator of inflammation and sepsis in toxemia of pregnancy and other infections (Billiau et al, 1991; Zentella, et al., 1991). These cytokines have also been detected in situ in tissues in areas of inflammation, and by molecular techniques such as reverse transcription of mRNA, followed by PCR analysis of cytokine cDNA in tissue extracts and blood cells.

All of the cytokines in this group can be analyzed by commercial ELISA assays, available from several sources. None of them are normally detectable in human serum, so any measurable levels (about 50 pg/ml or more) may be clinically significant. Some therapies with biological response modifiers can induce these cytokines, which become in this instance a means of monitoring the immunological effects of therapy.

Table 1. Assignment of cytokines to activity categories based on major effector activities.

I. Pro-inflammatory Cytokines

        Interleukin-1 alpha (IL-1 alpha)
        Interleukin-1 beta (IL-1 beta)
        Interleukin-6 (IL-6)
        Interleukin-8 (IL-8, NAP-1)
        Tumor Necrosis Factor-alpha (TNF-alpha)
        Tumor Necrosis Factor-beta (TNF-beta)

II. Hematopoietic Cytokines

        Interleukin-3 (IL-3)
        Interleukin-7 (IL-7)
        Interleukin-11 (IL-11)
        Stem Cell Factor (SCF, kit ligand)
        Granulocyte Colony Stimulating Factor (G-CSF)
        Granulocyte-Macrophage CSF (GM-CSF)
        Macrophage CSF (M-CSF, CSF-1)
        Erythropoietin (EPO)

III. Immunostimulatory Cytokines

        Interleukin-1 (IL-1, alpha and beta)
        Interleukin-2 (IL-2)
        Interleukin-4 (IL-4)
        Interleukin-5 (IL-5)
        Interleukin-6 (IL-6)
        Interleukin-9 (IL-9)
        Interleukin-12 (IL-12)
        Interferon-gamma (IFN-gamma)

IV. Suppressive Cytokines

        Transforming Growth Factor-beta (TGF-beta)
        Interleukin-10 (IL-10)
        IL-1 Receptor Antagonist (IL-1ra)
        [Soluble Cytokine Receptors]

V. Chemotactic Cytokines

        Interleukin-8 (IL-8)
        NAP-2
        MCAF
        MGSA/GRO
        MCP-1

THE HEMATOPOIETIC CYTOKINES

Among the most immediately useful cytokines for therapy are those factors which affect the production and/or maturation of hematopoietic cells from bone marrow (Gordon, 1991; Metcalf, 1984). In particular, erythropoietin is already licensed to relieve depressed erythropoiesis associated with renal malfunctions and some infectious diseases, such as AIDS. Oncologists have found several other factors, particularly G-CSF and GM-CSF, useful in patients whose marrow is depressed by cancer chemotherapy (Williams, et al., 1991). One newly described cytokine, IL-11, may have thrombopoietic activity, which would also be of great use in the oncology setting. Many of the cytokines in this group are in advanced clinical trials (e.g., IL-l, IL-3), while others are still in the developmental stages (e.g., SCF, IL-7).

The role of the clinical lab in developmental trials is to monitor cytokines in serum and other fluids to determine pharmacokinetic parameters, effective dose levels, and appropriate administration schedules. Commercial ELISA kits are available for all of the cytokines in this group. Based on experiences with EPO, it is unclear whether or not cytokine levels will need to be monitored clinically in patients receiving routine care. The role of monitoring may be restricted to research studies, and investigations of deficiencies and/or inhibitors resulting in distinct clinical sequelae. Such deficiency diseases have not as yet been described.

THE IMMUNOSTIMULATORY CYTOKINES

The largest group of cytokines includes factors involved in the initiation and amplification of immune responses. These cytokines are probably present during any ongoing immunological response. However, the greatest use of clinical monitoring is to measure the levels of exogenously introduced cytokines, used therapeutically. IL-2 has recently been licensed for use in the treatment of certain types of cancer, and it is important, considering the marked side effects of this material, to know serum levels, and to make sure safe doses are used.

In addition, it has been proposed that these cytokines can be partitioned into two groups, produced by different sub-populations of T cells, which effect primarily either the cell-mediated or the humoral arms of the immune response (Mossman, 1991). One group, produced by T_H1 helper cells, includes IL-2, IFN-gamma and TNF-beta, which are viewed as promoters of the cell-mediated responses. The other group, produced by T_H2 helper cells, includes promoters of the antibody response, such as IL-4, IL-5, IL-6. Although these classifications in humans are not absolute, laboratory monitoring could theoretically indicate differential effects of cytokine treatment, vaccine administration, or other therapy on immune responses.

Most of the cytokines in this group can be measured by ELISA assay, although commercial tests for IL-9 and IL-12 are just now being developed.

SUPPRESSIVE CYTOKINES

An important area of cytokine biology, which did not initially attract much attention, concerns the ability of cytokines to inhibit or control the extent of immune responses. This activity is of obvious interest in the therapy of immune stimulatory states leading to tissue damage, seen in acute and chronic inflammatory conditions and autoimmune diseases. Cytokines involved in these suppressive responses include TGF-beta and IL-10. But, as can be seen in Table 1, other cytokine-related factors can also be immunosuppressive in vivo (Broxmeyer, 1992). These include specific antagonists, such as the IL-1 receptor antagonist, and cytokine receptors shed from the surfaces of stimulated cells. Studies indicate that measurement of these soluble cytokine receptors shed into the serum may be as accurate a measure of immunological activity in vivo as measurement of the cytokine itself. These shed receptors act as inhibitors of ongoing responses by competing for available cytokine. Assays for these suppressive factors have been reported, but are not yet readily available in the cases of TGF-beta and IL-10. However, ELISA-based tests for soluble IL-2 receptor, soluble TNF-receptor and IL-1 receptor antagonist are commercially produced.

Another potential suppressor of cytokine action is anti-cytokine antibody, which can develop after the injection of genetically-engineered cytokines. No standard assay for evaluating these antibodies is yet developed.

CHEMOTACTIC CYTOKINES

The newest group of cytokines consist of small protein factors which are chemotactic for macrophages, neutrophils, or other cells (Oppenheim, et al., 1991; Yoshimura, et al., 1987). Although none of these factors have been used clinically, they are of interest as mediators of inflammatory responses. Antagonists to these factors may play a role in controlling inflammation, which would be very significant from a clinical standpoint. Several of these factors can be measured by commercial ELISA-based tests, but the significance of serum levels of these cytokines is still being investigated.

SPECIAL CONSIDERATIONS IN CYTOKINE MONITORING

Several special problems arise in the area of cytokine monitoring, most of which relate to the natural physiologic roles of these mediators. For example, the cytokines usually do not work in isolation, but are generated at various points at the sites of immune or inflammatory responses, act as required, and disappear. Thus, the timing of cytokine monitoring becomes important. The serum half-life of most cytokines is very short after exogenous administration, ranging from minutes to hours.

A second consideration is that during immune or inflammatory responses, one cytokine may induce the production of a different cytokine, and this may continue, resulting in a "cascade" effect. Therefore, when devising monitoring protocols, it may be preferable to monitor action of a primary cytokine by measuring one of the induced cytokines. This concept is illustrated in Figure 2.

It is well-established that treatment with some individual cytokines result in the appearance of other factors, in an orderly and predictable manner. These interactions are the ones invoked in the normal conduct of immunological responses. Thus, for example, therapeutic administration of IL-2 results, in a short time, in the appearance of the cytokine Gamma Interferon, as well as TNF and IL-6. Similarly IL-1 administration leads to detectable levels of CSF's, IL-2, IL-3 and IL-6 (among others). These sequential

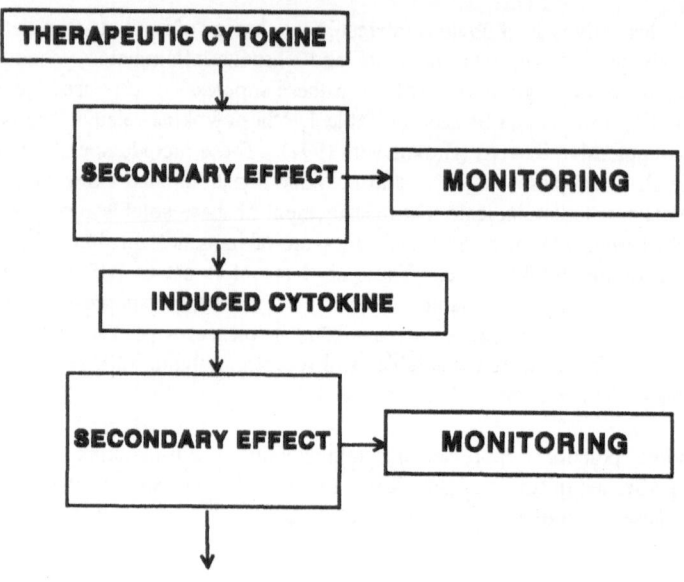

Figure 2. Secondary induction of cytokines.

inductions of successive cytokines are not surprising; indeed, it would be surprising if they were not seen. However, from the standpoint of the laboratory, it gives some flexibility in choosing which cytokines to monitor. If a lab has experience with a certain test, such as the detection of IL-6, it may suffice to measure IL-6 as a secondary cytokine following treatment with IL-1, IL-2, or TNF (for example), rather than measuring the primary cytokine at all. Also, since it is expensive and cumbersome to measure all cytokines, a more limited panel can be maintained in the laboratory by taking advantage of cascade induction of secondary and tertiary factors.

Many of the cytokine assays can be complicated by the presence of inhibitors in serum or other body fluids (Arend, et al., 1991). Many cytokines appear to be associated with serum proteins, although not covalently bonded to them. Still, this may limit their availability to some assay systems. Any material which could competitively inhibit the attachment of a cytokine to antibody could interfere with an ELISA or RIA. This may include antibodies to the cytokine present after treatment with exogenous cytokine or in the case of autoimmune antibodies. Also, the presence of soluble cytokine receptor, which is very well-characterized in the case of IL-2, and is becoming more well-understood for other cytokines, will effectively prevent the detection of serum cytokine (Dower, et al, 1990; Fernandez-Bostran, 1991). In these two cases, results will be lower than the true value of bioactive material present. There have been few comprehensive studies as to the utility of biochemical pre-processing of sera to release cytokine bound by serum protein, antibody or receptors (Canon, et al, 1988).

SELECTION OF CYTOKINE ASSAYS

At least 5 general classes of cytokine assays should be considered, depending on the type of data desired and the clinical samples involved. They are listed in Table 2.

Table 2. Cytokine Assay Formats

I.	Elisa/Radioimmunoassay
II.	Bioassay
III.	Western Blot
IV.	Northern Blot ± PCR
V.	In Situ Methods

There are pros and cons to each of the assay formats listed in the Table. As with other assay systems, considerations of reliability, sensitivity, specificity, and ease of use must be balanced against each other when choosing a test (Backwill, 1991; Beckmann, et al., 1991).

ELISA is in many cases the test of choice for the clinical laboratory, especially when large numbers of samples must be assessed. Most clinical labs are familiar with the ELISA format, and own a suitable spectrophotometer for reading the plates. The cytokine ELISA test market is broad, and there are many sources of kits, all of which come complete with all required reagents to perform the assay. Sensitivity is usually about 20-100 pg/ml cytokine protein, or roughly 1 unit/ml. Assays require from a few hours to overnight, but the actual technician time spent manipulating reagents is small.

The negative side of ELISA testing has both theoretical and practical components. On a theoretical basis, the ELISA may detect cytokine protein which is no longer biologically active. That is, if cytokine is degraded or damaged such that the biological activity is lost, the epitopes detected by the ELISA may not be affected. In practice, there have been few reports of this problem. On a more practical level, one should realize that not all cytokine ELISA kits are equal. Some kits may have problems detecting genetically engineered cytokines, as opposed to naturally occurring cytokines. Some kits may be better at detecting material in human serum than others which may be more suitable for tissue culture media. It is well worth the time of any laboratory to investigate carefully several manufacturers' kits for suitability. There are no FDA-licensed kits at the moment, so all ELISA's are for research purposes only. That is, no uniform standard of quality or reliability is enforced at this time. The buyer must beware.

RIA kits are less common now, but are available for some cytokines. Laboratories which are used to performing RIA's and have the necessary radiation counting equipment, safety equipment and licensing may prefer RIA to ELISA. Again, no uniform standards exist for kit producers, so run quality control testing in advance of large reagent purchases.

The classical methods for cytokine measurement involve assessing the actual biological effects of the cytokine, such as induction of cell proliferation, cell killing, inhibition of ongoing reactions, etc. (Gearing et al, 1988). The only assays accepted by the FDA for licensing of cytokine preparations for clinical or laboratory use are bioassays. These assays have been well-characterized in a number of sources, and will not be reviewed here.

The major advantages of bioassays are, first, that they measure actual bioactivity, as opposed to the presence of immunological epitopes (as in ELISA or RIA). Second, the bioassays are generally more sensitive than ELISA or RIA, often by more than an order of magnitude. On the negative side, these tests require the maintenance of many tissue culture cell lines or establishment of primary cultures. Most require three days to several weeks to complete. They are labor intensive, and expensive to implement and control. Unless cytokine assays are done on a frequent basis, the clinical laboratory can probably not afford to perform most bioassay procedures.

Since serum is convenient to obtain, most published information regarding cytokine levels in humans with various disease conditions, or who are receiving cytokine therapy, describe measurement of serum cytokine levels. These levels may not truly reflect the amount of cytokine present at the site of an immunological reaction, which is the critical measurement in most cases. Measurements of cytokines in tissue can be made, if the tissue samples are available. The last three methods in Table 2 are used for such monitoring.

Western blot of cell-associated protein is performed in many labs, and can be equally applied to cytokine product. Many good monoclonal and polyclonal antibody preparations are available to probe such blots.

Northern blots and/or PCR can also be used to detect cytokines in tissue samples. The methods are well-known for probing cytokine-specific mRNA (Dallman et al, 1991). There is, of course, an assumption that any RNA detected will be translated into protein and secreted, which may not be uniformly true. PCR technology will allow mRNA to be reverse-transcribed into cDNA, and then amplified. This allows detection of very tiny amounts of message, but is difficult to control, and is not quantitative. However, laboratories which are familiar with PCR technology and its pitfalls may want to add these cytokine detection methods to their repertoire (O'Garra, 1992).

Finally, cytokines can be detected on frozen sections or paraffin-embedded sections of tissue. This can be done with protein probes, or by in situ hybridization of cytokine mRNA. Both of these methods have been used successfully, although they are quite labor-intensive, and must be well-controlled (Sander et al., 1991).

CYTOKINE STANDARDS

There has been some difficulty in comparing cytokine preparations from various sources, such as extracts of tissue, E. coli-produced material (non-glycosylated), material from yeast, baculovirus, or human cells. Manufacturers would each assign specific activities to their preparations based on in-house tests or standards.

Now, this situation has been, for the most part, resolved. The World Health Organization, through its National Institutes for Biological Standards and Control in England, along with the National Cancer Institute's Biological Response Modifiers Program, the National Institute for Allergy and Infectious Diseases, and the U.S. Food and Drug Administration have joined to establish standard cytokine preparations of defined unitage. These standards have been made available to any manufacturer or research laboratory interested in cytokine research. At present, WHO-certified International Standards or Interim Reference Reagents (the step preliminary to acceptance as an International Standard) are available for most of the cytokines. For a current list, contact the NIBSC (Blanche Lane, Potters Bar, Hertfordshire, England EN6 3QG) or, for North Americans, contact the BRMP (National Cancer Institute, Biological Resources Branch, Frederick, Maryland 21702). The standards are distributed in small amounts for only a service charge, and are intended to be used to calibrate laboratory standards. Then, all laboratories can speak the same language when referring to cytokine unitage.

CONCLUSION

Most hospital laboratories will be measuring cytokines in patient samples in the near future (Aggarwal et al., 1992). At this moment, some cytokines are already well into clinical trials, and some are licensed for use (Henderson, 1992). Laboratory testing reagents will soon be licensed as well. Many other cytokines are in various stages of study; many of these will also be available for patient treatment or diagnosis within a few years. Lab heads must be aware of these new developments in the cytokine area, and must accommodate to the demands for new testing as we gain a better understanding of how to monitor and control immune responses using cytokines.

ACKNOWLEDGEMENTS

Research sponsored, at least in part, by the National Cancer Institute, DHHS, under contract NO1-CO-74102 with Program Resources, Inc./DynCorp. The contents of this publication do not necessarily reflect the views or policies of the DHHS, nor does mention of trade names, commercial products, or organizations imply endorsement by the U.S. Government.

REFERENCES

Aggarwal, B.B. and Gutterman, J.U., 1991, "Human Cytokines: Handbook for Basic and Clinical Research," Blackwell Scientific Publications, Boston.

Aggarwal, B.B. and Pocsik, E., 1992, Cytokines: From clone to clinic, *Arch. Biochem. Biophys.* 292:335.

Arend, W.P., Malyak, M., Bigler, C.F., Smith Jr., M.F. and Janson, R.W., 1991, The biological role of naturally-occurring cytokine inhibitors, *Brit. J. Rheumatol.* 30:49.

Backwill, F.R., 1991, "Cytokines. A Practical Approach," IRL Press, New York.

Beckmann, M.P. and Morrissey, P.J., 1991, Assays for lymphokines, cytokines and their receptors, *Curr. Opin. Immunol.* 3:247.

Billiau, A. and Vandekerckhove, F., 1991, Cytokines and their interactions with other inflammatory mediators in the pathogenesis of sepsis and septic shock, *Eur. J. Clin. Invest.* 21:559.

Broxmeyer, H.E., 1992, Suppressor cytokines and regulation of myelopoiesis. Biology and possible clinical uses, *Am. J. Pediatr. Hematol. Oncol.* 14:22.

Cannon, J.G., Van der Meer, J.W.M., Kwiatkowski, D., Endres, S., Lonneman, G., Buirke, J.F. and Dinarello, C.A., 1988, Interleukin-1 beta in human plasma: Optimization of blood collection, plasma extraction, and radioimmunoassay methods, *Lymphokine Res.* 7:457.

Clemens, M.J., Morris, A.G. and Gearing, A.J.H., eds., 1987, "Lymphokines and Interferons: A Practical Approach," IRL Press, Oxford.

Coligan, J.E., Kruisbeek, A.M., Margulies, D.H., Shevach, E.M. and Strober, W., eds., 1991, "Current Protocols in Immunology," John Wiley & Sons, New York.

Dallman, M.J., Montgomery, R.A., Larsen, C.P., Wanders, A and Wells, A.F., 1991, Cytokine gene expression: Analysis using northern blotting, polymerase chain reaction and in situ hybridization, *Immunol. Rev.* 119:163.

Dinarello, C.A., 1990, The pathophysiology of the pro-inflammatory cytokines, *Biotherapy* 2:189.

Dawson, M.M., "Lymphokines and Interleukins," 1991, CRC Press, Inc., Boca Raton.

Dower, S.K., Smith, C.A. and Park, L.S., 1990, Human cytokine receptors, *J. Clin. Immunol.* 10:289.

Fernandez-Botran, R., 1991, Soluble cytokine receptors: Their role in immunoregulation, *Faseb J.* 5:2567.

Gearing, A.J.H. and Hennessen, W., eds., 1988, "Developments in Biological Standardization. Cytokines: Laboratory and Clinical Evaluation," Vol. 69, S. Karger, Basel.

Gordon, M.Y., 1991, Hemopoietic growth factors and receptors: Bound and free, *Cancer Cells* 3:127.

Henderson, B. and Blake, S., 1992, Therapeutic potential of cytokine manipulation, *Trends Pharmacol. Sci.* 13:145.

Metcalf, D., 1984, "The Hematopoietic Colony Stimulating Factors," Elsevier, New York.

Mossman, T.R., 1991, Cytokine secretion patterns and cross-regulation of T cell subsets, *Immunol. Res.* 10:183.

O'Garra, A. and Vieira, P., 1992, Polymerase chain reaction for detection of cytokine gene expression, *Curr. Opin. Immunol.* 4:211.

Oppenheim, J.J., Gearing, A.J.H. and Rossio, J.L., eds, 1992 (In Press), "Clinical Applications of Cytokines: Role in Pathogenesis, Diagnosis and Therapy," Oxford University Press, Oxford.

Oppenheim, J.J., Zachariae, C.O., Mukaida, N. and Matsushima, K., 1991, Properties of the novel proinflammatory supergene "intercrine" cytokine family, *Annu. Rev. Immunol.* 9:617.

Rossio, J.L., Rager, H.C., Goundry, C.S. and Crisp, E.A., 1992, Cytokine Testing in Clinical Trial Monitoring, *in*: "Manual of Clinical Immunology (4th Ed.), N. Rose and H. Friedman, eds., American Society for Microbiology, Washington, D.C.

Sander, B., Andersson, J. and Andersson, U., 1991, Assessment of cytokines by immunofluorescence and the paraformaldehyde-saponin procedure, *Immunol. Rev.* 119:23.

Thomson, A.W., ed., 1991, "The Cytokine Handbook," Academic Press, New York.

Wagstaff, J., 1990, Lymphokines and cytokines, *Cancer Chemother. Biol. Resp. Modif.* 11:204.

Williams, D.E., Fletcher, F.A., Lyman, S.D. and de Vries, P., 1991, Cytokine regulation of hematopoietic stem cells, *Semin. Immunol.* 3:391.

Yoshimura, T., Matsushima, K., Oppenheim, J.J. and Leonard, E.J., 1987, Neutrophil chemotactic factor produced by lipopolysaccharide (LPS)-stimulated human blood mononuclear leukocytes: Partial characterization and separation from interleukin-1 (IL-1), *J. Immunol.* 139:788.

Zentella, A., Manogue, K. and Cerami, A., 1991, The role of cachectin/TNF and other cytokines in sepsis, *Prog. Clin. Biol. Res.* 367:9.

IL-2-BASED CONSOLIDATIVE IMMUNOTHERAPY AFTER AUTOLOGOUS BONE MARROW TRANSPLANTATION

Alexander Fefer, Mark C. Benyunes, Carl Higuchi, Andrea York, Celso Massumoto, Catherine G. Lindgren, C. Dean Buckner, and John A. Thompson

Division of Oncology, University of Washington and Fred Hutchinson Cancer Research Center Seattle, WA 98195

The success of autologous bone marrow transplantation (ABMT) for advanced hematologic malignancies is limited largely by a high incidence of relapse of the malignancy after ABMT.[1, 2, 3, 4, 5, 6, 7] The relapses may reflect the failure of the chemoradiotherapy to eradicate all residual disease and, possibly, the outgrowth of clonogenic tumor cells contaminating the infused autologous marrow. Therapy with Interleukin-2 (IL-2), with or without lymphokine-activated killer (LAK) cells, has been reported to induce regressions of advanced cancer in some patients.[8, 9, 10, 11] There are several reasons for postulating that IL-2 +/- LAK cells administered as consolidative immunotherapy early after ABMT for hematologic malignancies might decrease the relapse rate. (a) Human acute leukemia or lymphoma cells are known to be susceptible to LAK cell-mediated lysis in vitro,[12, 13, 14] and some patients with advanced hematologic malignancies have been reported to respond to therapy with high-dose IL-2 with or without LAK cells.[8, 9, 15, 16] Indeed, a review of eight trials of IL-2 +/- LAK cells for malignant lymphoma in relapse reveals an overall 20% response rate.[17] Moreover, some patients with acute myelogenous leukemia (AML) refractory to chemotherapy have also responded to IL-2 therapy.[18, 19, 20, 21] (b) Such immunotherapy is potentially non-cross-resistant with chemoradiotherapy. (c) A state of minimal residual disease is readily attained by the conditioning regimens used for ABMT--a setting in which immunotherapy should theoretically be more effective. (d) IL-2/LAK therapy after ABMT should theoretically be able to eradicate whatever clonogenic malignant cells might be present in the stored marrow and thus should obviate the need for purging the marrow of tumor cells. (e) The possibility exists that a graft-versus-leukemia (GVL) effect may exist in recipients of autologous marrow and might be amplified by IL-2 and/or lymphocytes.

Combination Therapies 2, Edited by A.L. Goldstein and E. Garaci   Plenum Press, New York, 1993

Since relapses most often occur within a few months after ABMT,[1, 2, 3, 4, 5, 6, 7] consolidative IL-2 +/- LAK cell therapy would have to be administered early, before the relapses are likely to occur. We have previously reported that IL-2-responsive LAK precursor cells are detectable in the peripheral circulation as early as 3 weeks after ABMT.[22] Patients thus have the capacity to respond immunologically to IL-2 during this early post-transplant period. However, high-dose chemoradiotherapy and ABMT may render patients more susceptible to IL-2-associated toxicities. Major toxicities of IL-2 and LAK therapy have included a "capillary-leak" syndrome characterized by oliguria, weight gain, azotemia, and hypotension sometimes leading to respiratory distress, cardiac arrhythmias, myocardial infarction, and even death.[8, 9, 10, 23, 24] Moreover, potential myelosuppression by IL-2 was of particular concern after ABMT, since IL-2-induced anemia and thrombocytopenia has been reported.[25]

PHASE IB TRIAL OF IL-2 AFTER ABMT FOR HEMATOLOGIC MALIGNANCY

Thus, the possibility was considered that early after ABMT patients might be too susceptible to IL-2 toxicity--especially in terms of the viability of the marrow graft and the capillary leak syndrome--and/or might not be able to respond immunologically to IL-2 administration. Therefore, a Phase Ib trial was performed to determine the toxicity and immunomodulatory effects of IL-2 administered early after ABMT for hematologic malignancies. Patients who recovered from ABMT and met the eligibility criteria for IL-2 were sequentially assigned to escalating (Roche) IL-2 "induction" doses of 0.3-4.5 x 10^6 U/m^2/day on day 1-5 of the IL-2 protocol. After a rest period, all patients received a low-dose "maintenance" infusion of IL-2 at 0.3 x 10^6 U/m^2/day on day 12-21. Patients received induction IL-2 in the hospital and maintenance IL-2 as outpatients in the clinic. The trial design was based on our experience with non-transplant cancer patients[11] and on the anticipated design of a subsequent trial of IL-2 plus LAK cells.

For the Phase Ib clinical trial of IL-2 after ABMT, 16 patients who had undergone ABMT for a variety of hematologic malignancies including eight with acute myelogenous leukemia (AML) in first relapse or beyond began IL-2 therapy a median of 33 days (range, 14 to 91) after ABMT.[26] Patients had had a variety of of pretransplant conditioning and marrow purging regimens. All had recovered from ABMT-associated acute toxicities, and had trilineage marrow engraftment documented by marrow aspiration. Eligibility requirements included: adequate BM function (a neutrophil count $\geq$ 500/mL; platelets > 20,000/mL with or without transfusion support); adequate renal and hepatic function and absence of infection off antibiotics.

Dose-related toxicities consisted largely of fever, nausea, diarrhea, skin rash and mild fluid retention. Dose-limiting toxicities were hypotension and thrombocytopenia. All toxicities reversed quickly after stopping IL-2. The maximal tolerated induction dose was identified as 3 x 10^6 U/m^2/day. No neutropenia but modest neutrophilia was noted during IL-2 therapy. The IL-2 regimen induced an initial lymphopenia followed by a marked "rebound" lymphocytosis representing a significant increase in cells expressing CD16 and CD56, with a concomitant increase in circulating LAK activity.[26]

FEASIBILITY TRIAL OF IL-2 + AUTOLOGOUS LAK CELLS AFTER ABMT FOR MALIGNANT LYMPHOMA (ML)

Once patients recovered from ABMT and met the eligibility criteria for IL-2, they received IL-2 at the maximal tolerated dose of 3×10^6 U/m^2/day by continuous intravenous infusion on days 1-5 of the IL-2 protocol. The patients underwent leukapheresis daily on days 7-9. The cells were incubated with IL-2, 1,000 U/ml for 5 days, and the resultant LAK cells were infused daily on days 12-14. A low maintenance dose of IL-2 at 3×10^5 U/m^2/day was administered on days 12-21. The details of pheresis, LAK cell generation and LAK cell harvesting have been previously described.[11]

Sixteen patients with malignant lymphoma were treated with ABMT plus IL-2 and autologous LAK cells.[27] They were heterogeneous in regards to diagnosis (12 with non-Hodgkin lymphoma and 4 with Hodgkin's disease), stage at ABMT (7 less advanced; i.e., in first relapse, and 9 advanced; i.e., second relapse or later), conditioning regimen (4 with chemotherapy alone and 12 with chemotherapy and total body irradiation). The marrow from patients with NHL were all purged with a cocktail of anti-B cell antibodies prior to reinfusion. All protocols and consent forms were approved by the Institutional Review Committee of the Fred Hutchinson Cancer Research Center.

Patients on this trial exhibited the same toxicity during the induction IL-2 cycle as did patients receiving the same IL-2 dose on the reported Phase I IL-2 trial. Maintenance IL-2 therapy was well tolerated. Leukapheresis was associated with marked exacerbation of thrombocytopenia. A median total of 1.4×10^{11} cells were infused per patient. Phenotypically, the cells infused were predominantly CD3$^+$, CD8$^+$ and CD56$^+$ and were highly lytic to Daudi cells. LAK cell infusions were generally well-tolerated, with only transient fever, rigors, and dyspnea which rapidly reversed.

IL-2/LAK therapy was associated with modest neutrophilia, significant thrombocytopenia and marked lymphocytosis. The thrombocytopenia was clearly more severe during the pheresis days. The immunologic changes observed with IL-2 + LAK therapy were comparable to those previously reported with IL-2 alone.[27]

CLINICAL FOLLOWUP OF PATIENTS TREATED WITH ABMT + IL-2 FOR AML

The clinical characteristics of the eight AML patients on the Phase I trial of IL-2 after ABMT have been described.[26] All underwent ABMT + IL-2 in first relapse or beyond. The median duration of their first CR was 11 months. Five patients were conditioned with busulfan 8 mg/kg, cyclophosphamide 60 mg/kg, and total body irradiation (TBI), and three with busulfan 16 mg/kg and cyclophosamide 200 mg/kg without TBI. Marrows from four patients were treated with 4-hydroxycyclophosphamide (4-HC) prior to cyropreservation. Four of the eight patients received the IL-2 at the MTD while four received lower doses of IL-2. Two patients have relapsed at 4 and 10 months, while 6 remain in CR 26+ to 40+ months after ABMT.

A historical control group was generated which consisted of all patients with AML in 1st relapse or beyond who underwent ABMT at our institution during the same time period with the same preparative and purging regimens as the IL-2 group, who met the eligibility criteria for IL-2 therapy but did not receive IL-2 either because they refused, or because IL-2 was temporarily unavailable to them. No patient who was eligible for IL-2 therapy was excluded from the control group.

The 15 controls thus selected did not differ significantly from the eight patients who received IL-2 with respect to age, FAB class, number of cycles of induction and consolidation chemotherapy, duration of first CR, use of 4-HC-treated marrow, type of preparative regimen or time to engraftment.

Table 1 compares the results of the "controls" with those of the "experimental" group. Two of the 15 control patients died of infection at 6 and 11 months, 9 relapsed, with a median of four months, while 4 remain in CR 7+ to 40+ (median = 26+) months after ABMT.

Table 1. ABMT + IL-2 for AML in ≥ First Relapse versus Historical Controls (ABMT Without IL-2)

Group	No. Relapsed (mos)	No. Alive in CR (mos)
IL-2 (n=8)	2 (4, 10)	6 (26+ to 40+)
No IL-2	9 (2 - 16)	4 (7+ to 36+)
(n=15)*	(median=4)	(median=26+)

*Two died of infections at 6 and 11 months.

Despite the very small number of patients involved, the long-term clinical follow-up results of the eight patients treated with ABMT and IL-2 forAML in first relapse or beyond are encouraging. They are better than would be expected from previous reports,[2, 28, 29, 30] and compare favorably with results reported after allogeneic BMT for AML beyond first CR.[31] Moreover, they are significantly better than those in our concurrently-transplanted historical controls who met the eligibility criteria for IL-2 but did not receive it because of patient refusal or IL-2 non-availability.

CLINICAL FOLLOW-UP OF 16 PATIENTS TREATED WITH ABMT AND IL-2/LAK FOR ML

Of the 16 patients treated in first relapse or beyond beginning a median of 31 days after ABMT, 5 relapsed 3 to 19 (median=5) months after ABMT, while 11 remain in CR at 6+ to 21+ months (median, 10+). These preliminary results compare favorably with our past experience in similar patients.[7]

The ML patients in this trial were considered to be at a high risk of post-transplant relapse. Despite the heterogeneity of the patients, these preliminary clinical results are encouraging, given that, historically, such patients have had a 60-80% probability of early relapse (median, 3-4 months).[7] The additional toxicity associated with the pheresis and LAK cell infusions was sufficiently great to lead to the conclusion that although LAK generation and infusion is feasible, it is not recommended.

Overall, these preliminary clinical results of IL-2 for AML and IL-2/LAK for ML after ABMT suggest that consolidative immunotherapy with IL-2 (+/- LAK cells) administered early after ABMT for patients with AML or ML known to be at high risk for early relapse may decrease the relapse rate. The data provide a basis for initiating prospectively randomized controlled trials of IL-2 versus no IL-2 after ABMT to establish definitively whether this approach will, indeed, reduce the relapse rate and ultimately improve disease-free survival in such patients.

ACKNOWLEDGEMENTS

Supported in part by Grants PO1 CA-47748, CA-18029, CA-15704 and T32 CA-09515, awarded by the National Cancer Institute, Department of Health and Human Services, the Jose Carreras International Leukemia Foundation and the Jennie Zoline Foundation.

REFERENCES

1. N. Gorin, P. Herve, P. Aegerter, et al,, Autologous bone marrow transplantation for acute leukaemia in remission, *Br J Haematol.* 64:385 (1986).
2. A. Yeager, H. Kaizer, G. Santos, et al, Autologous bone marrow transplantation in patients with acute nonlymphocytic leukemia, using *ex vivo* marrow treatment with 4-hydroperoxycyclophos-phamide, *N Engl J Med.* 315:142 (1986).
3. T. Philip, J. Dumont, F. Teillet, et al, High dose chemotherapy and autologous bone marrow transplantation in refractory Hodgkin's disease, *Br J Cancer.* 53:737 (1986).
4. T. Philip, J. Armitage, G. Spitzer, et al, High dose therapy and autologous bone marrow transplantation after failure of conventional chemotherapy in adults with intermediate grade or high grade non-Hodgkin's lymphoma, *N Eng J Med.* 316:1493 (1987).
5. T. Takvorian, G. Canellos, J. Ritz, et al, Prolonged disease-free survival after autologous bone marrow transplantation in patients with non-Hodgkin's lymphoma with a poor prognosis, *N Eng J Med.* 316:(1987).
6. B. Barlogie, R. Alexanian, K. Dicke, et al, High-dose chemoradiotherapy and autologous bone marrow transplantation for resistant multiple myeloma, *Blood.* 70:869 (1987).
7. F. Petersen, F. Appelbaum, R. Hill, et al, Autologous marrow transplantation for malignant lymphoma: A report of 101 cases from Seattle, *J Clin Oncol.* 8:638 (1990).
8. S.A. Rosenberg, M.T. Lotze, L.M. Muul, et al, A progress report on the treatment of 157 patients with advanced cancer using lymphokine-activated killer cells and interleukin-2 or high-dose interleukin-2 alone, *N Eng J Med.* 316:889 (1987).
9. W.H. West, K.W. Tauer, J.R. Yannelli, et al, Constant-infusion recombinant interleukin-2 in adoptive immunotherapy of advanced cancer, *N Eng J Med.* 316:898 (1987).

10. M. Lotze, A. Chang, C. Seipp, et al, High-dose recombinant interleukin-2 in the treatment of patients with disseminated cancer: Responses, treatement-related morbidity, and histologic findings, *JAMA.* 256:3117 (1986).

11. J. Thompson, K. Shulman, M. Benyunes, et al, Prolonged continuous intravenous infusion interleukin-2 and lymphokine-activated killer cell therapy for metastatic renal cell carcinoma, *J Clin Oncol.* 10:960 (1992).

12. K. Oshimi, Y. Oshimi, M. Akutsu, et al, Cytotoxicity of Interleukin 2-activated lymphocytes for leukemia and lymphoma cells, *Blood.* 68:938 (1986).

13. E. Lotzová, C.A. Savary, and R.B. Herberman, Induction of NK cell activity against fresh human leukemia in culture with Interleukin 2, *J Immunol.* 138:2718 (1987).

14. A. Adler, P. Chervenick, T. Whiteside, et al, Interleukin-2 induction of lymphokine-activated killer (LAK) activity in the peripheral blood and bone marrow of acute leukemia patients. I. Feasibility of LAK generation in adult patients with active disease and in remission, *Blood.* 71:709 (1988).

15. M.A.K. Allison, S.E. Jones, and P. McGuffey, Phase II trial of outpatient interleukin-2 in malignant lymphoma, chronic lymphocytic leukemia, and selected solid tumors, *J Clin Onc.* 7:75 (1989).

16. J. Weber, J. Yang, S. Topalian, et al, The use of Interleukin-2 and lymphokine-activated killer cells for the treatment of patients with non-Hodgkin's lymphoma, *J Clin Oncol.* 10:33 (1992).

17. M.C. Benyunes, and A. Fefer, IL-2 in the Treatment of Hematologic Malignancies, *in:* "Therapeutic Applications of Interleukin 2," Atkins and Mier, eds. Marcel Dekker, Inc., New York (in press).

18. R. Foa, M.T. Fierro, S. Tosti, et al, Induction and persistence of complete remission in a resistant acute myeloid leukemia patient after treatment with recombinant interleukin-2, *Leuk & Lym.* 1:113 (1990).

19. R. Foa, G. Meloni, S. Tosti, et al, Treatment of acute myeloid leukaemia patients with recombinant interleukin 2: a pilot study, *Brit J Haematol.* 77:491 (1991).

20. R. Foa, G. Meloni, S. Tosti, et al, Treatment of residual disease in acute leukemia patients with recombinant interleukin 2 (IL2): Clinical and biological findings, *Bone Marrow Transplantation.* 6:98 (1990).

21. D. Maraninchi, D. Blaise, P. Viens, et al, High-dose recombinant Interleukin-2 and acute myeloid leukemias in relapse, *Blood.* 78:2182 (1991).

22. C. Higuchi, J. Thompson, T. Cox, et al, Lymphokine-activated killer function following autologous bone marrow transplantation for refractory hematologic malignancies, *Cancer Res.* 49:5509 (1989).

23. R. Lee, M. Lotze, J. Skibber, et al, Cardiorespiratory effects of immunotherapy with interleukin-2, *J Clin Oncol.* 7:7 (1989).

24. E. Gaynor, L. Vitek, L. Sticklin, et al, The hemodynamic effects of treatment with interleukin-2 and lymphokine-activated killer cells, *Ann Intern Med.* (1988).

25. S.E. Ettinghausen, J.G. Moore, D.E. White, et al, Hematologic effects of immunotherapy with lymphocyte-activated killer cells and recombinant Interleukin-2 in cancer patients, *Blood.* 69:1654 (1987).

26. C.M. Higuchi, J.A. Thompson, F.B. Petersen, et al. Toxicity and immunomodulatory effects of Interleukin 2 after autologous bone marrow transplantation for hematologic malignancies. *Blood.* 77:2561 (1991).

27. M. Benyunes, A. York, C. Lindgren, et al, IL-2 ± LAK cells as consolidative therapy after autologous BMT for hematologic malignancies: A feasibility trial. *Proc Amer Soc Clin Oncol.* 11:319 (1992).

28. P. Stewart, C. Buckner, W. Bensinger, et al, Autologous marrow transplantation in patients with acute nonlymphocytic leukemia in first remission, *Exp Hematol.* 13:267 (1985).

29. R. Chopra, A. Goldstone, A. McMillan, et al, Successful treatment of acute myeloid leukemia beyond first remission with autologous bone marrow transplantation using busulfan/cyclophosphamide and unpurged marrow: The British Autograft Group experience, *J Clin Oncol.* 9:1840 (1991).

30. N. Gorin, P. Aegerter, B. Auvert, et al, Autologous bone marrow transplantation for acute myelocytic leukemia in first remission: A European survey of the role of marrow purging, *Blood.* 75:1606 (1990).

31. R. Clift, C. Buckner, E. Thomas, et al, The treatment of acute non-lymphoblastic leukemia by allogeneic marrow transplantation, *BMT.* 2:243 (1987).

TUMOR IMMUNOGENICITY INDUCED BY
THE LOCAL OCCURRENCE OF IL-2

Federica Cavallo[1], Francesco Di Pierro[1],
Mirella Giovarelli[1], Alessandra Vacca[3],
Alberto Gulino[3], Antonella Soppacciaro[4],
Andrea Modesti[5], and Guido Forni[2]

[1]Institute of Microbiology, University of Turin,
[2]CNR-Immunogenetics and Histocompatibility Center
10126 Turin,
[3]Department of Experimental Medicine, University
of L'Aquila,
[4]Department of Human Biopathology, University of Rome,
[5]Chair of Experimental Pathology, University of Chieti,
Italy

INTRODUCTION

Tumor as Immunological Trap

In natural situations, few immunogenic tumors escape destruction by immune reaction on the part of the host. Nevertheless, spontaneous tumors may often be antigenic owing to the abnormal proteins or peptides expressed on their cell membrane. They are not immunogenic, however, because their cells produce several suppressor factors that hamper local and systemic immune reactions. Attraction and paralysis by a tumor of a large variety of leukocytes through the local release of cytokines and chemotactic factors[1] means that spontaneous tumors are often found to be heavily infiltrated by leukocytes of several kind. It is uncertain, however, whether the reactive infiltrate impedes the growth of a tumor or is of prognostic significance[2].

It has been shown in fact, that infiltrating T-lymphocytes and those in tumor-draining lymph nodes are unable to react against the tumor, and also display a depressed response even to polyclonal activators. Long culture in particularly stimulating conditions is needed to rescue the activity of tumor associated leukocytes (TAL)[3], and they may even increase tumor proliferation. By releasing angiogenic factors and further suppressing lymphocyte reactivity tumor-trapped macrophages facilitate tumor growth[4]. Tumor immunosuppressive activity is completed by the kind of tumor-borne extracellular matrix and the factors released by tumor-interacting fibroblasts and tumor-sequestrated leukocytes[1].

This sponge feature allows tumors to absorb the host reaction and makes the immune system unable to mount a significant response, since the weak cellular reactions sometimes elicited during the early stages of tumor growth are progressively impaired.

Combination Therapies 2, Edited by A.L. Goldstein
and E. Garaci   Plenum Press, New York, 1993

Interleukin-2 (IL-2)-induced tumor immunogenicity

This natural scenario dictated by a tumor's suppressive capabilities can be drastically modified by the local addition of exogenous cytokines or their release by engineered tumor cells[5]. These cytokines do not affect tumor proliferation directly. Rather, they interfere with the control mechanisms of the immune system in a way that could surmount tumor-borne immunosuppression. This interference may be directly due to a cytokine or depend on its ability to induce the secretion of many other cytokines and factors, as in the cascade type of reactions[6].

In the present studies, IL-2 was chosen from the various cytokines whose presence affects tumor growth, since it plays a crucial regulatory role in the immune response. IL-2 was first characterized as an in vitro progression factor for T-helper and T-cytotoxic lymphocytes, and has since been shown to participate in B-lymphocyte activation, boost NK cells, generate lymphokine activated killer (LAK) activity, and trigger non-specific cytotoxicity in macrophages[7],[8].

In vivo, four consecutive i.p. injections of as little as 150 unit (U) of IL-2 reverse T-lymphocyte unresponsiveness in *Mycobacterium bovis* BCG-infected mice[9]. Moreover, the solid, long-lasting tolerance induced by i.v. injection of newborn mice with semiallogenic lymphoid cells can be nullified by IL-2 administration. When neonatal mice carrying tolerated healthy skin allografts received 1,200 U i.p. on days 58 and 59 after graft, there was a significant acceleration of rejection[10]. The possibility that exogenous IL-2 converts a non-immunogenic into an immunogenic stimulus is further supported by experiments showing that injection of 200 U of IL-2 transform a stimulus causing unresponsiveness (picrylated spleen cells injected i.v.) into one causing contact hypersensitivity[11]. Moreover, immunization of low responder mice with the antigen mixed with 100,000 U of IL-2 in complete Freund's adjuvant augments the antibody response to levels similar to those in high responder mice. IL-2 had no effect in congenic, high-responder mice, suggesting that it enhances suboptimal T-lymphocyte help in low-responders, whereas T-lymphocyte help is not a limiting factor in high-responders[12].

These findings suggest that IL-2 may affect several aspects of the tumor-host immune relationship and lead to enhanced tumor immunogenicity. Several experimental studies with exogenous recombinant IL-2 (rIL-2) injected at the tumor growth site, as well as with IL-2 released by IL-2 gene engineered tumor cells[1], indicate that IL-2 does indeed provide helper signals leading to a specific antitumor reaction. In clinical practice, intratumoral and perilymphatic infiltration of rIL-2 in patients with head and neck squamous cell carcinomas, and recurrent bladder carcinomas leads to tumor regression and the elicitation of tumor-specific T-cell mediated reactions[6].

Here we compare in mice the efficacy of the antitumor reaction activated by peritumoral infiltration with exogenous rIL-2 with that activated by the injection of rIL-2 releasing tumor cells.

MATERIALS AND METHODS

Mice and Tumors. Female BALB/cnAnCr (BALB/c) mice were from Charles River Lab., Calco, Italy. When sublethal whole body irradiation was required, mice received 4.5 Gy from a ^{137}Cs source providing a dose rate of 0.5 Gy/min. Irradiated mice were challenged 48 hours later. TS/A parental cells (TS/A-pc) are a tumor cell line from the first in vivo transplant of a moderately differentiated mammary adenocarcinoma that spontaneously arose in a 20-mo-old multiparous BALB/c mouse. CE-2 is a poorly immunogenic methylcholanthrene-induced sarcoma of BALB/c mice. 4×10^4 and 2×10^3 are respectively the minimal 100% TS/A-pc and CE-2 tumor-inducing dose in BALB/c mice[13]. Mice were challenged with either 4×10^4 or 1×10^5 TS/A-pc injected sc in the middle of the left (primary challenge) or right (secondary challenge) flank. Neoplastic masses were measured with calipers in the two perpendicular diameters for 60 days twice weekly. Mice tumor-free at the end of this period were classed as survivors.

rIL-2 injection. Mice were challenged in the left inguinal flank with the minimal 100% tumor inducing dose of TS/A. Starting 1-48 hours after challenge, some mice received ten daily injections of 0.2 ml of Hanks basal salt solution (HBSS) supplemented with 2% fetal bovine serum (FBS) alone (controls), or with 10 BRMP U of rIL-2 (EuroCetus, Amsterdam, The Netherlands).

IL-2 gene transfection. TS/A-pc were transfected by electroporation with 20 μg of linearized BCMGneo or BCMGneo-IL-2 plasmids (kindly provided by Dr. Karasuyama) as previously described in detail[13]. Various IL-2 releasing clones were isolated. The clone B6.3600 used in these experiments releases 3600 IL-2 BRMP $U/10^5$ cells/48 hours.

RESULTS

Rejection of B6.3600 cells

To investigate reaction mechanisms associated with IL-2 release, mice were killed 24 h, 3, 5 and 10 days after challenge with 1×10^5 B6.3600 cells. After 24 h, a poorly cohesive tissue nodule of neoplastic cells in active proliferation was already evident in both TS/A-pc and B6.3600 challenged mice. After 3 days, TS/A-pc formed solid tumors with many mitotic figures and a small reactive infiltrate that progressively invaded the fibroadipous tissue and epidermis. A massive infiltrate, mostly composed of neutrophils, was already evident around and within B6.3600 cells. At day 5, B6.3600 masses consisted of isolated neoplastic cells in various stages of degeneration surrounded by neutrophils. A massive neutrophil and lymphomononuclear cell reaction was apparent around the tumor and the perivascular areas. At day 10, neoplastic cells were no longer detectable, and the tumor was replaced by a granulation tissue infiltrated by macrophages and few leukocytes (not shown). This rejection pattern is very close to that which followed peritumoral injection of rIL-2. There, too, tumor mass was infiltrated by eosinophils and neutrophils, whereas few lymphocytes were present. No istological or ultrastructural distinction, however, could be drawn between the two patterns[13,14].

Primary rejection of TS/A-pc

The ability to inhibit the growth of TS/A-pc by rIL-2 and B6.3600 cells, after injection around the area in which TS/A-pc cells have been injected was compared. Starting 48 hours after tumor challenge, mice received daily injection of 0.5 ml of HBSS supplemented with 2% FBS or containing 10 BRMP U of rIL-2. Previous studies have shown that this is the most efficacious dosage in tumor inhibition. Forty-eight hours after challenge, other groups of mice received a single injection of 1×10^5 B6.3600 cells (Table 1).

rIL-2 injection elicits 30% TS/A-pc inhibition, whereas complete inhibition was found following B6.3600 rejection. In both cases, inhibition does not take place if mice are first sublethally irradiated, showing that this rejection pattern depends on radiosensitive reaction mechanisms.

Memory induction

The morphological findings show that B6.3600 rejection rests on the recruitment of several predominantly nonspecific and local cell-reaction mechanisms. A similar nonspecific pattern was previously described during TS/A-pc rejection induced by rIL-2. To see whether these immune reactivities lead to a tumor-specific immune memory, untreated mice and mice that rejected TS/A-pc 30 days earlier in the left flank were challenged in the right flank with either TS/A-pc and CE-2 tumors in a criss-cross experiment.

Table 1. Anti-tumor activity of rIL-2 and B6.3600 cells.

Mice		Tumor challenge	Surviving/total challenged mice.
Immunosuppression	Treatment		
None	HBSS	B6.3600	10/10 (100%)
4.5 Gy	HBSS	B6.3600	1/10 (10%)
None	HBSS	TS/A-pc	0/10 (0%)
None	rIL-2	TS/A-pc	12/40 (30%)
4.5 Gy	rIL-2	TS/A-pc	2/12 (17%)
None	B6.3600	TS/A-pc	0/19 (0%)
4.5 Gy	B6.3600	TS/A-pc	0/10 (0%)

As shown in Table 2, a substantial number of mice surviving the first TS/A-pc challenge after rIL-2 and B6.3600 cell treatment were specifically protected against a second lethal TS/A-pc inoculum, but not against the unrelated CE-2 cells. Comparison of the efficacy of the protective immunity shows that elicited by the rejection of B6.3600 cells is higher than that elicited by rIL-2 injections.

Table 2. Tumor-specific immune memory elicited by rIL-2 and B6.3600 cells.

First challenge (left)		Second challenge (right)	
Tumor	Treatment	Tumor	Surviving/total mice.
None	none	TS/A-pc	0/10 (0%)
None	rIL-2	TS/A-pc	0/10 (0%)
TS/A-pc	rIL-2	TS/A-pc	6/12 (50%)
TS/A-pc	rIL-2	CE-2	0/ 6 (0%)
None	B6.3600	TS/A-pc	10/10 (100%)
TS/a-pc	B6.3600	TS/A-pc	9/ 9 (100%)
TS/A-pc	B6.3600	CE-2	0/ 9 (0%)

DISCUSSION

The local introduction of rIL-2 has offered a new way of boosting NK cells and allowed the generation of LAK cells. The adoptive transfer of LAK cells and the systemic administration of high doses of rIL-2 are now a medical strategy for a few tumors[15]. These nonspecific approaches have assumed that human tumors do not express tumor associated antigens[8]. The possibility of using rIL-2 to expand TAL *in vitro* was next tested in both an experimental system and clinical studies. Besides their higher ability to reach the tumor and cause its regression, TAL can establish a long-lasting immune memory. The growing evidence that human tumors are often antigenic justifies this specific immunotherapeutic approach[8]. The results here reported further support the notion that most tumors are potentially immunogenic, and envisage completely new strategical use of IL-2 as a component of a new tumor vaccine.

The local availability of IL-2 near to an incipient TS/A-pc challenge leads to two distinct situations, namely tumor rejection through non-specific mechanisms and the induction of tumor-specific reactivity. The outcome of such specific and T-lymphocyte mediated memory is not simply related to tumor shrinkage, since it takes place against a spontaneous and apparently non-immunogenic tumor, in which surgical excision, radiation- and chemotherapy-induced regression have failed to elicit an anti-tumor immune response[13,14].

Memory induction rests upon the unique conditions occurring during the rejection. Intense tumor cell destruction, and the release and phagocytosis of dead tumor cell remnants, build up the conditions for an efficient indirect presentation of tumor antigens to T-lymphocytes. Moreover, the presence of IL-2 provides accessory signals of importance in T-lymphocyte activation[5-11]. These cytokines also up-modulate the expression of adhesion molecules and major histocompatibility complex glycoproteins on leukocytes, fibroblasts and endothelia, thus facilitating cell-to-cell interactions and antigen presentation[1].

The observation that the local availability of exogenous rIL-2 is enough to significantly affect the growth of a tumor and increase its immunogenicity holds out the prospect of new medical procedures[16]. By avoiding most of the side-effects associated with systemic injection of large rIL-2 doses, local rIL-2 administration can be easily undertaken with tumor patients. Clinical trials have shown that the infiltration of low doses of rIL-2 around lymph nodes draining primary and recurrent squamous cell carcinomas of the head and neck, and IFN-γ around lymph nodes draining bladder carcinomas, induces a substantial number of complete or partial responses[6].

With primary and accessible tumor, peritumoral infiltration with rIL-2 is a simple and inexpensive procedure. However, when the efficacy of peritumoral rIL-2 administration has been compared with the utilization of IL-2 gene engineered tumor cells, it was clear that transfected cells are more efficacious and more easily handled in order to elicit a systemic immunity. The numerous technical problems connected with the preparation of IL-2 gene transduced tumor cells should be carefully explored in a human context.

Studies are currently in progress to determine whether tumor immunogenicity stemming from the presence of a single cytokine or the combination of a few cytokines is powerful enough to activate an efficient immune response, even in conditions of minimal residual disease or initial metastatic spread.

Acknowledgments

We thank Dr. J. Iliffe for careful review of the manuscript. This work was supported by grants from ISS Italy-USA special project on cancer immunotherapy and AIDS, the Italian Association for Cancer Research (AIRC), and the CNR PF-ACRO and Invecchiamento.

REFERENCES

1. M.P. Colombo, A. Modesti, G. Parmiani, and G. Forni. Local cytokine availability elicits tumor rejection and systemic immunity through granulocyte-T-lymphocyte cross-talk. *Cancer Res.* 52:1(1992).

2. W.E. Clark, D.E. Elder, G. Du Pont IV, L.E. Braitman, B.J. Trock, D. Schultz, M. Synnestved, and A.C. Halpern, Model prediciting survival in stage I melanoma based on tumor progression. *J. Natl. Cancer. Inst.*, 81:1823(1989).

3. T.L. Whiteside, S. Miesher, J. Hurlimann, L. Moretta, and V.Von Fliedner, V. Separation, phenotyping and limiting-dilution analysis of T lymphocyte infiltrating human solid tumors. *Int. J. Cancer* 37:803(1986).

4. A. Mantovani, Tumor associated macrophages. *Curr. Opinion Immunol.* 2:689(1990).

5. G. Forni, H. Fujiwara, F. Martino, T. Hamakoa, C. Jemma, P. Caretto, and M. Giovarelli. Helper strategy in tumor immunology: Expansion of helper lymphocytes and utilization of helper lymphokines for experimental and clinical immunotherapy. Cancer Met. Rev. 7:289(1988).

6. G. Forni, F. Pericle, M. Giovarelli. Effects of local cytokine therapy, *in*: "Clinical Application of Cytokines: Role in Pathogenesis, Diagnosis, Therapy" J.L. Rossio, J.J. Oppenheim, A.J.H. Gearing eds, Oxford University Press, Oxford 1993.

7. K.A. Smith, Cytokines in the nineties. *Eur Cytokine Net* 1:7(1990).

8. F. Cavallo, M. Giovarelli, F. Novelli, and G. Forni. Tumor immunogenicity induced by exogenous interleukins *in*: "Lymphohaematopoietic Growth Factors in Cancer Therapy II", R. Mertelsmann , ed., Springer-Verlag, Berlin (1992).

9. V. Colizzi. In vivo and in vitro administration of interleukin-2 containing preparations reverses T-cell unresponsiveness in Mycobacterium bovis BCG-infected mice. *Infect Immunity* 45:25(1984).

10. M. Malkowsky, P.B. Medawar, D.R. Thatcher, J. Toy, R. Hunt, L.S. Rayfield and C. Dore', Acquired immunological tolerance of foreign cells is impaired by recombinant interleukin 2 or vitamin A acetate. *Proc. Natl. Acad. Sci. USA* 83:536(1984).

11. V. Colizzi, M. Malkowsky, G. Lang and G.L. Asherson. In vivo activity of interleukin-2: conversion of a stimulus causing unresponsiveness to a stimulus causing contact hypersensistivity by injection of interleukin-2. *Immunology* 56:653(1985).

12. H. Kawamura, S.A. Rosenberg and J.A. Berzofsky, Immunization with antigen and interleukin 2 in vivo overcomes Ir gene low responsiveness. *J Exp. Med.* 162:381(1985).

13. F. Cavallo, M. Giovarelli, A. Gulino, A. Vacca, A. Stoppacciaro, A. Modesti, Role of Neutrophils and CD4+ T lymphocytes in the primary and memory response to nonimmunogenic murine mammary adenocarcinoma made immunogenic by IL-2 gene transfection. *J. Immunol.* 1992 (*in press*).

14. G. Forni, M. Giovarelli, A. Santoni, A. Modesti and M. Forni: Interleukin-2 activated tumor inhibition in vivo depends on the systemic involvement of host immunoreactivity. *J. Immunol*, 138:4033(1987).

15. S.A. Rosenberg, B.S. Packard, P.M. Aebersold, P. Solomon, S.L.

Topalian, S.T. Toy, P. Simon, M.T. Lotze, J.C. Yang, A.A. Seipp, C. Simpson, C. Carter, S. Bock, D. Schwartzetruber, J.P. Wei and D.E. White. Use of tumor-infiltrating lymphocytes and interleukin-2 in the immunotherapy of patients with metastatic melanoma. *N. Engl. J. Med.* 318:1676(1988).

16. C. S. McCune and D.M. Marquis. Interleukin 1 as an adjuvant for active specific immunotherapy in a murine tumor model. *Cancer Res* 50:1212(1990).

THYMOSIN α_1: CHEMISTRY, MECHANISM OF ACTION AND CLINICAL APPLICATIONS

Allan L. Goldstein

Department of Biochemistry and Molecular Biology, The George Washington University School of Medicine, Washington, D.C. 20037

INTRODUCTION

Thymosin α_1 is a 28 amino acid, 3108 molecular weight acidic peptide isolated from thymosin fraction 5 (1). Its amino acid sequence is homologous in murine, bovine and human species (2) and a chemically synthesized version (3) has shown activity similar to the native peptide in modulating T-cell maturation (1).

In vivo, thymosin α_1 is involved in the conversion of pluripotent cells to thymocytes and in the subsequent production of activated T-lymphocytes including helper, memory, effector, killer and suppressor T-cells (4). Thymosin α_1 also influences immunoregulatory T-cell function and promotes the production of cytokines such as alpha interferon (αIFN), gamma interferon (αIFN) and interleukin-2 (IL-2) by activated lymphocytes (5-7). Thymosin α_1 has also been shown to increase the expression of high affinity IL-2 receptors on the surface of activated lymphocytes (5-6,8-10).

There is evidence to suggest that thymosin α_1 may influence the recruitment of pre-natural killer (NK) cells which then become cytotoxic after exposure to interferon (5,11). Thymosin α_1 may also directly influence the lytic activity of mature NK cells (11). Recent investigations have shown that thymosin α_1 enhances both allogenic and autologous human mixed lymphocyte reactions by activation of T4 (helper/inducer) cells (12). This provides additional evidence that T4 cells may be a significant target for the biological effects of thymosin α_1 (5,12).

Clinical trials of thymosin α_1 as primary or adjunctive therapy indicate that it may be of potential utility for the treatment of chronic hepatitis B infections, certain forms of cancer and AIDS. It has also been shown to enhance immunoresponsiveness to both hepatitis B and influenza vaccines in immune-depressed individuals. The number of human subjects who have received thymosin α_1 now totals more than 600. No significant adverse constitutional, local or systemic effects have been observed to date.

BIOCHEMISTRY

Chemical Description

Thymosin α_1 is an acetylated 28 amino acid peptide hormone. The amino acid sequence is shown below in Figure 1.

Ac-Ser-Asp-Ala-Ala-Val-Asp-Thr-Ser-Ser-Glu-Ile-Thr-Thr-Lys-
-Asp-Leu-Lys-Glu-Lys-Lys-Glu-Val-Val-Glu-Glu-Ala-Glu-Asn-OH

Figure 1

Chemical synthesis of thymosin α_1 has been achieved by both solution phase peptide synthesis and by solid phase synthesis. By using recombinant DNA methods, the gene for thymosin α_1 has been isolated and expressed in E. coli, which produces desacetyl-thymosin α_1, not the desired product thymosin α_1 itself.

BIOLOGICAL CHARACTERIZATION

Mechanism of Action

Although the mechanism of action of thymosin α_1 has not been totally defined, it acts primarily to increase the efficiency of T-cell maturation and to increase the ability of T-cells to produce lymphokines such as αIFN, αIFN, IL-2 and IL-3 following antigen and/or mitogen activation and to upregulate and express high affinity lymphokine receptors (Figure 2) (13). Thymosin α_1 is classified as a biological response modifier on the basis of these effects on lymphocyte markers and lymphocyte functional activity both in vivo and in vitro. Initial studies demonstrated that thymosin α_1 induced markers of mature T-cell differentiation on lymphocytes from the bone marrow of adult thymectomized mice (14). Subsequent studies defined a post-differentiation activity with respect to the induction of lymphokine and lymphokine receptors on peripheral blood lymphocytes. This dual activity is perhaps the reason why thymosin α_1 exhibits such a wide range of bioactivities and may explain its synergism with lymphokines in tumor model systems (see below).

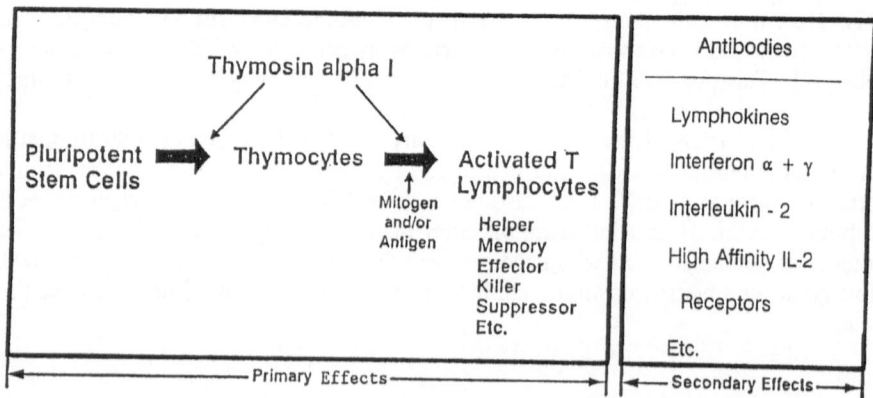

Figure 2

Thymosin α_1 interacts with mitogens to increase the production by lymphocytes of IL-2 and aIFN and to increase the number of high affinity receptors for IL-2. In the receptor studies, thymosin α_1 at 50 μg/ml was incubated with non-adherent peripheral blood lymphocytes for 30 minutes without serum followed by addition of PHA at optimal (1.0 μg/ml) and suboptimal (0.2 μg/ml) concentrations and pooled human AB serum (8). Following three days in culture, the cells were harvested, washed and the presence of high affinity IL-2 receptors evaluated using ^{125}I-labelled recombinant IL-2 in standard receptor binding assays with Skatchard analysis. Increases in high affinity receptors due to incubation with thymosin α_1 above that induced by the mitogen treatment alone were demonstrated for both mitogen concentrations.

The induction of IL-2 and total IL-2 receptors (as defined using the anti-Tac antibody) were demonstrated under similar conditions as those used for the high affinity receptors alone (5,10). The major difference was that receptor induction as measured by the anti-Tac method (which measures both high and low affinity receptors) was only observed at the suboptimal mitogen concentrations. The induction of IL-2 and total IL-2 receptors was demonstrated not only in non-adherent PBL's but on mitogen stimulated large granular lymphocytes (LGL) as well. In the LGL studies, thymosin α_1 induction of aIFN (measured by RIA) was also demonstrated as well as an enhancement of natural killer cell activity (as defined by the lysis of K562 targets). These observations are consistent with those of Huang et al., (15) and Hsai et al., (16).

In vivo studies with thymosin α_1 by Frasca et al (13) using an aging mouse model confirmed the in vitro observations on lymphokine and lymphokine receptor induction. Lymphocytes from older mice have lower IL-2 production and IL-2 receptor expression when cultured with mitogen. Administration of thymosin α_1 at 10 μg/mouse to 12-18 month old mice seven days before harvesting the spleens resulted in an increase in Con A (2 μg/ml Con A) stimulated IL-2 compared to saline injected controls. Immunizing 12-18 month old mice with TNP-SRBC three days after thymosin treatment resulted in an increase in TNP specific plaque forming cells in spleens isolated from the old mice four days later, thus demonstrating the functional utility of thymosin α_1 administration.

Ohta et al (17) demonstrated that thymosin α_1 administration at 0.5 μg/ml to nude mice twice a week for three weeks resulted in an increase in colony formation and IL-3 secretion by bone marrow cells. Since IL-3 is a growth factor for many kinds of hemopoietic precursor cells, this activity may also contribute to the functional utility of thymosin α_1.

In Vivo Animal Studies

Combination Therapy with thymosin α_1. Thymosin α_1 administered to mice in combination with IL-2 and cyclophosphamide (Cy) significantly enhanced the anti-tumor activity of this therapeutic regimen (18,19). Thymosin α_1 was administered at 200 μg/kg/day starting 10 days after tumor inoculation, IL-2 was administered at 50,000 units three times daily starting 14 days after tumor inoculation, and Cy was given as a single injection of 200 mg/kg on day 8 after tumor inoculation. The major observation was that addition of thymosin α_1 to the Cy/IL-2 therapy regimen prevented the relapse which often occurs with this mode of therapy. The addition of thymosin α_1 also permitted the induction of tumor regression with a lower non-toxic dose of IL-2.

Thymosin α_1 also was effective in enhancing the anti-tumor activity of an α/β IFN/Cy combination in a mouse tumor model (20). Thymosin α_1 was administered at 200 μg/kg/day for four days starting 10 days after tumor inoculation, α/β IFN was given as a single injection of 30,000 units/mouse 13 days after tumor inoculation, and

Cy was given as a single injection of 200 μg/kg on day 8 after tumor inoculation. The most significant effects observed from the addition of thymosin α_1 was a prolongation of survival time and an increase in the number of survivors.

Thymosin α_1 as a Vaccine Adjuvant. When thymosin α_1 was administered to old mice, the antibody response following tetanus toxoid vaccination was restored to the level seen with young animals (21). In this study thymosin α_1 was administered to old (23-month) and young (2-3 month) mice on the day of vaccination and for four additional days after vaccination. The thymosin-treated mice were then compared to similar groups of untreated mice. The old mice that were not treated with thymosin α_1 had a significantly lower antibody response than the young mice. However, with thymosin α_1 treatment, the old mice responded as well as the young mice. In contrast, treatment with thymosin α_1 had no effect on the antibody response of the young mice.

Enhanced Resistance to Infection with thymosin α_1. Thymosin α_1 administered at 1 μg/mouse/day from day 7 pre-infection to day 3 post-infection with herpes simplex virus (HSV-1) increased the survival time of 12-week-old susceptible mice (22). If the mice were immunosuppressed with a chemotherapeutic agent such as 5-fluorouracil prior to HSV-1 infection, the resulting enhanced infection rate and decreased survival time were reversed by treatment with thymosin α_1. In a related study, Effros et al. (23) demonstrated that pretreatment with thymosin α_1 enhanced the capacity of old mice to mount an effective cytotoxic response against influenza infection.

Using a mouse model where enhanced opportunistic infection rates can be induced by 5-fluorouracil immune suppression, thymosin α_1 was shown to be effective in protecting the immune-suppressed animals (24). Thymosin α_1 was administered to immune-suppressed mice at 40 μg/kg/day beginning seven days before intraperitoneal infection with L. monocytogenes, C. albicans, or P. aerugenosa. In all instances a significant increase in the number of surviving mice was noted. Similar studies have also been reported by Bistoni et al. (25) and Salvin et al. (26).

Thymosin α_1 in a Woodchuck Hepatitis Model. The Woodchuck hepatitis virus is closely related to the human hepatitis B virus and chronic hepatitis infection in woodchucks is one of several animal models for human chronic hepatitis B infection. Unlike its human counterpart, there is little inflammatory liver disease associated with a chronic woodchuck hepatitis infection. However, most chronically infected animals progress to hepatocellular carcinoma. In the study reported by Korba, et al. (27), twelve animals ranging from 9 to 24 months of age were randomized to receive no treatment or thymosin α_1 (10 μg/kg) twice weekly for six months. At the end of treatment, the serum viral titers remained at constant high levels in the no treatment controls, while viral titers were not measurable in four of six treated animals and were reduced to 1% of entry values in the remaining two animals. Twelve weeks post-treatment, viremia had returned in two of the four animals that had no measurable virus at the end of treatment. In the two animals with reduced viremia at the end of treatment, virus titers progressively declined to undetectable levels within the twelve weeks.

CLINICAL STUDIES

Over 600 subjects have been treated with thymosin α_1 in clinical trials. The initial trials were aimed at the treatment of various cancers and the use of thymosin α_1 as an antiviral vaccine adjuvant in immunedepressed subjects. The more recent trials have been aimed at treatment of infectious diseases such as chronic hepatitis B and AIDS. Each of these trials is summarized below. No significant adverse effects from thymosin α_1 treatment have been observed in any of these trials.

Phase I Trials

Malignant Glioma Patients. The first clinical trial with thymosin α_1 was reported in 1982 (28). In this trial, 11 patients with incurable malignant gliomas received doses ranging from 300 to 900 mg/m2 of thymosin α_1 subcutaneously twice a week for four weeks. There were no obvious signs of clinical toxicity, nor changes in blood cell counts or T-cell levels during treatment or during four weeks of followup. Levels of alpha 2HSglycoprotein and prealbumin increased from depressed baselines during treatment and followup.

NonLeukemic Cancer Patients. In a second study (29), escalating doses of thymosin α_1 (0.6, 1.2, 2.4, 4.8, and 9.6 mg/m^2) were given intramuscularly to 20 advanced cancer patients. Doselimiting toxicity was not observed although three patients experienced minor toxicities that were possibly drug related (fever, mild nausea).

Phase II/Phase III Trials

Adjuvant for Influenza and Hepatitis Vaccines. Five Phase II trials have been completed evaluating the efficacy of thymosin α_1 as an adjuvant for antiviral vaccines. The results of these studies are summerized below.

Adjuvant for Influenza Vaccine in Elderly Subjects. a. In a 1985 study conducted at the Cornell Medical Center in New York City, thymosin α_1 was administered after influenza vaccination to nine elderly subjects who were previously nonresponsive to influenza vaccine (30). Six of the nine subjects responded with high levels of antiinfluenza antibodies, while only one of six vaccinated subjects who did not receive thymosin α_1 developed antibodies. No toxicity was observed in any of the thymosin α_1 treated patients.

b. In a 1986 trial conducted at the University of Wisconsin V.A. Medical Center, 94 veterans over 64 years of age were vaccinated with trivalent influenza vaccine and randomized to receive thymosin α_1 or placebo in a doubleblind study (31). The subjects were injected with thymosin α_1 or placebo twice weekly for four weeks commencing immediately after vaccination. Three patients dropped out and one died, leaving 90 patients, from whom sera of 85 were evaluable. Of the patients receiving thymosin α_1, 68% were effectively immunized (four fold or greater rise in antibody titer over three to six weeks as measured by ELISA) versus 46% of those receiving placebo. No toxicity was observed with thymosin α_1.

c. In 1987, a trial with a similar design to the Wisconsin V.A. Medical Center trial was conducted at the U.S Soldier's and Airmen's Home in Washington D.C. (32). In this study, the effect of four versus eight injections of 900 μg/m^2 thymosin α_1 (given twice weekly) following vaccination with trivalent influenza vaccine were compared. A total of 337 patients initially participated, with 330 available for analysis. Analysis of the antibody responses in these patients revealed that the response to the A/H1N1 antigen was significantly greater (p=0.015) among all those who received eight injections of thymosin α_1 compared with those who received placebo. Among those 80 years and older, the response was greater to the B/Ann Arbor antigen (p=0.035) and the A/H3N2 Leningrad antigen (p=0.012) as well. There was no statistical difference between the placebo groups and the groups which received only four injections of thymosin α_1. No toxicity associated with thymosin α_1 injection was observed in any of the subjects.

d. In a separate study, Shen et al. (33) evaluated the efficacy of thymosin α_1 as a stimulant for influenza vaccine in another group of hemodialysis patients in a second randomized, doubleblind trial. Vaccination with monovalent A/Taiwan/1/86 (H1N1) vaccine was followed by eight injections of thymosin α_1 or placebo (given twice weekly). Sera was evaluated for antibody titer four weeks after vaccination. Thirtyfour out of fortyeight (71%) thymosin α_1 treated patients versus twentyone out of fortynine (43%) of placebo treated patients exhibited a four fold or higher titer of specific antibody as determined by ELISA. No patient exhibited any signs or symptoms of toxicity due to injections of thymosin α_1.

Adjuvant for Hepatitis Vaccine in Hemodialysis Patients. Shen et al. (34) evaluated the effect of thymosin α_1 on increase the responsiveness of previously non-responding hemodialysis patients to Heptavax B vaccine. The trial was double blind and placebo controlled. Three vaccine injections were given one month apart and each was followed by five biweekly thymosin α_1 injections at a dose of 900 $\mu g/m^2$. Seven of eleven (64%) thymosin α_1 treated patients and two of twelve (17%) placebo treated patients developed sustained HBsAB titers. No toxicities associated with thymosin α_1 were noted.

Pilot Study in Advanced Cancer Patients. Dillman et al. (35) evaluated various doses of thymosin α_1 in 14 advanced cancer patients to determine its effect on immune restoration. A dose of 1.2 mg/m2 was associated with a substantial improvement in 46% of abnormal in vitro immune tests.

Trial in Head and Neck Cancer. A Veteran's Administration funded Phase II clinical trial involving 58 patients with head and neck cancer was completed in 1988 at the University of Michigan and VA Medical Center in Ann Arbor, MI. (36). The patients had advanced cancers that required treatment by a combination of surgery and postoperative radiation therapy. In most patients, the interval between treatment and tumor recurrence was short and was not significantly increased by thymosin α_1 treatment.

Trial in Post-Radiation Therapy NonSmall Cell Lung Cancer Patients. Schulof et al. (37) evaluated the use of thymosin α_1 in a randomized Phase II double blind placebocontrolled trial of 42 postradiation therapy patients with nonsmall cell lung cancer. Two regimens of thymosin α_1 therapy were employed commencing within one week of the completion of radiotherapy: twice weekly injections of 900 $\mu g/m^2$ or 14 daily injections of 900 $\mu g/m^2$ followed by twice weekly injections. Thymosin α_1 or placebo injections were continued for one year or until relapse. Patients receiving placebo or the initial 14 daily injections of thymosin α_1 exhibited a gradual decrease in percent OKT3 and OKT4 cells and in the OKT4/OKT8 ratio while patients receiving only twice weekly injections of Thymosin alpha 1 maintained mean percent OKT3 and OKT4 cells at nearly 90% of pretreatment values over 15 weeks of serial monitoring. Among 41 evaluable patients, there were statistically significant improvements in both relapsefree survival (p = 0.04) and overall survival (p = 0.009) for the thymosin treatment groups compared with the placebo group. The only toxic side effects noted were mild burning at the injection site in three patients and a mild transient loss of muscle mass in one patient. All four of these patients were receiving injections from a single lot of thymosin α_1. After switching to another lot of thymosin α_1, no further side effects were noted.

Chronic Hepatitis B. A Phase II study of thymosin α_1 and thymosin fraction 5 for the treatment of chronic active hepatitis B was reported by Mutchnick, et al. (38). Subsequently, Dr. Mutchnick has reported on the long term follow up and on additional patients enrolled in this trial (39). Overall, nine patients were given thymosin α_1 (two concentrations, 900 $\mu g/m^2$ and 1200 $\mu g/m^2$) twice per week for 26 weeks (four patients received 2 4 injections of thymosin fraction 5 instead of thymosin α_1 at the beginning of therapy). Seven of the nine (78%) who were treated for at least 24 weeks with thymosin α_1 responded to treatment and were in remission six months after cessation of treatment. Six of these seven responders are still in remission after a mean of 3.5 years.

Trial in Post-Radiation Therapy Non-Small Cell Lung Cancer Patients. A Phase III study of thymosin α_1 treatment postradiation therapy in nonresectable non-small cell lung cancer patients was sponsored by the National Cancer Institute and managed by the Radiation Therapy Oncology Group. The results of this randomized, doubleblind, placebo controlled study which enrolled 253 patients have not been published. However, it is known that there were no toxic effects attributable to thymosin α_1 injection (Paul Chretien, personal communication).

INFECTIOUS DISEASES

AIDS

Phase I/II Trial in HIV Seropositive Patients: Schulof et al. (40) reported a Phase I/II trial of thymosin α_1 and thymosin fraction 5 in the treatment of HIV seropositive patients. A total of 42 patients were treated in four consecutive studies of which 30 were considered evaluable. Thymosin α_1 (600 $\mu g/m^2$) was administered daily to 10 patients (10 evaluable) for 10 weeks followed by twice weekly injections for four weeks. No local, systemic, or laboratory toxicities were seen with thymosin α_1, although several patients receiving thymosin fraction 5 had mild erythema and skin reactions and two subjects had thymosin fraction 5 shots discontinued because of erythema and swelling at sites of prior injections. This trial was not of sufficient duration or size to determine efficacy, and no results relevant to efficacy were reported.

Combination Therapy with AZT and αIFN. Recently, Garaci et al. (41) have presented data on the combination of thymosin α_1, αIFN and zidovudine (AZT) in the treatment of HIVinfected patients with CD4 counts of 500 and lower. Patients were randomized to three arms; AZT alone (10 patients), AZT plus αIFN (6 patients), or AZT, αIFN, and thymosin α_1. The doses for the three drugs were AZT, 500 mg/day; αIFN, 2 MU s.c. twice weekly; and thymosin α_1, 1.0 mg s.c. twice weekly. After one year of therapy, the combination of thymosin α_1 with IFN and AZT was well tolerated and resulted in a statistically significant increase (paired test) in CD4+ counts compared with the groups receiving AZT alone or AZT plus αIFN. No adverse effects were associated with the combination therapy. In addition, the group receiving the combination therapy with thymosin α_1 and αIFN had a significantly lower viremia as measured by PCR testing.

REFERENCES

1. Low T.L.K., et al. I. Isolation, characterization, and biological activities of thymosin alpha-1 and polypeptide b1 from calf thymus. J. Biol. Chem. 1979, 254:981-86.

2. Low, T.L.K., et al., In: "The Year in Hematology," (1978) 281-319.

3. Wang, S.-S., Synthesis of Thymosin a1. U.S. Patent No. 4,148,788. 1979.

4. Schulof R.S., et al. Thymic Factors, In Biological Response Modifiers and Cancer Therapy, 1988, Marcel Dekker, Inc.

5. Serrate S.A., et al. Modulation of human natural killer cell cytotoxic activity, lymphokine production and interleukin 2 receptor expression by thymic hormones. J. Immunol. 1987, 139:2338-2343.

6. Baxevanis C.N., et al. Enhancement of human T lymphocyte function by prothymosin alpha: increased production of interleukin-2 and expression of interleukin-2 receptors in normal human peripheral blood T lymphocytes. Immunopharmac. and Immunotoxic. 1990, 12(4):595-617.

7. Hu S.-K., et al. Thymosin enhances the production of IL-1a by human peripheral blood monocytes. Lymphokine Res. 1989, 8(3):203-214.

8. Leichtling K.D., et al. Thymosin alpha 1 modulates the expression of high affinity interleukin-2 receptors on normal human lymphocytes. Int. J. Immunopharmac. 1990, 12:19-29.

9. Sztein M.B., et al. Modulation of interleukin 2 receptor expression on normal human lymphocytes by thymic hormones. Proc. Natl. Acad. Sci. U.S.A. 1986, 83:6107-6111.

10. Sztein, M.B., et al. Characterization of the immunoregulatory properties of thymosin alpha 1 on interleukin-2 production and interleukin-2 receptor expression in normal human lymphocytes. Int. J. Immunopharmac. 1989, 11(7):789-800.

11. Favalli C., et al. Modulation of natural killer activity by thymosin alpha 1 and interferon. Cancer Immunol. Immunother. 1985, 20:189-192.

12. Baxevanis C.N., et al. Immunoregulatory effects of fraction 5 thymus peptides. I. Thymosin enhances while thymosin B4 suppresses the human autologous and allogeneic mixed lymphocyte reaction. Immunopharm. 1987, 13:133-141.

13. Frasca, D., et al., Reconstitution of T cell functions in aging mice by Thymosin a1. Immunopharmacology (1986) 11:155-163.

14. Bach, J.F., et al., Appearance of T-cell markers in bone marrow rosette forming cells after incubation with thymosin, a thymic hormones. Proc. Natl. Acad. Sci., 68:2735-2738.

15. Huang, K.-Y., et al., Thymosin treatment modulates production of Interferon. J. Interferon Rsch. (1981) 1:3:411-420.

16. Hsai, J., et al., Peripheral blood mononuclear cell Interleukin-2 and Interferon-a production, cytoxicity, and antigen-stimulated blastogenesis during experimental rhinovirus infection. J. of Infectious Diseases. (1990) 162:591-597.

17. Ohta, Y., et al., Thymosin a1 enhances haemopoietic colony formation by stimulating the production of Interleukin 3 in nu/nu mice. Int. J. Immunopharmac. (1986) 8:7:773-779.

18. Mastino, A., et al., Thymosin a1 potentiates interleukin 2 induced cytotoxic activity in mice. Cell. Immunol., (1991) 133:196-205.

19. Mastino, et al., Combination therapy with thymosin alpha 1 potentiates the anti-tumor activity of Interleukin-2 with cyclophosphamide in the treatment of the Lewis lung carcinoma in mice. Int. J. Cancer (1992) 50:493-499.

20. Garaci et al., Combination treatment using thymosin alpha 1 and interferon after cyclophosphamide is able to cure Lewis lung carcinoma in mice. Cancer Immunol. Immunother. (1990) 32:154-160.

21. Ershler, et al., Effects of thymosin alpha 1 on specific antibody response and susceptibility to infection in young and aged mice. Int. J. Immunopharm. (1985) 7:465-471.

22. Shiau, et al., The effects of thymosin on experimental herpes simplex virus infections. J. Formoson Med. Assoc. (1988) 87:34-71.

23. Effros, et al., The effect of thymosin alpha 1 on immunity to influenza in aged mice. In Aging: Immunology and Infectious Disease. (1988) 1:31-40.

24. Ishitsuka, et al., Protective activity of thymosin against opportunistic infections in animal models. Immunol. Immunotherapy. (1983) 144-150.

25. Bistoni, et al., Increase of mouse resistance to Candida Albicar infection by thymosin alpha 1. Infect. Immun. (1982) 36:609-614.

26. Salvin, S.B., In vivo effects of Thymosin on cellular immunity. Clin. Immun. Newsletter. (1984) 5:9:129-135.

27. Korba, B.E., et al., Treatment of Chronic Woodchuck Hepatitis Virus Infection with Thymosin alpha 1. Hepatology (1990) 12:880;

Personal communication NIAID.

28. Baskies, A.M., et al., Thymosin Alpha-1: First clinical trial and comparison with thymosin fraction 5. Current Contents in Human Immunol. and Cancer Immunomodulation. (1982) 567-574.

29. Dillman, R.O., et al., Phase I trials of thymosin fraction 5 and Thymosin a1. J. of Biolog. Resp. Mod. (1982) 1:35-41.

30. McConnell, L.T., et al., Augmentation of influenza antibody levels and reduction in attach rates in elderly subjects by thymosin alpha 1 (TA1). The Gerontologist (1989) 29:188A.

31. Gravenstein, S., et al., Augmentation of influenza antibody response in elderly men by Thymosin alpha one, A double-blind placebo-controlled clinical study. JAGS (1989) 37:1-8.

32. McConnell, L.T., Influenza vaccine and adjuvant thymosin alpha-1: A double-blind placebo-controlled trial. (Unpublished report).

33. Shen, S.Y., et al., Age-Dependent enhancement of influenza vaccine responses by thymosin in chronic hemodialysis patients. In: Biomedical advances in aging. (1990) 523-530.

   Shen, S.Y., et al., Increases in specific antibody responses to influenza vaccine responses with adjuvant thymosin alpha 1 in chronic hemodialysis patients. (Unpublished report).

34. Shen, S., et al., Effects of thymosin alpha 1 (TA1) on peripheral T-cell and heptavax-B vaccination (V) in previously non-responsive hemodialysis (HD patients (Pts). Hepatology (1987) 7:1120.

35. Dillman, R.O., et al., In vivo immune restoration in advanced cancer patients after administration of thymosin fraction 5 or thymosin a1. J. of Biolog. Resp. Mod. (1983) 2:139-149.

36. Wolfe, G.T. Prospective randomized trial of thymosin alpha (Ta1) immune reconstitution in patients with advanced head and neck squamous carcinoma (HNSC): 5 year results. In: Proceedings of the American Association for Cancer Research (1989) 30:261.

37. Schulof, R.S., et al., A randomized trial to evaluate the immunorestorative properties of synthetic thymosin-a1 in patients with lung cancer. J. Biolog. Resp. Mod. (1985) 4:147-158.

38. Mutchnick, M.G., et al., Thymosin treatment of chronic hepatitis B a placebo-controlled pilot trial. Hepatology (1991) 14:3:409-415.

39. Mutchnick, M., et al., Sustained response to thymosin therapy in patients with chronic active hepatitis B (CAHB). Second International Symposium on Combination Therapies. (1992) 36.

40. Schulof, R.S., et al., Phase I/II Trial of thymosin fraction 5 and thymosin alpha one in HTLV-111 Seropositive Subjects. J. Biolog. Resp. Mod. (1986) 3:429-443.

41. Garaci, E., et al., Combined therapy with zidovudine -thymosin alpha 1 - alpha interferon in the treatment of HIV-infected patients. Second International Symposium on Combination Therapies. (1992) 33.

COMBINATION THERAPY WITH THYMOSIN α1 AND CYTOKINES IN THE

TREATMENT OF CANCER AND INFECTIOUS DISEASES

Enrico Garaci, Antonio Mastino, Francesca Pica, and Cartesio Favalli

Department of Experimental Medicine and Biochemical Sciences, University of   Rome "Tor Vergata", Via O. Raimondo 00173 Rome, Italy

INTRODUCTION

During recent years, many studies have stressed the importance of new approaches in the use of biological response modifiers (BRMs) in the treatment of cancer and infectious diseases. Although there is general agreement on the therapeutical potential of these agents, their clinical use did not yield the expected results. As a consequence, in the attempt to improve the efficacy of these molecules, many groups are trying different approaches, including combination therapies with various cytokines. In particular, it seems likely that combinations of different BRMs can result in a more potent effect than single treatments (1-4) The rationale of this new approach stems from the observations that immune physiologic responses involve cascades and feedback networks in which the release of one cytokine modulate both cytokine and cytokine-receptor production. Moreover, combination of BRMs could affect different immune effector cells.

Regarding to the possible combinations of cytokines, it is important to mention that some authors have focused their attention on the capacity of thymic hormones (THs) to stimulate the production of cytokines by peripheral blood lymphocytes (PBL). This has been shown for the migration inhibition factor (MIF) (5) and for colony stimulating factors, for the granulocyte/ macrophage GM-CSF (6,7) and for the B-cell growth factor (8), for interferon (IFN) (9-11) and for interleukin 2 (IL-2) (12,13). Thymosin α1 (Tα1) has been also shown to induce IFN-α after in vivo administration (9). However, an attentive analysis of these results and our data indicate that THs principally

Combination Therapies 2, Edited by A.L. Goldstein
and E. Garaci Plenum Press, New York, 1993

act as super-inducing accessory signals in the induction of cytokines. Because of these interesting interactions, combined treatment with THs and the above mentioned cytokines could be considered as a possible approach. In fact, our studies during the last recent years have demonstrated that combination treatments with THs and IFN or IL-2 exert powerful biological effects. It has been shown that Tα1 can upregulate the expression of high-affinity IL-2 receptors in mitogen-stimulated human PBL or LGL, and enhance IL-2 production (14,15). On the other hand, it is well known that IL-2 is able to augment MHC-restricted and -unrestricted cytotoxic activities (16). Thus, we have studied the possibility of potentiating the IL-2-induced cytotoxic activity of spleen cells in vitro, obtained from normal mice and from tumor- or CY-suppressed mice, by in vitro or in vivo pretreatment with Tα1. We have observed that IL-2 action on cytotoxic activities is effectively modulated by Tα1. In fact, pretreatment, either in vitro or in vivo, with this synthetic polypeptide enhanced the IL-2-induced cytotoxic activity against both NK-sensitive YAC-1 cells and NK-resistant MBL-2 cells (17). One possible explanation of these results could be the effect of Tα1 on the activation/differentiation of non-cytolytic and/or IL-2-low-responsive progenitor cells. Indeed, results, previously obtained by our group in bone marrow chimera experiments, suggest that Tα1 can influence the in vivo process of maturation of bone marrow progenitor cells to cytolytic effectors (18). In addition, we have studied the effect of administration of an immunotherapeutic protocol with Tα1 and IL-2, on the cytotoxic activities in vivo. Our results clearly show how a treatment with Tα1 and IL-2 in vivo can exert a powerful and impressive synergistic action on cytotoxic functions of immune cells from normal mice or from 3LL tumor-bearing mice, with or without chemotherapy treatment (19). Since IL-2 induced killer cells play a critical role in the defense against tumors, we have performed experiments on the effects of Tα1 and IL-2, alone or in combination, directly on tumor growth in 3LL tumor-bearing mice, treated or not with CY. In addition, it has been demonstrated the capacity of THs to enhance the expression of specific receptors for IL-2 in mitogen-stimulated PBL or LGL (13,20,21). On the basis of these results, it was interesting to verify whether treatment with THs could be able to enhance the functional response to IL-2. In fact, we demonstrated that in vitro or in vivo pretreatment with Tα1 potentiates IL-2-induced cytotoxic activity of spleen cells from normal mice and tumor- or CY-suppressed mice. Enhanced cytotoxic activity was directed against both NK sensitive YAC-1 cells and NK-resistant MBL-2 cells, thus indicating a LAK-type phenomenon (17). The following step was studying the effect of in vivo administration of an immunotherapeutic protocol with THs and IL-2 on the cytotoxic activities of 3LL tumor-bearing mice, with or without chemotherapy treatment. The results have shown that a combination treatment with Tα1 followed by human recombinant IL-2 caused an evident increase in cytotoxic activity against both NK-sensitive and NK-resistant target cell lines, and also against fresh 3LL autologous tumor cells (19). These effects were associated to a powerful antitumoral action, when THs and IL-2 were associated to chemotherapy, as reported below in the section on cancer. Regarding to the interaction between THs and IFN, some years ago we demonstrated that Tα1 and IFN-α,ß are able to perform a synergic stimulatory action on the NK activity of animals immunodepressed by cyclophosphamide (22).

The studies on the other approach with Tα1 and IFN-α,ß demonstrated that the combination treatment can powerfully stimulate the cytotoxic response also during the NK activity depression associated with experimental tumor growth in mice (23). Also in this experimental model, animals are in a state of non-responsiveness to the treatment with IFN alone. Thus, we have tried to verify whether THs and IFN combination treatment could prove effective if administered in combination with chemotherapy. In fact, such a kind of combination immunotherapy strongly stimulated NK activity and cytotoxicity against autologous 3LL tumor cells, in 3LL tumor bearing mice treated with CY, whereas treatments with either agent alone did not, or slightly, modify the cytotoxic activity towards Yac-1 or 3LL target cells. The killer cells stimulated by combination chemoimmunotherapy treatment bear the phenotypic characteristics of asialo-GM1 positive cells. A histological study has shown a high number of infiltrating lymphoid cells in the tumors obtained from mice treated with combination chemoimmunotherapy.

COMBINATION THERAPY WITH THYMOSIN α1 AND CYTOKINES IN INFECTIOUS DISEASES

Considering the important role of immune response in the control of infectious diseases, immunotherapeutic treatments have a rational application particularly in controlling infectious agents, which are poorly, if not at all, aggredible by conventional direct antimicrobial chemotherapy. This is the case of antibiotic-resistant bacterial or fungal agents and of viruses. Moreover, the number of immunocompromised hosts is increased lately, due to the spread of AIDS epidemic, cancer chemotherapy and immunosuppressive therapy. As a consequence, increased attention is concentrated on the prevention and treatment of the infections that affect these individuals. One of the most interesting clinical approaches in these patients is immunotherapy with a number of substances reconstituting the immune functions. The list of substances, currently under careful experimentation in order to ascertain their effectiveness in the stimulation of immune response, increased considerably during the recent years. Among them the cytokines have been extensively studied. These substances share the common characteristic of being physiologically involved in the regulation of ontogenesis and of activation of different immune cells, and are considered to exert a certain selective action on the immune response. Furthermore, most of them are now available in large quantities through biotechnological techniques. Results obtained using these substances in controlling infectious diseases, although encouraging, appear limited and strictly related to the experimental model employed (24-27). Moreover, it might be considered that immunosuppression is quite usual for patients affected by infectious diseases, and that in some cases, as in HIV infection, immunosuppression is strictly connected with the infection itself. It is also known that in immunosuppressed patients effector immune cells can be refractory to cytokines, thus causing an additional problem to the immunotherapeutic control of infectious diseases. Since, on the basis of the current knowledge, the physiologic way cytokines act is cooperation, another cause of their partially unsuccessful use could be attributed to their utilization as single agents. These considerations open the way for the rational use of combination therapies with cytokines, with or without conventional antimicrobial therapy, in the treatment of infectious diseases. Here we report the results of our studies on HIV and Hepatitis infections.

Regarding HIV infection, increasing evidence shows that: i) anti-retroviral therapy with zidovudine (ZVD) alone slows down, rather than preventing totally HIV replication and disease progression to late AIDS; ii) impaired functions of the remaining uninfected immune cells plays an important role in immunodeficiency associated with HIV infection (27). Combination treatment with Tα1 plus IFN would therefore be a possible candidate as immunotherapy in adjunction to ZVD antiretroviral therapy. In a preliminary experiment, in order to test this hypothesis, PBL collected from HIV-positive patients, either treated or not with ZVD, were cultured for 24 hours in the presence of human recombinant IFN-α, with or without pretreatment with Tα1. At the end of the culture, cytotoxic activity against an NK-sensitive cell line was tested. Results show that in most cases pretreatment with Tα1 was able to potentiate the cytotoxic activity of PBL collected from HIV-positive patients. PBL from all healthy controls responded to Tα1 pretreatment. PBL from ZVD-treated patients in advanced disease did not respond so well to combination treatment. Considering our preliminary results and the fact that IFN has been shown to be synergistic against HIV when combined with ZVD, a clinical study has been designed to examine the potential beneficial effects of a combination regimen, which includes Tα1 plus IFN in conjunction with ZDV. The results of these experiments are reported in detail in an other chapter of this book. In addition, as previously reported, combined immunotherapy treatment with Tα1 and IL2 after CY inoculation resulted the most efficacious combined treatment, inducing 100% of surviving tumor-free mice in 3LL tumor experimental model. The conclusion of this series of experiments is that the enhancement of the response of effector cells to IL-2 with Tα1 may enable lower doses of IL-2 to be effective, and could overcome the problem of toxicity of IL-2 when administered at high doses. IL-2, indeed, was found to enhance HIV replication in vitro, suggesting, some years ago, the abandonment of its possible use in AIDS patients. These data make us extremely cautious in hypothesizing the possibility of also transferring this protocol to HIV-infected patients. However, we must consider that HIV-infection in vitro is very

TABLE 1. Treatment schedule for HBCAH patients

Inductive treatment, first week:
Thymosin alpha 1: 1mg/day, s.c. days 1-4
natural alpha-IFN: 3 MUI/day, i.m. day 4.
Maintaining treatment, successive 25 weeks:
thymosin alpha 1: 1mg/day, s.c. days 1,4
alpha-IFN: 3 MUI/day,i.m. days 1,4

---

different from in vivo infection, when, even in an advanced phase, only a minority of immune cells seems to contain the virus, and that ZVD treatment seems to be really effective, at least in an initial period, in controlling viral replication. Moreover, the possibility of utilizing low doses of IL-2 after a

Tα1-pretreatment could reduce the risk of the activation of viral replication. Further preclinical studies must, in any case, be performed before examining the hypothesis of the clinical use of Tα1, in combination with IL-2, in ZVD-treated HIV-patients. On the other hand, combination treatment with Tα1 and IL-2 could be useful in infections different from that caused by HIV.

TABLE 2. Results of 11 evaluable HBCAH patients after 6 months of combination treatment with thymosin α1 and IFN.

Pat.	DAYS					
	0	180	0	180	0	180
	HBV/DNA pg/ml		CD4+ abs.No.		ALT	
1	5.1	<1.8	258	415	116	32
2	2.0	<1.8	1080	2150	192	101
3	30.0	6.5	698	877	34	31
4	16.9	<1.8	927	577	48	43
5	48.4	27.6	545	762	119	78
6	18.1	7.1	732	716	158	90
7	35.1	<1.8	751	925	150	62
8	23.4	9.5	658	836	120	50
9	27.5	<1.8	681	859	180	25
10	34.8	26.8	702	710	87	137
11	10.0	<1.8	451	603	137	26

Patients affected by viral hepatitis represent other potential candidates to combination immunotherapies. In fact IFN has been already used with a certain efficacy in the therapy of HBsAg- chronic-active-hepatitis (HBCAH); however IFN treatment does not always induce a favorable clinical response. As consequence we evaluated the possibility that Tα1 could potentiate the effect of IFN in HBCAH patients. To this purpose we started a clinical trial in order to evaluate the systemic effects of combination therapy with Tα1 plus IFN on HBCAH patients who failed to respond to IFN alone. Here we report the results of the first 11 evaluable patients after 6 months of therapy. The clinical diagnosis of HBCAH in these patients was confirmed in all cases by liver biopsy. All patients were previously treated for six months with recombinant IFN-α2 alone and were enrolled after a pause of at least six months starting from the end of the previous therapy. Each patient underwent a thorough medical and laboratory evaluation on days 0, 5, 15, 60, 120, 180 starting from the beginning of the trial. The following parameters have been evaluated: serum levels of aspartate aminotransferase (AST) and alanine aminotransferase (ALT), serologic markers of hepatitis B infection (HBsAg, anti-HBs, HBeAg, anti-HBe, HBV-DNA), immunological monitoring (flow cytometry analysis of lymphocyte subsets, NK activity). The following exclusion criteria were utilized: diagnosis of cirrhosis, malignancies, hiv or other severe infections, hematological or immunological disorders. The preliminary results indicate that all (100%) patients did respond to the combination therapy. Positive/negative (<1.8) conversion of HBV-DNA was observed in 6 of 11 patients (55%) and reduced values in the remaining of 5 patients (45%); in all patients a decrease in ALT was detected (in 6 to normal values). This result correlated with an absolute and relative increase in T lymphocytes, and particularly of the CD4+ subset, in most of the cases. Table 1 and 2 summarize the treatment schedule and part of the results, respectively. These results seem to be encouraging, suggesting, by now, to program a prospective randomized phase III clinical trial in untreated HBCAH patients. In addition, on the basis of the results obtained in the pilot study in HBV patients, a clinical trial is now in progress also in C hepatitis patients.

COMBINATION THERAPY WITH THYMOSIN α1 AND CYTOKINES IN CANCER

One of the potentially most important applications of BRMs is in the area of immunotherapy of cancer. The rationale for the use of these agents in treating tumors includes their supposed ability to restore the immune system of cancer patients leading to a reduction or an arrest in the growth of cancer cells, to enhance the cancer patient's ability to repair normal cells damaged by chemotherapy or radiation, and to stimulate their immune resistance so preventing secondary infections. As a consequence, during the last few years different research groups have tested various BRMs in animal experimental models and in humans. In fact, a series of studies demonstrated the efficacy of the BRMs in stimulating the immune response and in inhibiting, at least in part, the development of neoplasias. Among the BRMs, besides the products of microbial origin, a new category of substances, that includes interferons, interleukins, tumor necrosis factors and synthetic thymic hormones are potentially the most efficacious. As previously referred, the results of the immunotherapic approach has been not always positive and often inferior to expectations. In order to improve the efficacy of these agents, we are trying the route of combination therapies. As previously reported, we studied the combination therapy with Tα1 with IFN or IL-2. The results of the combined treatment with Tα1 and IFN without chemotherapy caused an increase in survival time, but no long-term survivors were observed (28). As a result, we have attempted to find out whether THs and IFN treatment would prove more effective if administered in combination with chemotherapy. As a consequence we performed experiments which demonstrated that combination treatment with Tα1 followed by a single injection of murine IFN-αß, starting after CY treatment, caused a rapid disappearance of the tumor burden in 3LL tumor bearing mice. The chemo-immunotherapy protocol was effective even in the long-term survival of 75% of the animals, and results were significantly different when compared to treatment with the single agents in conjunction with chemotherapy, or to chemotherapy itself. The antitumoral results were associated with immunological modifications, as reported before. After having observed that in vitro or in vivo pretreatment with Tα1 potentiates IL-2-induced cytotoxic activity in spleen cells from normal mice and tumor or CY suppressed mice, we have performed experiments regarding the effects of Tα1 and IL-2, alone or in combination, directly on 3LL tumor growth (19). The results of these experiments showed that combined immunotherapy treatment with Tα1 and IL-2 can significantly slow tumor growth and prolong survival time, as compared to all the other groups. The efficacy is more evident when immunotherapy was combined to chemotherapy. In fact, in these experiments, long-term survivors were observed when immunotherapy was associated with CY-treatment, as well as tumor disappearance, in 100% of mice. More recently we extended our studies to mice injected with highly metastatic Friend erythroleukemia cells. Particularly we utilized the 3Cl-8 Friend erythroleukemia cell line variant, which is highly IFN-α,β resistant. These tumor cells have been widely used to investigate the antitumor effects of high doses of IFN α,β (29-32), IL-1 and IL-2 (33-34), and are highly metastatic to the liver and spleen when transplanted into syngeneic mice (35). Results of combined treatment with Tα1 plus IFN or Tα1 plus IL-2 after CY resulted in a

TABLE 3. Effects of systemic administration of Tα1 plus IFN or plus IL-2 in combination with cyclophosphamide on survival time in DBA/2 mice injected subcutaneously with 3Cl-8 Friend leukemia cells.

Treatment	M.S.T.± S.D.[a] (days)	
	without Tα1	plus Tα1
Control	35.6 ± 5.5	N.D.
IFN	N.D.	33.2 ± 3.6
IL-2	N.D.	46.5 ± 2.5
CY	56.5 ± 10.5	53.7 ± 10.2
CY+IFN	55.5 ± 11.4	70.6 ± 13.6[b]
CY+IL-2	57.3 ± 10.8	69.2 ± 12.1[c]

[a] Results are expressed as mean survival time ± SD (calculated only for dead mice in the groups in which a curative effect was observed). Each group consisted of 10 mice.
[b] Mean from 6 dead mice. Four mice were definitively cured in this group.
[c] Mean from 7 dead mice. Three mice were definitively cured in this group.

powerful antitumor effect in mice inoculated with 3Cl-8 Friend leukemia cells. These treatments induced the complete regression of the primary s.c. tumor in all the mice and completely cured a significant percentage of them. Interestingly, treatments were started when tumors were fully developed and tumor cells had already started to metastasize to liver and spleen in most of the mice. Moreover, the same treatments also produced a significant increase in mean survival time in mice injected intravenously with the 3Cl-8 leukemia cell line. When leukemia cells are injected by this route the tumor is much more aggressive, owing to a rapid spread to different vascularized organs, with an early and inevitable death of mice. The antitumor effect was associated with: a) a powerful stimulation of cytotoxicity against both NK-sensitive cells and NK-resistant 3Cl-8 leukemia cells, b) a high lymphoid cell infiltration at the site of tumor inoculation and in the livers. In addition the selective depletion of CD4, CD8 or asialo-GM1 positive cells abrogated the antitumor action of chemoimmunotherapy. All these data indicate a clear involvement of the immune system, and demonstrate that the efficacy of combined immunotherapy with Tα1 plus IFN or IL-2 in association with chemotherapy is not restricted to a single experimental model. The detailed results of these experiments have been recently published (36).

TABLE 4. Effects of systemic administration of Tα1 plus IFN or plus IL-2 in combination with cyclophosphamide on survival time in DBA/2 mice injected intravenously with 3Cl-8 Friend leukemia cells.

Treatment	M.S.T.± S.D.[a] (days)	
	without Tα1	plus Tα1
Control	10.1 ± 1.1	N.D.
IFN	N.D.	10.4 ± 1.5
IL-2	N.D.	12.9 ± 3.8
CY	22.0 ± 4.6	23.2 ± 5.4
CY+IFN	24.0 ± 4.9	37.0 ± 8.5
CY+IL-2	24.4 ± 5.6	34.9 ± 8.5[b]

[a] Results are expressed as mean survival time ± SD (calculated only for dead mice in the groups in which a curative effect was observed). Each group consisted of 10 mice.
[b] Mean from 9 dead mice. One mouse in this group survived over 60 days. At that time it was sacrificed and the presence of metastases was evidenced.

Considering that the results of the experiments on the effect of combination therapy with chemotherapeutic agents and Tα1 plus IFN in tumor bearing mice proved to be very encouraging, we have decided to extend our studies on combination chemoimmunotherapy to humans. For ethical reasons and in order to compare the results obtained with combination chemoimmunotherapy treatment to those obtained with chemotherapy alone, we selected two neoplastic diseases, quite common and quite refractory to chemotherapy treatment. Standard chemotherapy regimens were not altered, but the combination immunotherapy treatment was inserted between the courses of chemotherapy itself. These clinical studies are currently in progress. In particular we are performing two pilot clinical studies in inoperable, stage III & IV, non small cell lung carcinoma (NSCLC) and in metastatic melanoma patients. The main objectives of these studies are: 1) the evaluation of systemic effects of combination therapy with Tα1 plus IFN in association with chemotherapy on the immune response of NSCLC and metastatic melanoma patients; 2) the evaluation of the possibility that immunotherapy with Tα1 plus IFN could potentiate the effect of chemotherapy in NSCLC and metastatic melanoma patients. Chemotherapic drugs were cisplatin+etoposide for NSCLC and dacarbazine for melanoma, respectively, utilized according to standard protocol as previously described (37)

No major side-effects attributable to the immunotherapy have been observed up until now in patients affected by both neoplastic diseases, and treated with the new chemoimmunotherapy regimens. The immunological monitoring of the cancer patients has shown a cyclic variation in the cytotoxicity, with a dramatic decline after chemotherapy and an evident boosting after immunotherapic treatment, which occurs repeatedly during each cycle. Patients classified as non-responders seem not to be stimulated by immunotherapy which demonstrate a relationship between immunological response to thymic hormone plus IFN and the progression of the neoplastic disease. Moreover, both in melanoma and NSCLC patients, immunotherapy treatment induced the stimulation of cytotoxic response against DAUDI, NK resistant target cells, in about 20% of cases. The study of CD4+ and CD8+ subpopulations, by flow cytometry, demonstrated that in patients treated with combination immunotherapy there was an increase either in percentage or in absolute number of CD4+ subpopulation, an absolute increase of CD8+ cell population, and an increase of CD4+/CD8+ ratio. The clinical results of patients treated with chemotherapy plus combination immunotherapy are promising both in terms of tolerance and efficacy of treatment. The clinical trial on NSCLC has been recently concluded and definitive results are reported in another chapter of this book. The clinical trial in melanoma patients is in progress, and definitive results will be obtained within few months.

In conclusion, since efficacy of the immune response, and in particular of some cytotoxic cells towards tumor and microbial agents has been well documented, the use of cytokines in the therapy of cancer and infectious diseases has a clear theoretical indication. In any case, preclinical and clinical therapeutical results are currently quite limited. This could be due to the complexity of the immune system and the restricted knowledge we have at present on the rational use of immunotherapy schemes. Our studies, which demonstrate that Tα1 combined with IFN or IL-2 exerts a synergistic action in stimulating effector immune cells, indicate a new direction in the immunotherapy of cancer as well as of infectious diseases. The efficacy of combination therapies based on this hypothesis, will be confirmed by our studies which are now in progress.

Acknowledgements: This work was in part supported by CNR, Special Projects "FATMA", "ACRO" and "Aging".

REFERENCES

1. Brunda MJ, Bellantoni D, Sulich V. In vivo anti-tumor activity of combinations of interferon α and interleukin-2 in a murine model. Correlation of efficacy with the induction of cytotoxic cells resembling natural killer cells. Int. J Cancer 1987; 40:365-71.

2. Ciolli V, Gabriele L, Sestili P, et al. Host antitumor mechanism in the combined IL-1/IL-2 therapy in mice injected with highly metastatic Friend leukemia cells. Effects on rstablished metastases. J Exp Med 1991; 173:313-22.

3. Iligo M, Sakurai M, Tamura T, Saijo N, Hoshi A. In vivo antitumor activity of multiple injections of recombinant interleukin-2, alone and in combination with three different types of recombinant interferon, on various syngenic murine tumors. Cancer Res 1988; 48:260-4.

4. McIntosh JK, Mulè JJ, Krosnick JA. Rosenberg SA. Combination cytokine immunotherapy with tumor necrosis factor α, interleukin 2, and α-interferon and its synergistic antitumor effects in mice. Cancer Res 1989; 49:1408-14.

5. Thurman GB, Seals C, Low TLK, and Goldstein AL. Restorative effects of thymosin polypeptides on purified protein derivative-dependent migration inhibition factor production by peripheral blood lymphocytes of adult thymectomized guinea pigs. J. Biol. Resp. Mod. 1984; 3: 160.

6. Ohta Y, Sueki K, Kitta K, Takemoto K, Ishitsuk H, and Yagi Y. Comparative studies on the immunosuppressive effect among 5-deoxy-5-fluorouridine, ftorafur, and 5-fluorouracil. Gann. 1980; 71: 190.

7. Ohta Y, Tezuka E, Tamura S, and Yagi Y. Thymosin alpha 1 exerts protective effect against the 5- FU induced bone-marrow toxicity. Int. J. Immunopharmac. 1985; 7: 761. N. Y. Acad. Med. 1989; 65: 111.

8. Kouttab NM, Goldstein AL, Lu M, Lu L, Campbell B, and Maizel AL. Production of human B and T cell growth factor is enhanced by thymic hormones. Immunopharmacology 1988; 16: 97.

9. Haung KY, Kind PD, Jagoda EM, Goldestein AL. Thymosin treatment modulates productions of interferon. J. Int. Res. 1981; 1: 411.

10. Shoham J, Eshel I, Aboud M, Salzberg S. Thymic hormonal activity on human peripheral blood lymphocytes, in vitro. II. Enhancement of the production of immune interferon by activated cells. J. Immunol. 1980; 125: 54.

11. Svedersky LP, Hui A, May L, McKay P, and Stebbing N. Induction and augmentation of mitogen-induced immune interferon production in human peripheral blood lymphocytes by α-desacetyl thymosin α1. Eur. J. Immunol. 1982; 12: 244.

12. Sztein MB, Serrate SA. Characterization of the immunoregulatory properties of thymosin α1 on interleukin-2 production and interleukin-2 receptor expression in normal human lymphocytes. Int J. Immunopharmac. 1989; 11: 789.

13. Sztein MB, Serrate SA, and Goldstein AL. Modulation of interleukin 2 receptor expression on normal human lymphocytes thymic hormones. Proc. Natl. Acad. Sci. USA 1986; 83: 6107.

14. Leichtling KD, Serrate SA, Sztein MB. Thymosin alpha 1 modulates the expression of high affinity interleukin 2 receptors on normal human lymphocytes. Int. J. Immunopharmac. 1990; 12: 19-29.

15. Sztein MB, Serrate SA. Characterization of the immunoregulatory properties of thymosin α1 on interleukin-2 production and interleukin-2 receptor expression in normal human lymphocytes. Int J. Immunopharmac. 1989; 11: 789-80.

16. Mule' JJ, Shu S, Rosenberg SA. The anti tumor efficacy of lymphokine-activated killer cells and recombinant interleukin- 2 in vivo. J. Immunol. 1985; 135: 646-652.

17. Mastino A, Favalli C, Grelli S, Innocenti F, Garaci E. Thymosin α 1 potentiates interleukin 2-induced cytotoxic activity in mice. Cell. Immunol. 1991; 133: 196-205.

18. Favalli C, Jezzi T, Mastino A, Rinaldi-Garaci C, Riccardi   C, and Garaci E. Modulation of natural killer activity by   thymosin alpha 1 and interferon. Cancer Immunol. Immunother. 1985; 20:189-192.

19. Mastino A, Favalli C, Grelli S, Rasi G, Pica F, Goldstein AL, Garaci E. Combination therapy with thymosin α1 potentiates the anti-tumor activity of interleukin-2 with cyclophosphamide in the treatment of the Lewis lung carcinoma in mice. Int.J.Cancer 1992; 50: 1-7.

20. Leichtling KD, Serrate SA, and Sztein MB. Thymosin alpha 1 modulates the expression of high   affinity interleukin 2 receptors on normal human lymphocytes. Int. J. Immunopharmac. 1990; 12: 19.

21. Serrate SA, Schulof RS, Leondaridis L, Goldstein AL, and Sztein M. Modulation of   human natural killer cell cytotoxic activity: limphokine production, and interleukin 2 receptor expression by thymic hormones.J. Immunol. 1987; 139: 2338.

22. Favalli C, Jezzi T, Mastino A, Rinaldi - Garaci C,   Riccardi C, and Garaci E. Modulation of natural killer   activity by thymosin alpha 1 and interferon. Cancer Immunol.   Immunother. 1985; 20: 189.

23. Favalli C, Mastino A, Jezzi T, Grelli S, Goldstein AL, and Garaci E. Synergistic effect of thymosin   α1 and alpha- beta Interferon on NK activity in tumor-bearing mice. Int. J. Immunopharmac. 1989; 11: 443.

24. Bistoni F, Marconi P, Frati L, Bonmassar E, Garaci E. Increase of mouse resistance to Candida Albicans infection by   thymosin alpha 1 . Infect. Immun. 1982; 36: 6O9-614.

25. Fujiki T, Tanaka A. Antibacterial activity of recombinant murine beta interferon Infect. Immun. 1988; 56:548-551.

26. Jeevan A, Asherson GL. Recombinant interleukin-2 limits the replication of mycobacterium lepraemurinum and mycobacterium bovis BCG in mice. Infect. Immun. 1988; 56: 660-664.

27. Phinching AJ. HIV/AIDS pathogenesis and treatment: new twists and turns. Cur. Opin. Immunol. 1991; 3: 537-542.

28. Garaci E, Mastino A, and Favalli C. Enhanced immune response and antitumor immunity with combinations of biological response modifiers. Bull.

29. Belardelli F, Gresser I, Maury C, Duvillard D, Prade M, Maunoury MT.

antitumor effects of interferon in mice injected with interferon-sensitive and inteferon-resistant Friend Leukemia cella. III Inhibition of growth and necrosis of tumor implanted subcoutaneously. Int J Cancer 1983; 31: 649-653.

30. Gresser I, Maury C, Wooddrow D, et al. Interferon treatment markedly inhibits the development of tumor metastases in the liver and spleen and increases survival time of mice after intravenous inoculation of Friend erythroleukemia cells. Int J. Cancer 1988; 41: 135-142.

31. Grasser I, Maury C, Carnaud C, De Maeyer E, Maunoury MT, Belardelli F. Antitumor effects of interferon in mice injected with interferon-sensitive and interferon-resistant Friend erythroleukemia cells. VIII. Role of the immune system in the inhibition of visceral metastases. Int J. Cancer 1990; 46: 468-474.

32. Gresser I, Carnaud C, Maury C. et al. Host humoral and cellular mechanisms in the continued suppression of Friend erythroleukemia metastases after interferon $\alpha\beta$ treatment in mice. J. Exp. Med. 1991; 173: 1193-1203.

33. Belardelli F, Ciolli V, Testa U, et al. Antitumor effects of interleukin-2 and interleukin-1 in mice transplantated with different syngeneic tumors. Int. J. Cancer 1989; 44: 1108-16.

34 Belardelli F, Gabriele L, Proietti E, et al. Sinergistic antitumor effects of combined IL-1/IFNα/β therapy in mice injected with metastatic Friend erythroleukemia cells. Int. J. Cancer 1991; 49: 274-278.

35. Belardelli F, Ferrantini M, Maury C, Santurbano L, Gresser I. On the biologic and biochemical differences between in vitro and in vivo passaged Friend erythroleukemia cells. Tumorigenicity and capacity to metastaside. Int. J. Cancer 1984; 34: 389-395.

36. Garaci E, Pica F, Mastino A, Palamara AT, Belardelli F, Favalli C. Antitumor effect of thymosyn α1/Interleukin-2 or thymosyn α1/Interferonα/β following cyclophosphamide in mice injected with highly metastatic friend erythroleukemia cells. J Immunother. 1993; 13: 7-17.

37. Garaci E and Favalli C. Combination therapy with thymic hormones and cytokines after chemotherapy in cancer treatment. Combination Therapies, Ed. by A.L. Goldstein and E. Garaci, N. York, 1992.

EFFECT OF THYMOSIN α 1 ON COCAINE-INDUCED INHIBITION OF T-CELL DEPENDENT MURINE IMMUNE RESPONSE

Giampietro Ravagnan[1], Roberto Falchetti[1], Paolo Di Francesco[2], Roberta Gaziano[2], Giulia Lanzilli[1], Cartesio Favalli[2] and Enrico Garaci[2]

[1] Institute of Experimental Medicine, CNR, Viale Marx 14
I-00137 Rome, Italy
[2] Department of Experimental Medicine and Biochemical Sciences
University of Rome, Tor Vergata, Via O. Raimondo, I-00173
Rome, Italy

INTRODUCTION

The effect of cocaine use/abuse on immune responses has recently received strong impulse from epidemiological data that have demonstrated a high prevalence of AIDS in poly-drug users[1]. In experimental models, administration of cocaine suppressed the antibody response to sheep red blood cells (SRBC)[2], measured with plaque forming cells (PFC) assay, as well as Natural Killer (NK) cell activity and T lymphocyte-induced cytotoxycity[3]. In addition, in vivo cocaine administration suppresses the ability of spleen lymphocytes to produce Interferon (IFN)-γ, Interleukin (IL)-2 and IL-4, following in vitro stimulation by mitogens[4]. Phagocitic activity of peritoneal macrophages was inhibited by a single injection of cocaine, while short term administration induced a significant reduction of spleen and thymus weight[2].

A recent study demonstrated that in vivo administration of Thymosin alpha one (Tα1), a synthetic peptide of thymic origin[5], restored different T-cell responses depressed

Combination Therapies 2, Edited by A.L. Goldstein
and E. Garaci   Plenum Press, New York, 1993

by cocaine treatments[6]. In particular, $T\alpha_1$ accelerates the recovery of normal cytotoxicity when administrated continously during cocaine treatment and for five days after the suspension of cocaine administration[6]. In the present study we further evaluated the effect of $T\alpha_1$ treatment on cocaine-induced immunodepression by measuring the primary in vivo immune response against the T-dependent antigen SRBC. The antibody response was evaluated by using a recently developed methodology[7] which permits fast, accurate and reproducible measure of spleen cell-mediated SRBC hemolysis.

MATERIALS AND METHODS

Animals and drugs

Four-week-old inbred males BALB/c mice (Charles River, Como, Italy) were used. Cocaine hydrochloride (S.A.L.A.R.S., Como, Italy) was dissolved, just before use, in Hank's balanced salt solution (HBSS, Flow Laboratories) and diluted so that each mouse received 0.2 ml volume of the drug solution. Thymosin α_1 (Alpha One Biomedicals, Inc., Washington, D.C.; a generous gift from Dr. A.L. Goldstein, The George Washington University, Washington D.C.) was dissolved in sterile phosphate buffered solution (PBS) at the concentration of 1 mg/ml and stored at -20°C. The endotoxin level was less than 0.03 pg per mg of $T\alpha_1$, as measured by a standard limulus lysate assay.

Treatment schedule

Mice were weighed before treatment and injected intraperitoneally (i.p.) with: a) cocaine (1mg/kg/day) on days -5,-4,-3,-2,-1,0; b) $T\alpha_1$ (200 µg/kg/day) administered daily during cocaine treatment and for 5 days after suspension of cocaine. A group of animals received $T\alpha_1$ alone. When $T\alpha_1$ was administered with cocaine, 8 hrs elapsed before the thymic hormone was given; c) control diluent (PBS) at the same time as treated animals. On day 0, all mice were immunized i.p. with 0.2 ml of a 2,5 % SRBC suspension. Five days later the animals were sacrificed, spleens were removed and cell suspensions were prepared by teasing individual spleens. Cell counting was performed by using a Coulter Counter ZM (Coulter Elect., U.K.).

Determination of lymphocyte-mediated SRBC hemolysis

Lymphocyte-mediated SRBC hemolysis was quantified according to the following method: 0.05 ml of the spleen cell suspension (30×10^6 cells/ml) and 0.05 ml of the SRBC suspension were mixed in a microtiter plate and 0.05 ml of 1:10 guinea pig complement was added. The plate was incubated in a humidified chamber at 37°C for 1 hr, and than centrifuged at 500xg for 10 min. 100 µl each of the supernatants was transferred to a fresh microtiter plate and the optical density (O.D.) was measured using a 414 nm narrow bandpass filter in a ELISA plate reader (Multiskan MCC/340-Labysistem-Finland).

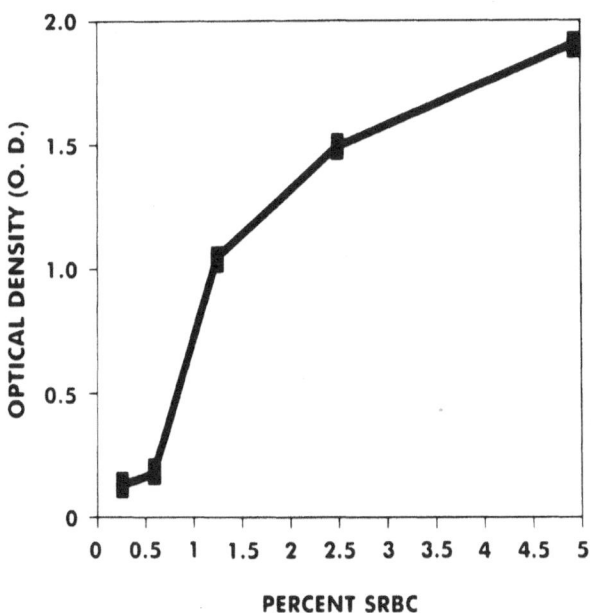

Figure 1. Four-week-old BALB/c mice were immunized i.p. with different concentrations of SRBC. Mice were sacrificed 5 days later and the spleen cell-mediated hemolytic response to SRBC was measured. The extent of the response is expressed as optical density values.

RESULTS

In vivo responsiveness to varied SRBC concentrations

BALB/c mice were immunized i.p. with different concentrations of SRBC, ranging from 0,3 to 5%. Five days later, spleen cells were assayed for reactivity to SRBC, according to the described method. The results in Figure 1 show a correlation between the amount of immunogen injected and the spleen cell-mediated hemolytic response measured as optical density. All the subsequent experiments were carried out using the SRBC concentration of 2,5 %.

Effect of Tα1 treatments on spleen cell-mediated SRBC hemolysis in cocaine-treated mice

The results are reported in Figure 2. Cocaine impaired the response to SRBC in 46% of the animals treated with the drug (1mg/kg/day) for 5 consecutive day. The decrease of SRBC responses in cocaine-treated mice was statistically significant when compared to control mice (P<0.001).Tα1 (200 μg/kg) administered during and for 5 days after cocaine treatment completely restored the response to immunogen. Finally, Tα1 *per se* did not induce significant varations in the responsiveness to SRBC.

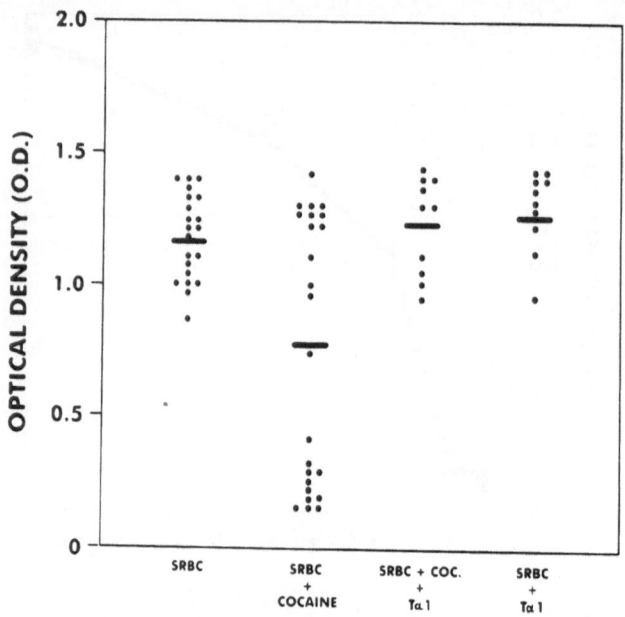

Figure 2. Four-week-old BALB/c mice were treated with cocaine, cocaine plus $T\alpha_1$ or $T\alpha_1$ alone, as described in the Methods, and were individually tested for their response to SRBC (2.5%) stimulation. Linear bars between points are the mean values. Statistical analysis by Mann Whitney U Test:
SRBC *vs* SRBC+Cocaine: $P<0.001$
SRBC+Cocaine *vs* SRBC+Cocaine+$T\alpha_1$: $P<0.05$
SRBC *vs* SRBC+$T\alpha_1$: not significant.
SRBC+Cocaine+$T\alpha_1$ *vs* SRBC+ $T\alpha_1$: not significant.

Effect of treatments on spleen cellularity

The above described treatments did not induce significant changes in spleen cellularity, which largely suggests that the inhibitory effect of cocaine was not correlated to a not specific loss of effector cells (Fig. 3). In addition, cocaine-treated mice were healthy and no weight loss was observed (data not shown).

DISCUSSION

The results presented in this paper indicate that cocaine administered daily to BALB/c mice from day -5 to day 0 (the day of immunization) induces a significant impairment of the antibody response to the T-dependent antigen SRBC. This agrees with the findings by Ou *et al.*, [2] showing that the maximum inhibition of PFC responses was obtained when the drug was administered early in the immunization schedule. The authors suggest that cocaine exerts its inhibitory effect during the inductive phase of antibody production, in which the cooperation of both T-helper cells and macrophages is required for the presentation of

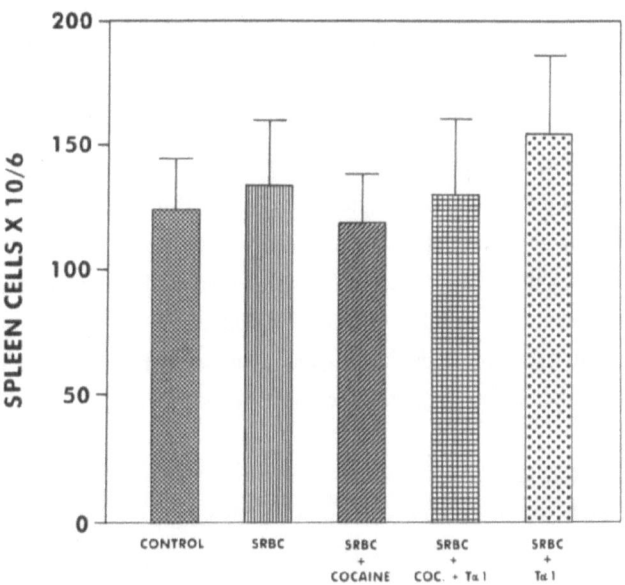

Figure 3. Effect of cocaine, cocaine plus $T\alpha_1$ or $T\alpha_1$ alone on the number of spleen cells. The differences are not statistically significant.

cooperation of both T-helper cells and macrophages is required for the presentation of antigens to B-cells. The impairment of the antibody response to SRBC may therefore be due to an effect of cocaine on B-cells, T-cells or macrophages. It would therefore be interesting to know what subset of cells represents the main target of cocaine activity. Recent data indicate that $T\alpha_1$ admininistration can restore a specific T-cell response [*i.e.*, allogenic cytotoxic T-lymphocyte (CTL) generation] depressed by cocaine administration[6]. The results presented here extend these findings. They show that $T\alpha_1$ also restores the antibody response to the T-dependent antigen (SRBC) in animals treated with an immunosuppressive dose of cocaine, confirming that the main target of cocaine effect is the T-cell subset response.

It must be noted that no changes in spleen cellularity were found in the animals treated with cocaine, $T\alpha_1$, or cocaine plus $T\alpha_1$. In addition, $T\alpha_1$ did not induce appreciable varations in the immune response when administered to normal animals. Therefore, the restorative activity of $T\alpha_1$ seems to be due to an effect on a specific T-cell subset more than an overall effect on the different cell populations.

Thymic hormones have been used successefully in humans and in experimental models to improve the decrease of T-cell functions associated with aging, cancer and several immunodeficencies[9,10] (see also Garaci *et al.* in this book). The mechanisms involved in the modulation of lymphocyte functions by $T\alpha_1$ are not fully understood. In fact, no conclusive information is avalaible regarding both the effect of $T\alpha_1$ on the different T-cell subsets and the maturation and activation stage of the cells affected by its activity. A consistent number of reports, however, suggest an activity of $T\alpha_1$ on T-helper cells. Frasca *et al.*,[8] demonstrated that $T\alpha_1$ when administered to aging animals was able to amplify helper T-cell activity by increasing the frequency of precursor T-cells. Our results suggest that the use of immunomodulating agents could have a practical therapeutic value in controlling adverse effects of cocaine on the immune system. This could be of additional help in the rescue of drug addictis. In fact, the possibility of controlling infections and improving the quality of life without resorting to massive debilitating antimicrobial treatments could hold significant value for the success of detoxification and rehabilitation therapies.

ACKNOWLEDGMENTS

We would like to thank Enrico Salvatore Pistoia for his excellent technical assistance. This work was supported by CNR, CT04 and M.U.R.S.T., grant 60%. Corresponding author: Paolo Di Francesco, Ph. D.

REFERENCES

1. R. Pillai, B.S. Nair and R.R. Watson, Aids, drugs of abuse and the immune system: a complex immunotoxicological network. *Arch.Toxicol.*, 65: 617, (1991).

2. D.W. Ou, M.L. Shen and Y.D. Luo, Effects of cocaine on the immune system of Balb/c mice. *Clin. Immunol. Immunopathol.* 52: 305, (1989).

3. P. Di Francesco, F. Pica, C. Croce, C. Favalli, E. Tubaro, E.Garaci, Effect of acute or daily cocaine administration on cellular immune response and virus infection in mice. *Nat. Immun. Cell Growth Regul*, 9: 397 (1990).

4. P. Di Francesco, S. Marini, F. Pica, C. Favalli, E. Garaci, In vivo cocaine administration influences lymphokine production and humoral immune response. *Immunol. Res.* 11, 74-79, (1992).

5. A.L. Goldstein, Low, T.L., Adoo, M., Mc Clure, J., Thurman, G.B., Rossio, G., Lay, C.Y., Chang, D., Wang, S.S., Harwey, C., Ramel, A.H. and Meienhofer, J. Thymosin alpha one: isolation and sequence analysis of immunological active polypeptide. *Proc. Natl. Acad. Sci.*, 74: 725 (1977).

6. P. Di Francesco, F. Pica, S. Marini, C. Favalli, and E. Garaci, Thymosin alpha one restores murine T-cell-mediated respones inhibited by *in vivo* cocaine administration. *Int. J. Immunopharmacol.*, 14 (1): 1 (1992).

7. T.B. Poduval, Quantitation of lymphocyte-madiated sheep red blood cell hemolysis using an Elisa reader. *J. Immunol. Methods*, 142:137 (1991).

8. D. Frasca, L. Adorini and G. Doria, Enhanced frequency of mitogen-responsive T cell precursor in old mice injected with thymosin alpha 1. *Eur. J. Immunol.*, 17: 727, (1987).

9. K.K. Oates and M.C. Coss, The role of thymosins as biological response modifiers. *Med. Sci. Res.*, 17: 793, (1989).

10. E. Garaci, Mastino, A. Pica, F. and Favalli, C. Combination treatment using thymosin alpha one and interferon after cyclosphamide is able to cure Lewis lung carcinoma in mice. *Cancer Immunol. Immunother.*, 32: 154 (1990).

REGULATION OF GENE EXPRESSION BY INTERFERONS

Santo Landolfo, Marisa Gariglio, Mirella Gaboli, David Lembo, Cristina Mana, Paola Foresta, Alessandra Angeretti and Rossana Cavallo

Institute of Microbiology, Medical School, University of Torino and Immunogenetics and Histocompatibility Center, CNR, 10126 - Torino

SUMMARY

IFNs are proteins produced by cells following stimulation with biological or synthetic inducers. The interaction with the membrane receptor is followed by the activation of the expression of particular genes that are responsible for their antiviral, antiproliferative and immunomodulatory properties. In this review we will briefly discuss the mechanisms exploited by IFNs to control at transcriptional level the expression of inducible genes. In particular we will focus on some characteristics of cis-acting DNA elements that are located upstream from the initiation site for RNA transcription and of nuclear trans-acting factors that are required for modulation of gene expression by IFNs.

TRANSCRIPTIONAL GENE ACTIVATION

Studies with cDNA and genomic clones coding for IFN inducible proteins revealed that gene expression, although not solely, is mainly regulated at the transcriptional level[1]. Although it is not yet clear whether IFNs themselves act as second messengers by directly binding nuclear receptors or send second messengers after receptor binding, it has been demonstrated that in cells exposed to IFNs there is a rapid increase in transcription of IFN-activatable genes[1]. In this regard using nuclear transcription assays, some investigators[2,3] have shown in isolated nuclei that RNA synthesis of some IFN-regulated genes (e.g. pIF-1, pIF-

2, 1-8) doubles in 5-10 min after exposure of cells to IFN-α/β, reaches the maximum (10-50 folds) between 30 and 180 min and decreases again after 4-6 hours to reach basal levels at 12-24 hours. However, if IFN is removed after 8 hour exposure, transcription rate falls rapidly below the basal levels. Transcription of class I HLA, β-microglobulin and metallothionein IIA genes following IFN-α/β treatment appears independent on protein synthesis since it takes place even in the presence of cycloeximide and it is blocked by α amanitine, indicating that this transcription requires RNA polymerase II[4].

Since in the initiation of transcription at least two different levels of control are involved, the frequency and the site of initiation[5], two questions can be asked: what are the DNA cis acting elements that control transcription? What is the nature of the cellular factors which interact with the cis-elements and thereby regulate transcription?

Promoter elements essential for mRNA synthesis by RNA polymerase II upon IFN-treatment have been identified in the region surrounding transcription initiation sites (cap site) of many IFN-inducible genes[5]. These promoter elements have been defined by transiently transfecting hybrid genes consisting of the 5' flanking region of an IFN-responsive gene (e.g. 202 gene) fused to the coding region of a reporter gene (e.g. chloramphenicolacetyltransferase, CAT)[6]. Transcription of the CAT gene in the recipient cells was increased upon exposure of these cells to IFNs. The gene segment rendering the expression of the CAT gene inducible by IFN has also enhancer-like characteristics: it can activate heterologous promoters, it is active in both the direct and the inverted orientation, and in either upstream or downstream locations from the activated promoter[7].

Recent reports from different laboratories revealed that highly homologous elements termed IFN-stimulated regulatory elements (ISREs) (consensus sequence: NGGAAA(N) TGAAACT) are present in the 5' regions of most IFN-inducible genes. This consensus sequence was first detected in the 5' flanking region of human class I HLA and metallothionein genes[4] and later on in the promoter region of the murine class I H-2K gene[8]. A number of other IFN-responsive genes have now been cloned and characterized and comparative sequence analysis have defined IFN-stimulated response elements in the promoters of these genes[1]. However the responsiveness of these enhancer elements seems to be conditioned by the cellular contest, since it has been observed that in nuclear run on assays the 2'-5' oligoadenylate synthetase and H-2L genes, driven by promoters containing the IRSEs, are differentially activated by IFNs depending on the transfected cell type (e.g. T- vs. B-lymphhocytes and fibroblasts)[9]. Using different strains of mice[10] have demonstrated an impaired transcription of the poly rI:rC- and IFN-activatable 202 gene in mice and cell lines from the C57BL/6 strain. Taken as a whole, these findings imply that cell- and strain-specific factors modulate the IFN action at the transcriptional level.

Identification of the ISREs has made it possible to search for and identify proteins that bind and activate these minimal required elements. The techniques used for detection are gel-retardation assays and protein footprintings, that allow detection of proteins specifically interacting with a labeled DNA probe[5]. It has been shown in the case of the IFN-activatable gene 6-16[11], that induction of transcription by IFN-alpha is likely to be regulated by binding of induced factors to the ISRE and 5'-upstream sequences. The IFN-induced complexes, termed E, M, L or C1/C2 depending on the cell type as source of nuclear extracts, appear a few minutes or a few hours after treatment with IFN-α, migrate relatively slowly in gel-retardation assays and in the case of the E complex no protein synthesis is required. For the induction of two other genes (ISG-54 and -15) by IFN-alpha[12], constitutive (ISGF-1, ISGF-2) and inducible (ISGF-3) DNA-protein complexes could be detected that display molecular charateristics similar to those previously described. Further purification and isolation of IFN-induced transcription factors and of the genes encoding them will allow definitive assessement of the role of these trans-acting factors in transcriptional activation, and of the mechanisms of signal transduction from cell surface to the nucleus of target cells.

ACKNOWLEDGMENTS

The experimental work performed by the group of S.L. and reviewed in this paper was supported by grants from the CNR (P.F. "Biotecnologie e Biostrumentazione" and "Applicazioni Cliniche nella Ricerca Oncologica"), from the A.I.R.C. and from the M.U.R.S.T. (40%).

REFERENCES

1. J.E. Darnell. Variety in the level of gene control in eukaryotic cells. Nature 297:365 (1982).
2. A.C. Larner, G. Jonak, Y-S.EE. Cheng, B. Korant, E. Knight and J.E. Darnell. Transcriptional induction of two genes in human cells by β-interferon. Proc. Natl. Acad. Sci USA 81:6733 (1984).
3. R.L. Friedman, S.P. Manly, M. McMajon, I. Kerr and G.R. Stark. Transcriptional and post-transcriptional regulation of interferon induced gene expression in human cells. Cell 38:745 (1984).
4. R.L. Friedman and G.R. Stark. α-Interferon-induced transcription of HLA and metallothionein genes containing homologous upstream sequences. Nature 314:637 (1985).
5. T. Maniatis, S. Goodbourn and J.A. Fischer. Regulation of inducible and tissue-specific gene expression. Science 236:1237 (1987).
6. H. Samanta, D.A. Engel, H.M. Chao, A. Thakur, M.A. Garcia-Blanco and P. Lengyel. Interferon as gene activators. Cloning of the 5' terminus and the control segment of an interferon activated gene. J. Biol. Chem. 261:11849 (1986).

7. G. Gribaudo, E. Toniato, D.A. Engel and P. Lengyel. Interferon as genes activators. Characteristics of an interferon-activatable enhancer. J. Biol. Chem. 262:11878 (1987).

8. A. Israel, A. Kimura, A. Fournier, M. Fellous and P. Kourilsky. Interferon response sequence potentiates activity of an enhancer in the promoter region of a mouse H-2 gene. Nature 322:743 (1986).

9. G. Gribaudo, M. Gariglio, M. Giovarelli, C. Iemma, G. Cavallo and S. Landolfo. Cell and type specificity of interferon action. Unusual characteristics of the transcriptional control of gene expression by interferon-gamma in T cells. Eur. J. Immunol. 20:124 (1990).

10. M. Gariglio, S. Panico, G. Cavallo, C. Divaker, P. Lengyel and S. Landolfo. Impaired transcription of the poly rI:rC- and interferon-activatable 202 gene in mice and cell lines from the C57BL/6 strain. Virology 187:115 (1992).

11. T.C. Dale, A.M. Ali Imam, I.M. Kerr and G.R. Stark. Rapid activation by interferon α of a latent DNA binding protein present in the cytoplasm of untreated cell. Proc. Natl. Acad. Sci USA 86:1203 (1989).

12. D.E. Levy, D.S. Kessler, R. Pine, N. Reich and J.E. Darnell. Interferon-induced nuclear factors that bind a shared promoter element correlate with positive and negative transcriptional control. Genes Dev. 2:383 (1988).

INTERACTIONS BETWEEN TUMOR NECROSIS FACTOR ALPHA AND GLUCOCORTICOID HORMONES IN THE REGULATION OF TUMOR CELL GROWTH *IN VITRO*

Ildo Nicoletti, Graziella Migliorati[1], M. Cristina Pagliacci, Fausto Grignani and Carlo Riccardi[1]

Institutes of Clinica Medica I and Farmacologia Medica[1], Perugia University Medical School, 06100 Perugia, Italy

INTRODUCTION

Tumor necrosis factor-alfa (TNF-α) is a multifunctional cytokine with an important role in inflammation, tissue repair and immune reactions[1,2,3]. This molecule also exerts a cytocidal activity against some tumor cell lines but not against normal cells "in vitro"[4]. Several tumor cells are or become resistant, however, to the growth-inhibiting activity of TNF-α[4,5,6] and the cytokine can also stimulate the growth of normal human fibroblasts as well as of some trasformed cells in culture[7,8]. Little is known about the mechanisms responsible for TNF-α mediated cytotoxicity[9] and cytostatic, cytolytic and apoptotic[4,10] effects have been reported in different cellular models.

Steroid hormones are key regulators of cell growth. Depending on the cell type and nature of the steroid, cell growth or cell death can be implemented with physiological levels of these substances. Androgens and estrogens promote growth of prostate and breast tumors by both enhancing cell proliferation and reducing programmed or apoptotic death of tumor cells[11]. Another aspect of steroid effect on cell growth is the destruction of lymphoid precursors by glucocorticoids[12]. This response is dependent on the presence of functional glucocorticoid receptors, which in the presence of a glucocorticoid turn on the synthesis of specific mRNA and proteins leading to cell death. Interleukins (IL-1, IL-2 and IL-4) antagonize the glucocorticoid-induced apoptosis of T-cell precursors, suggesting that a finely tuned balance between cell growth factors and steroid hormones regulates cell number and survival[13]. Glucocorticoid hormones have been recently reported to reduce TNF-α cytotoxicity in rodent tumor models, but the mechanism of their activity is still an open question[14,15].

To better define the interactions between steroid hormones and cytokines in cell growth control, we analyzed the effects of TNF-α and dexamethasone (DEX), a synthetic glucocorticoid hormone, either used alone or together, on proliferation and death of tumor cells *in vitro*.

Combination Therapies 2, Edited by A.L. Goldstein and E. Garaci Plenum Press, New York, 1993

MATERIALS AND METHODS

Cells and cell culture

MCF-7 cells (kindly supplied by Dr. Laura del Senno, Department of Biochemistry, University of Ferrara, Italy) were cultured in DMEM supplemented with 10% FBS, 50 U/ml penicillin, 50 µg/ml streptomycin and 300 mg/l l-glutamine. L-929 cells (kindly supplied by Dr. Francesco Colotta, Istituto Mario Negri, Milan, Italy) were grown in RPMI-1640 plus 10% FCS, non-essential aminoacids, sodium pyruvate, HEPES and mercaptoethanol. GH3 cells (Flow ICN, Irvine, U.K.) were cultured in Ham's F-10 medium supplemented with 15% horse serum and 2.5% FCS. Cultures were performed in humified atmosphere of 95% air and 5% CO_2 at 37° C.

Analysis of cell growth

Exponentially growing cells from stock cultures were washed twice with sterile Hank's BSS and removed from the dishes with 0.05% trypsin and 0.02% EDTA. The cells were then collected by centrifugation, washed, and dispersed by gentle passages through a Pasteur pipette. Cells were seeded at 20000/ml in the above reported media either in 35-mm diameter culture dishes for flow cytometric analyses or in 96-well culture plates (2000 cells/100 µl) for 96-hours experiments.. At the selected time, TNF-α in PBS-BSA, or the same volume of PBS-BSA alone, was added to the wells until the pre-established final concentration of TNF-α was reached. Cells were counted directly in an hemocytometer after trypsinisation and dispersion or indirectly by a 3-(4,5-dimethyl-thyazol-2-yl)-2,5-diphenyltetrazolium bromide colorimetric assay (MTT-assay) that measures the reduction of MTT to formazan by living cells[16] The test was performed in 96-well plates as previously described[17] and showed a good concordance (r 0.98) with the cell number in a wide range of cell concentrations.

Analysis of TNF-α-induced cytotoxicity

For assay of TNF-α cytotoxicity MTT-dye reduction micro assay was used according to Green et al.[18]. Briefly, $5 \cdot 10^3$ cells were incubated in 100 µl of appropriate media with or without pre-established concentrations of TNF-α in 96/well microplates. After a 72h incubation period 10 µl MTT was added for 3 h and absorbancy read as described. The percentage of dead cells was calculated as the ratio of OD in wells with and without TNF-α.

Cell cycle analysis and flow cytometric evaluation of cell death

A quantitative measure of cell cycle distribution was obtained by flow cytometric analysis of DNA histograms, according to Fried et al.[19] as previously described[20]. Briefly, cells were cultured in 35-mm plastic wells in appropriate media with and without the pre-established concentrations of TNF-α. At the pre-established times, cells were washed twice with cold PBS and 2 ml fluorochrome solution (propidium iodide 0.05 mg/ml dissolved in 0.1% Na citrate with 0.1% Triton-X 100) added. The plates were placed at 4°C in the dark for 60-90 min, the adherent cells dislodged by repeated pipetting and the stained cells transferred to test tubes for DNA analysis. Cell fluorescence was measured in a FACSCAN flow cytometer (Becton Dickinson, Mountain View, USA) and the percentage of nuclei in the different phases of cell cycle (G0/G1, S and G2/M) was calculated from the histogram of DNA fluorescence area with DNA cell-cycle analysis software (Cell-Fit, Becton Dickinson).

Statistical analysis

All data are the mean±SE. Due to the non-normal distribution of the data, non-parametric tests (Wilcoxon's rank sum test and Kruskal-Wallis' and Friedman's analysis of variance) were adopted for statistical evaluation of the results.

RESULTS

Different responses of tumor cell lines to growth inhibition exerted by TNF-α

The addition of TNF-α to culture media of exponentially growing MCF-7 human breast cells resulted in an evident growth-inhibitory effect. The inhibition was dose dependent in a 3-day MTT-growth assay and was maximal with TNF-α concentrations around 1000 U/ml (Figure 1). The sensitivity of L-929 mouse fibrosarcoma cells was more pronounced, and the percentage of surviving cells was under 20% of controls at the greatest TNF-α concentration. On the contrary, GH3 rat pituitary tumor cells showed a complete resistance to TNF-α inhibition.

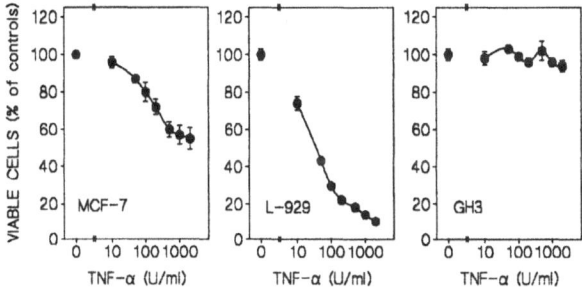

Figure 1. Effect of different TNF-α concentrations on growth of MCF-7, L-929 and GH3 tumor cell lines. Cells were cultured for 72 h and viable cells measured by MTT-reduction assay. Results (mean±SD) are the percentage of viable cells with respect to controls incubated in the same conditions without TNF-α.

TNF-α exerts cytostatic, cytolytic and apoptotic effects on tumor cells

The TNF-α effect on cell cycle progression, DNA content and chromatin structure in individual nuclei was evaluated by flow-cytometric techniques as described[15]. Time course analysis of TNF-α treated MCF-7 cultures, revealed a progressive reduction in the percentage of S-phase cells which was appreciable after 6h and reached the nadir after 24h of treatment. The decrease in the percentage of S-phase, DNA-synthesizing cells was followed by a reduction in the G2/M compartment. Conversely, there was a progressive accumulation of cells in the G0/G1 phase (Figure 2 A). The cytostasis (G1/S block) was followed by unequivocal cytotoxic effects (increase in the percentage of trypan-blue positive cells, reduction in the number of viable cells by the MTT-reduction assay). The same TNF-α dose did not produce any relevant effect on cell-cycle distribution in L-929 cells (Figure 2 B), except a slight and transient increase in G2/M cell percentage.

The reduction in number of viable cells induced by TNF-α was associated to a large increase in the percentage of nuclei with flow-cytometric characteristics of apoptosis (i.e.

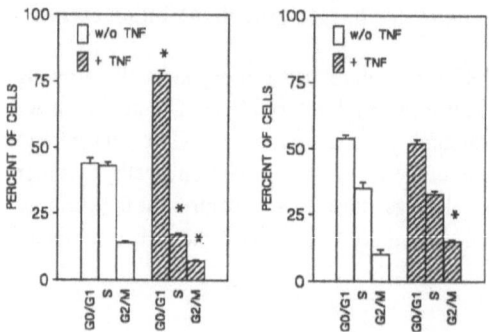

Figure 2. Effect of 24h TNF-α treatment (1000 U/ml) on cell cycle distribution of MCF-7 (left panel) and L-929 (right panel) cells. A clear cytostatic effect (increase in G0/G1 and reduction in S-phase and G2/M cell percentage) was observed in MCF-7 but not in L-929 cells.

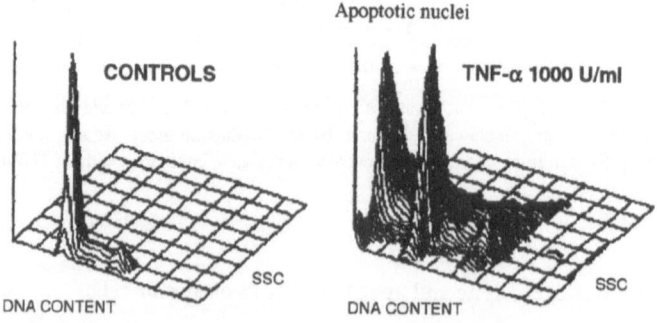

Figure 3. Effect of 24h TNF-α treatment (1000 U/ml) on DNA content and chromatin condensation (SSC) of L-929 nuclei in a computer-drawn three dimensional plot. A great percentage of TNF-α treated nuclei display the flow cytometric characteristics of apoptosis. Untreated L-929 cells, incubated in the same experimental conditions, are reported for comparison in the left panel.

reduced DNA content and enhanced chromatin condensation, Figure 3). Thus TNF-α can exert cytostatic, cytolytic and apoptotic effect in different targets.

Glucocorticoid hormones antagonize the effects of TNF-α in tumor cell lines

Glucocorticoid hormones (GCH) have been reported to reduce the TNF-α action in several "in vitro" models[14,15]. We investigated, therefore, the effect of synthetic GCH dexamethasone (DEX) against the growth-inhibitory activity of TNF-α in L-929 and MCF-7 cell lines. Dose-response experiments (Figure 4) showed a protective influence of high DEX concentrations (10^{-6} and 10^{-4} M) against the effects of 1000 U/ml TNF-α in a 48h MTT-growth-assay.

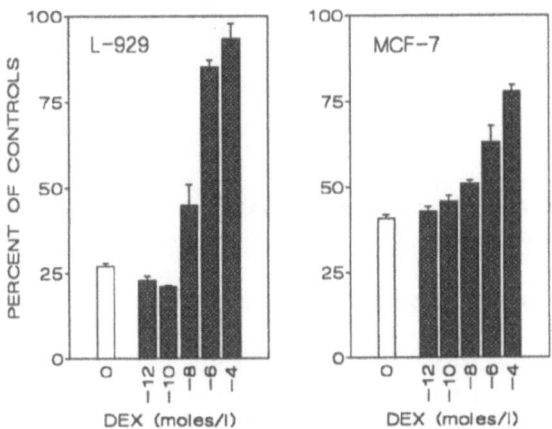

Figure 4. Dose-dependent protective effect of the GCH Dexamethasone against cytotoxicity exerted by 1000 U/ml TNF-α in L-929 and MCF-7 cell lines. Cell survival (expressed as percentage of control cultures incubated without TNF-α) was measured by MTT-reduction assay after a 48h incubation period. Results are the mean±SD.

Flow-cytometric analysis of parallel experiments showed that DEX did not counteract the cytostatic activity of TNF-α. The reduction in S-phase and the corresponding increase in G0/G1 percentages induced by TNF-α in MCF-7 cells were not modified by DEX (Figure 5). TNF-α did not produce any important cytostatic effect in L-929 cells (see Figure 2). Nevertheless, micromolar concentrations of DEX, strongly counteracted the growth inhibiting activity of TNF-α in L-929 cell line. Three-dimensional plots of DNA content and chromatin structure of L-929 nuclei demonstrated that the main effect of DEX against TNF-α was reduction of apoptosis. This confirms that TNF-α effect on tumor cell growth has both cytostatic and cytotoxic components and indicates that only the cytotoxic activity of TNF-α can be inhibited by glucocorticoid hormones.

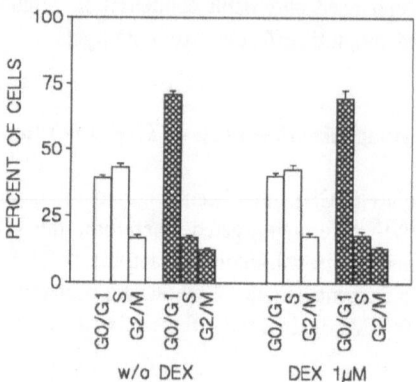

Figure 5. Effect of 24h TNF-α treatment (1000 U/ml) on cell cycle distribution of MCF-7 cells (crossed bars). Open bars are the percentages of parallel MCF-7 cultures incubated without TNF-α. The potent cytostatic effect (increase in G0/G1 and reduction in S-phase and G2/M cell percentage) exerted by TNF-α was not antagonized by 1 μM Dexamethasone.

The protective effect of glucocorticoid hormones against TNF-α cytotoxicity requires an intact protein synthesis machinery

The anti-inflammatory properties of GCH are mediated by synthesis of a 40 kDa protein (lipocortin)[21]. We investigated, therefore, whether the protective effect of DEX against the cytotoxicity of TNF-α in tumor cell lines was also dependent on protein neo-synthesis. At this purpose, we tested protective concentrations of DEX with and without the protein synthesis inhibitor cycloheximide, against the cytotoxicity exerted by 1000 U/ml TNF-α in L-929 cells. Inhibition of protein synthesis by increasing concentrations of cycloheximide, was followed by dose-dependent disappearance of the protective effect exerted by DEX (Figure 6).

DISCUSSION

The precise mechanism by which TNF-α kills tumor cells is still debated. Cytostatic, cytolytic and apoptotic effects have been reported in a number of experimental models, but the factors which are responsible for different sensitivity of tumors to TNF-α and the type of TNF-α action (i.e. cytostatic vs. cytotoxic) are not fully understood[1-4,9,10]. Our present results confirm that TNF-α can exert both cytostatic and cytotoxic effects in different tumor cell targets *in vitro*. The cytostatic effect of TNF-α appeared quite rapidly in MCF-7 cells, reaching the maximum at 24h of incubation, before any sign of cytotoxicity. Cytostasis was followed by a a clear cytolysis, as revealed by the MTT-assay and trypan-blue exclusion,

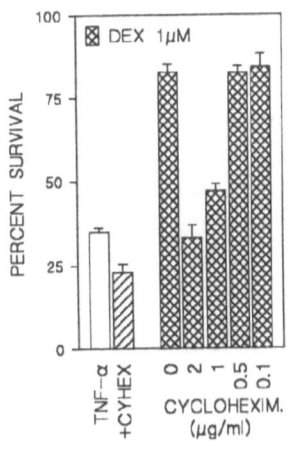

Figure 6. Effects of protein synthesis inhibition by cycloheximide on the protection afforded by DEX against TNF-α cytotoxicity in L-929 cells. Survival of cells incubated for a 48h period with 1000 U/ml TNF-α with and without the indicated substances was measured by MTT-assay. Two μg/ml cycloheximide completely abrogated the protective effect of DEX, confirming that active protein synthesis is essential for the action of GCHs.

indicating that the growth inhibiting activity of TNF-α in MCF-7 cells results from both inhibition of cell proliferation and enhancement of cell death.

On the contrary, the apoptotic effect of the cytokine in L-929 cell line was only preceded by a modest and transient increase in G2/M cell percentage, without any other sign of cytostasis at the cell cycle analysis. This finding confirms that different tumor cell lines can be killed by TNF-α through different mechanisms.

Although the exact mechanism by which TNF-α exerts its cytotoxic activity remains unknown, an activation of phospholipase-A2 has been demonstrated in L-929 rodent tumor cells[22]. Since glucocorticoid hormones are potent inhibitors of phospholipase A2[21] and have been reported to reduce TNF-α cytotoxicity in rodent tumor models[14,15], we tested the synthetic glucocorticoid dexamethasone against the growth inhibitory activity of TNF-α in tumor cell lines. Micromolar concentrations of DEX significantly inhibited the TNF-α effect on both MCF-7 and L-929 cell lines. Quite surprisingly, the cytostatic and cytotoxic effects of TNF-α in MCF-7 cells showed a different sensitivity to GCH, and DEX reduced cell death produced by TNF-α without modifying the antiproliferative activity of the cytokine. The apoptotic effect of TNF-α in L-929 cell line was also strongly inhibited by DEX. Thus, the protective effect of DEX appears to be selective against the cytotoxic activities of TNF-α.

Because the precise mechanisms of cytotoxic effects of TNF-α are still a matter of debate[9], it is very difficult to explain how glucocorticoid hormones can exert their protective effect. It is known, however, that cells metabolically crippled by inhibitors of protein synthesis or inhibitors of transcription (cycloheximide and D-actinomycin) are more sensitive to the cytotoxic activity of TNF-α[23]. This suggests that tumor cells synthesize protein(s) that actively protect them from the cytotoxic actions of TNF-α and that the cell response to the cytokine is regulated by a balance between lytic and protective events. Since the synthesis of protective proteins can be enhanced by heat stress, glucose starvation and TNF-α itself[24,25], it could be hypothesized that glucocorticoid hormones, which are classical transcriptional regulators[26], are also able to increase the synthesis of protective proteins. This view was indirectly supported by the observation that the protein-synthesis inhibitor cycloheximide exerted a dose-dependent reduction of the protective effect of DEX. Cycloheximide concentrations above 1 μg/ml produced a complete abrogation of DEX protection against TNF-α cytotoxicity in L-929 tumor cells.

In conclusion our results demonstrate that the growth inhibitory effects of TNF-α on tumor cells *in vitro* are exerted through multiple mechanisms. Glucocorticoid hormones counteract the cytotoxic activity of TNF-α without any antagonism on the cytostatic effect. Although preliminary, the present findings suggest that different activities of TNF-α against tumor cell targets can be separately modulated by both natural (i.e. hormones) or synthetic molecules.

Acknowledgments

The work was supported by Italian Association against Cancer (AIRC) and by P.F. ACRO, CNR, Italy

REFERENCES

1. Beutler B and Cerami A. Cachectin (Tumor Necrosis Factor): a macrophage hormone governing cellular metabolism and inflammatory response. *Endocrine Reviews,* 9:57 (1988)
2. Beutler B and Cerami A. Cachectin: more than a tumor necrosis factor. *New Eng J Med* 316:379 (1987)
3. Akira S, Hirano T, Taga T and Kishimoto T. Biology of multifunctional cytokines: IL6 and related molecules (IL1 and TNF). *FASEB J* 4:2860 (1990)
4. Sugarman BJ, Aggarwal BB, Hass PE, Figari IS, Palladino MAJr and Shepard HM. Recombinant human tumor necrosis factor alpha: effects on proliferation of normal and transformed cells in vitro. *Science* 230:943 (1985)
5. Tsujimoto M, Yip YK and Vilcek J. Tumor necrosis factor: specific binding and internalization in sensitive and resistant cells. *Proc. Natl. Acad. Sci. USA* 82:7626 (1985)
6. Patek PQ and Ling Y. In vitro selection of a cell line for resistance to lysis by tumor necrosis factor-α selects for reduced tumorogenicity. *J. Immunol.* 146:3457 (1991)
7. Palombella VJ and Vilcek J. Mitogenic and cytotoxic actions of tumor necrosis factor in BALB/c 3T3 cells: role of phospholipase activation. *J. Biol. Chem.* 264:18128 (1989)
8. Lachman LB, Brown DC and Dinarello CA. Growth-promoting effect of recombinant IL-1 and tumor necrosis factor for a human astrocytoma cell line. *J. Immunol.* 138:2913 (1987)
9. Larrick JW and Wright SC. Cytotoxic mechanism of tumor necrosis factor-α. *FASEB J,* 4:3215 (1990)
10. Laster SM, Wood JC and Gooding LR. Tumor necrosis factor can induce both apoptotic and necrotic forms of cell lysis. *J. Immunol.* 141:2629 (1988)
11. Kyprianou N and Isaacs JT. Activation of programmed cell death in the rat ventral prostate after castration. *Endocrinology,* 122:552 (1988)
12. Willie AH. Glucocorticoid-induced thymocyte apoptosis is associated with endogenous endonuclease activation. *Nature,* 284:555 (1980)
13. Nieto MA. and Lopez-Rivas A. 1989. IL-2 protects T lymphocytes from glucocorticoid-induced DNA fragmentation and cell death. *J. Immunol.* 143:4166 (1989)
14. Suffys F., Beyaert R, Van Roy F and Fiers W. Reduced tumor necrosis factor-induced cytotoxicity by inhibition of arachidonic acid metabolism. *Biochem. Biophys. Res. Commun.* 149:735 (1987)
15. Tsujimoto M, Okamura N and Adachi H. Dexamethasone inhibits the citotoxic activity of tumor necrosis factor. *Biochem. Biophys. Res. Commun.* 153:109 (1988)
16. Pagé M, Bejaoui N, Cinq-Mars B, Lemieux P. Optimization of the tetrazolium-based colorimetric assay for the measurement of cell number and cytotoxicity. *Int. J. Immunopharm.* 10:785 (1988)

17. Pelicci G, Pagliacci MC, Lanfrancone L, Pelicci PG, Grignani F, Nicoletti I. Inhibitory effect of the somatostatin analogue octreotide (SMS 201-995) on rat pituitary tumor cells (GH3) proliferation "in vitro". *J. Endocrinol. Invest.* 13:657 (1990)

18. Green LM, Reade JL and Wave CF. Rapid colorimetric assays for cell viability: application to the quantitation of cytotoxic and growth inhibitory lymphokines. *J. Immun. Methods,* 20:257 (1984)

19. Fried J, Perez AG, Clarkson BD. Rapid hypotonic method for flow cytofluorometry of monolayer cell cultures. Some pitfalls in staining and data analysis. *J. Histochem. Cytochem.* 26:921 (1978)

20. Pagliacci MC, Tognellini R, Grignani F and Nicoletti I. Inhibition of human breast cancer cell (MCF-7) growth in vitro by the somatostatin analog SMS 201-995: effects on cell cycle parameters and apoptotic cell death. *Endocrinology,* 129:2555 (1991)

21. Flower RJ and Blackwell GJ. Anti-inflammatory steroids induce biosynthesis of a phospholipase A2 inhibitor which prevents prostaglandin generation. *Nature,* 278:456 (1979)

22. Clark MA, Chen MJ, Crooke ST and Bomalaski JS. Tumor necrosis factor (cachectin) induces phospholipase A2-activating protein in endothelial cells. *Biochem. J.* 250:125 (1988)

23. Kull FC jr and Cuatrecasas P. Possible requirement of internalization in the mechanism of in vitro cytotoxicity in tumor necrosis factor serum. *Cancer Res.* 41:4885 (1981)

24. Kusher DI, Ware CF and Gooding LR. Induction of the heat shock response protects cells from lysis by tumor necrosis factor. *J. Immunol.* 145:2925 (1990)

25. Sugawara S, Nowicki M, Xie S, Song HJ and Dennert G. Effects of stress on lysability of tumor targets by cytotoxic T cells and tumor necrosis factor. *J. Immunol.* 145:1991 (1990)

26. Beato M. Gene regulation by steroid hormones. *Cell,* 56:335 (1989)

BEHAVIOURAL, PYROGENIC AND ELECTROCORTICAL EFFECTS OF TUMOR
NECROSIS FACTOR - ALPHA GIVEN INTRACEREBRALLY IN RATS

G.B. De Sarro[1], D. Rotiroti[1], and G. Nistrico'[2]

[1]Chair of Pharmacology, Faculty of Medicine
Univerity of Reggio Calabria, Italy
[2]Department of Biology, University of Roma
"Tor Vergata", Italy

INTRODUCTION

Cytokines are peptides synthesized by immunecompetent cells
which are released during inflammatory states, acting as
local response coordinators, but also mediate distant acute
phase responses in an endocrine manner. There is clear
evidence that cytokines may also have a hypotalamic site of
action. Interleukin-1 beta, interleukin-3 and tumor necrosis
factor- α (TNF-α) also affect the hypothalamic regulation of
body temperature and may induce pyrexia (Dinarello, 1986;
Nistico' and De Sarro, 1991a).
Recent evidence has demonstrated that cytokine mRNAs occur in
both neuronal cell bodies and astrocytes in the brain (see
Nistico' and De Sarro, 1991b). Furthermore TNF-α has been
detected in the brain (Grau et al., 1987) and has been
reported to cause astroglia surface expression of maior
histocompatibility complex molecules (Massa et al., 1987) and
to induce capillary blood vessel formation in the rat cornea
(Leibovich et al., 1987). In addition human TNF-α
chronically administered to rats induces anorexia, weight
loss, depletion of whole-body protein and lipid stores
(Tracey et al., 1988). More recent evidence has shown that
TNF- αapplied on the membrane of neurons of Aplysia affects a
slow inward current associated with decrease in K+
conductance (Sawada et al., 1990).
Therefore, the present experiments were aimed to better
characterize the central effects of TNF- α after its
intracerebral microinjection. In particular, the
electrocortical (ECoG) activity, the behavioural and body
temperature changes, the variations of drinking and body
weight were studied after single or repeated intracerebral
administration of TNF-α.

METHODS

Adult male Wistar rats (200-250 g) were used. They were
stereotaxically implanted with stainless steel guide
cannulae, under chloral hydrate anaesthesia (400 mg/Kg i.p.),

according to the atlas coordinates of Paxinos and Watson (1982), to permit microinfusion into the third cerebral ventricle (ICV) or into the locus coeruleus (LC) or into the dorsal hippocampus (DH). After surgery, a minimum of 48 hr was allowed for recovery before experiments were carried out. At least 5 rats were used for each dose and area of the brain studied. Post-mortem histological examination confirmed the location of the guide cannulae. Body temperature was recorded on a Grant temperature recorder by means of a thermistor implanted beneath the skin of the interscapular region. ECoG activity was recorded (8 channel ECoG machine OTE Biomedica, Florence) through 4 chronically-implanted steel screw electrodes. The ECoG changes were computerized and statistically analysed as previously described (Nistico' and De Sarro, 1991a).

Chronic treatment with TNF-α lasted 10 days. Each morning TNF-α was administered i.c.v. in the rats and changes in body weight, food and water intake were recorded. A Kruskall-Wallis analysis of variance was first carried out and if this was significant a Student't test was used to compare control and drug-treated animals.

DRUGS: recombinant human TNF-α , a highly specific polyclonal rabbit anti-human TNF-α antibodies, anti IL-1 and anti-IL-2 receptor monoclonal antibodies were purchased from Genzyme-Omnia Res. (Cinisello Balsamo, Milano, Italy). Meclophenamic acid was obtained from Menarini (Firenze, Italy) wilst acetylsalicylic acid and ibuprofen were purchased from Sigma (St. Louis, Missouri, USA). All drugs were easily dissolved in 67 mM sodium phosphate buffer containing 5 mg of serum albumin for 1 ml.

RESULTS

Single treatment

TNF-α (0.29, 0.57, 1.14 and 2.28 pmol) injected into the III cerebral ventricle produced dose-dependent behavioural and ECoG sedative effects which were associated with an increase in body temperature. The latter effect was evident within 20 min after injection of TNF-α reached the maximum increase after 70-120 min and remained elevated for approx 180 min. ECoG synchronization lasted from 35 to 180 min and was characterized by an increase in total voltage power as well as in 0-3 and 3-6 Hz frequency bands. Lower doses of TNF-(30, 60 and 90 fmol) injected into the LC increased locomotor activity, produced behavioural stimulation and ECoG desynchronization lasting 20-30 min. This phase was followed by a period of behavioural sedation and ECoG synchronization lasted from 45 to 80 min which was characterized by an increase in total voltage power as well as in 0-3 and 3-6 Hz frequency bands (Fig. 1). A pretreatment (15 min before) with rabbit anti-human TNF-α (5 and 10 ng) was able to significantly antagonize the effects of TNF-α microinjected into the LC. On the contrary, a pretreatment with anti-IL-1 receptor monoclonal antibodies (10 ng, into LC) or anti-IL-2 receptor monoclonal antibodies (10 and 20 ng, into LC) was unable to significantly affect the stimulation of behaviour and ECoG desynchronizing effects elicited by a following

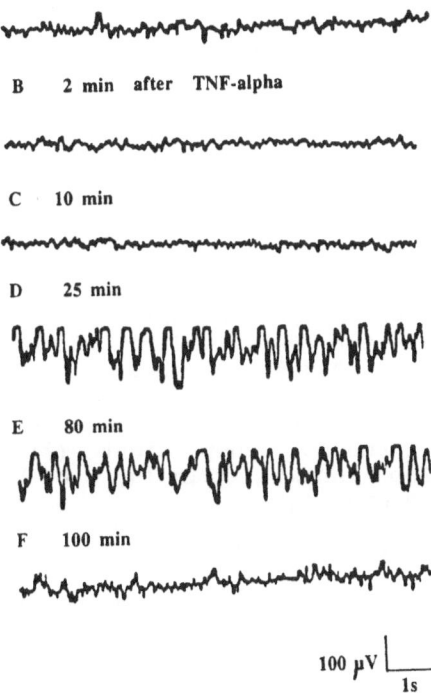

A   Control

B   2 min after TNF-alpha

C   10 min

D   25 min

E   80 min

F   100 min

100 µV
       1s

Fig. 1 Typical biphasic ECoG response following
the intra-LC microinfusion of TNF-α (30 fmol). Note
that after an initial state of ECoG desynchronization
(B and C) lasting approx 20 min, a longer lasting
(approx 1 h) period of high voltage slow waves (D
and E) was observed.

microinfusion of TNF-α into the LC. The same pretreatment
into the LC with anti-IL-1 or anti-Il-2 receptor monoclonal
antibodies was instead able to prevent the ECoG synchronizing
phase elicited by TNF-α (60 fmol) given into the same site. A
single microinjection of TNF-α (0.14, 0.28 or 0.42 pmol)
into the dorsal hippocampus elicited during the infusion a
specific ECoG pattern characterized by spiking activity
lasting from 12 to 30 min which was associated with some
episodes of wet dog shake or a frozen state of the rat. All
the ECoG and behavioural effects induced by the microinfusion
of TNF-α into the DH or ICV were antagonized by a pretreatment with polyclonal rabbit anti-human TNF-α antibodies (5,
10, 20 or 50 ng). Acetylsalicylic acid (0.4 and 0.8 umol),
meclophenamic acid (0.1 and 0.2 umol) and ibuprofen (1 and 2
umol) microinjected i.c.v. 15 min TNF-α attenuated or
completely abolished the fever induced by this cytokine.

Changes in food intake after repeated treatment

Intracerebroventricular administration of TNF-α induced a

statistically significant decrease in drinking compared to the same period with the vehicle-treated control group. In addition, chronic administration of TNF-α (0.14 or 0.42 pmol for 10 days) into the third cerebral ventricle induced anorexia. In fact as shown in Table 1, a significant decrease of food intake and a loss of body weight was observed in groups treated with TNF-α when compared to the same period with the sham operated control group or the vehicle treated group.

Table 1. The effect of intracerebral infusion of TNF-α on food intake and body weight after repeated administration for 10 days in rats.

	Total amount of food intake in 10 days (g)	Body weight gain (g)	(%) of changes of body weight in 10 days (a)
Control	239±5.40	+38.4±3.4	18.9±1.6
Vehicle	252±5.70	+40.2±3.8	21.8±2.3
TNF-α 0.14	171±4.80*	-8.6±2.6*	-14.9±5.3
TNF-α 0.42	152±5.10*	-15.9±4.3**	-26.8±5.8*

Data are expressed as means ± S.E.M. Vehicle group consisted in animals receiving vehicle (67 mM phosphate buffer containing 5 mg of serum albumin for 1 ml). (a)The comparison was made with values of the starting day of experiments. Ten animals were included in each group. *P< 0.05, **P< 0.01 vs each control group.

DISCUSSION

The present study indicates that intracerebral microinfusion of TNF-α produced specific and marked behavioural effects. When microinfused ICV TNF-α produced behavioural and soporific effects which were not different from those obtained with IL-1, IL-2 and IL-3. However, when microinjected into the LC TNF-α elicited specific effects. Thus, in comparison to other cytokines (IL1, IL2 and IL3) (Nistico and De Sarro, 1991a, 1991b; De Sarro et al., 1990) the ECoG profile of TNF-α given into the LC was different and due to stimulation of specific receptors. In fact, an initial phase of behavioural stimulation and ECoG desynchronization was followed by a second phase characterized by sedation and ECoG synchronization. However, highly specific polyclonal rabbit anti-human TNF-antibodies antagonize both phases, whereas the prior injection into the same site of selective monoclonal anti IL1 and IL2 antibodies prevented only the ECoG synchronizing and sedative effect. This suggests that the second phase could be due to the release of interleukins. In addition our results confirm that TNF-α plays a pivotal role in the pathogenesis of anorexia and fever (Tracey et al., 1988; Old, 1977; Beutler and Cerami, 1988). In fact, chronic ICV infusion of TNF-α induced significant inhibition of food intake and body-weight gain in rats.

Although animals with fever (Fontana et al., 1984) would increase drinking behaviour, we have obtained unexpectedly that drinking behaviour was also decreased after ICV administration of TNF-α . TNF-α mediated anorexia and inhibition of drinking may be mediated at hypothalamic level and thes effects may be operative during acute and chronic disease (Beutler and Cerami, 1988). Since protection against TNF-α induced changes in feeding and drinking were blocked by selective TNF-α polyclonal antibodies and were not antagonized by passive immunization with IL-1 and IL-2 monoclonal antibodies we may suppose that these phenomena are directly mediated by TNF-α . In conclusion, our results indicate that ECoG effects of TNF-α are, in part, different from those observed with other cytokines (i.e. IL-1, IL-2 and IL-3) and that TNF-α plays a pivotal role in the pathogenesis of the anorexia. In addition, the present experiments show that the prostanoids are almost certainly involved in the pathophysiology of pyrogenic responses elicited by TNF-α .

REFERENCES

Beutler B. and Cerami A., 1988, Tumor necrosis, cachexia, shock, and inflammation: a common mediator. Ann. Rev. Biochem. 57: 505.
De Sarro G.B., Masuda Y., Ascioti C., Audino M.G. and Nistico' G., 1990, Behavioural and ECoG spectrum changes induced by intracerebral infusion of interferons and interleukin-2 in rats are antagonized by naloxone. Neuropharmacol. 29: 167.
Dinarello C.A., 1986, Multiple biological properties of recombinant human interleukin-1(B). Immunology, 178: 301.
Fontana A., Weber E. and Dayer J.M., 1984, Synthesis in interleukin-1 endogenous pyrogen in the brain of endotoxin-treated mice: a step in fever induction? J.Immunol. 133: 1696.
Grau G.E., Fajardo L.F., Piguet P., Allet B., Lambert P. and Vassalli P., 1987, Tumor necrosis factor (cachectin) as an essential mediator in murine cerebral malaria. Science, 237: 1210.
Leibovich S.J., Polverini P.J., Shepard H.M., Wiserman D.M., Shively V. and Nuseir N., 1987, Macrophage-induced angio-genesis is mediated by tumor necrosis factor-alpha. Nature, 329: 630.
Massa P.T., Schimpl A., Wecker E. and Ter Meulen V., 1987, Tumor Necrosis factor amplifies measles virus-mediated Ia induction on astrocytes. Proc. Natl. Acad. Sci. USA, 84: 7242.

Nistico' G., De Sarro G.B., 1991, Is interleukin-2 a neuromodulator in the brain? Trend in Neurosci, 14: 146.

Nistico' G., De Sarro G.B., 1991, Behavioural and electrocortical spectrum power effects after microinfusion of lymphokines in several areas of the rat brain. Ann.New York Acad. Sci., 621: 119.

Old L.J., 1987, Polypeptide mediator network. Nature, 326: 330.

Paxinos F., Watson C., 1982, The rat brain in stereotaxic coordinates. Academic Press, London.

Sawada M., Hara N., and Maeno T., 1990, Extracellular tumor necrosis factor induces a decreased K+ conductance in an identified neuron of Aplysia kurodai. Neurosci. Lett. 115: 219.

Tracey K.J., Wei H., Manogue K.R., Fong Y., Hesse D.G., Nguyen H.T., Kuo G.C., Beutler B., Cotran R.S., Cerami A. and Lowry S.F., 1988, Cachectin/tumor necrosis factor induces cachexia, anemia, and inflammation. J. Exp. Med. 167: 1211.

BIOLOGICAL SIGNIFICANCE AND THERAPEUTIC POTENTIAL OF TUMOR-ASSOCIATED LEUKOCYTES

Alberto Mantovani, Barbara Bottazzi, Silvano Sozzani, Giuseppe Peri, Paola Allavena, Annunciata Vecchi and Francesco Colotta

Istituto di Ricerche Farmacologiche "Mario Negri"
Via Eritrea 62, 20157 Milan, Italy

INTRODUCTION

Macrophages are a major component of the lymphoreticular infiltrate of rodent and human tumors (Mantovani et al 1992a). Since these cells are situated at the very interface between tumor and host, they may represent a strategically located target for therapeutic intervention. Interest in these cells is stimulated by the knowledge that macrophages have the potential to kill neoplastic cells including drug-resistant variants surviving conventional chemotherapy (Allavena et al 1987).

Tumor-associated macrophages (TAM) derive from circulating monocytic precursors. Tumor-derived chemotactic factors (TDCF) have been identified (Bottazzi et al 1983).

In addition to releasing chemoattractants various human tumor lines release an inhibitor of chemotaxis antigenically related to the transmembrane protein P15E of murine retroviruses (Snyderman and Cianciolo 1984; Wang et al 1986). Hence the regulation of monocyte infiltration in tumors is complex and may involve a balance of factors with opposing influences on leukocyte migration.

The functional properties of macrophages infiltrating murine and human metastatic tumors have been characterized in an effort to obtain indications as to the role played by these cells in the immunobiology of neoplastic tissues (Mantovani et al 1992a). This analysis has indicated how TAM can contribute to important aspects of tumor tissue biology, such as fibrin deposition and angiogenesis.

Combination Therapies 2, Edited by A.L. Goldstein
and E. Garaci   Plenum Press, New York, 1993

Moreover TAM in certain tumors are a source of growth factors which actually provide the optimal conditions for tumor growth. More in general, this type of analysis has shown how TAM, within the mononuclear phagocyte system, represent a population with peculiar phenotypic and functional properties. Here, we will summarize recent work on molecules involved in the regulation of macrophage infiltration and function in neoplastic tissues.

MCP-1, A CYTOKINE INVOLVED IN THE REGULATION OF TAM

TAM originate from circulating monocytic precursors. Tumors vary widely in the size of their macrophage infiltrate although this is relatively stable for each neoplasm. For many murine tumors, the number of TAM is not affected by transplantation of the tumor into mice with defective T-cell-mediated immunity (thymectomized, nude or ultraviolet-irradiated). This suggests that, in many tumors, specific immunity is not an important determinant of macrophage infiltration, and that factors inherent to the tumor itself regulate macrophage levels in neoplastic tissues (for review, see Mantovani et al 1992a).

This consideration prompted us to search for monocyte chemoattractants released by tumor cells (Bottazzi et al 1983). We have identified a cytokine of about 12kDa, called tumor-derived chemotactic factor (TDCF), which is chemotactic for monocytes and is released by various murine and human tumor cells. Recently, the sequence and structure of this cytokine, which we now refer to as monocyte chemotactic protein-1 (MCP-1) have been determined (Furutani et al 1989, Yoshimura et al 1989, Van Damme et al 1989, Bottazzi et al 1990, Matsushima et al 1989). MCP-1 is a 76-amino-acid mature polypeptide with one N-linked glycosylation site. The gene encoding MCP-1 is identical to JE, a gene identified in activated fibroblasts, and is homologous to genes expressed in activated lymphocytes and mesenchimal cells (for a review see Oppenheim et al 1991). The structural hallmarks of these cytokines are four conserved cysteines, the first two of which are in tandem, and which are probably important for the three-dimensional structure. The same four-cysteine motif is shared by cytokines of the platelet factor (PF)4 family, except that the first two cysteines are interrupted by an intervening amino acid. The PF4 family includes interleukin (IL)-8 and melanocyte growth-stimulating activity (MGSA/gro), which are chemotactic for neutrophils. Thus, MCP-1 belongs to an emerging superfamily of cytokines, some of which are involved in the regulation of leukocyte recruitment and activation. The term intercrines and, more recently, chemokines, has been proposed for these mediators. MCP-1 is produced by a variety of cell types, including lymphocytes, mononuclear phagocytes and fibroblasts. Particularly significant in the context of monocyte recruitment is the fact that it is produced by vascular smooth muscle cells and endothelial cells (Valente et al 1984, Sica et al 1990).

As expected from its in vitro chemotactic activity, injection of MCP-1 in vivo induces extravasation of monocytes (Zachariae et al 1990). There is also evidence that it has an important role in the regulation of TAM levels in vivo. In a series of murine tumors, in tumor biopsies from ovarian carcinomas, and in human tumor variants transplanted into nude mice, a significant, though far from absolute, correlation was found between the number of TAM and the MCP activity produced by the tumor cells (Bottazzi et al 1983; Walter et al 1991). Finally, MCP-1 gene transfer resulted in higher levels of TAM in a murine melanoma (Bottazzi et al 1992).

The metastatic capacity of clones expressing the human MCP-1 gene was studied by injecting tumor cells i.v. MCP-1 expressing clones were more metastatic than control cells in terms of lung involvement (number or weight) and of the occurrence of extrapulmonary lesions (Table 1). This observation is in line with a higher tumorigenicity at low tumor inocula in spite of a slower in vivo growth rate (Bottazzi et al 1992). Mononuclear phagocytes recruited by MCP-1 may help the initial implantation and outgrowth of the small number of cells that ultimately give rise to metastasis.

PARACRINE REGULATION OF TAM SURVIVAL AND PROLIFERATION

The mechanisms involved in the maintenance of constant levels of macrophages in growing tumors are complex and involve various factors. It has been reported that TAM have increased proliferative capacity (e.g. Evans and Cullen 1984, Mahoney and Heppner 1987, Bottazzi et al 1990) and in situ proliferation may contribute to the macrophage content of tumor tissues.

The proliferative capacity of TAM from two murine sarcomas was investigated by cytofluorography: the frequency of cells in the S phase of the cell cycle was 7-11% for TAM and 1-2% for resident or elicited macrophages. The proliferation and differentiation of mononuclear phagocytes is regulated by the growth factor M-CSF which is also active on differentiated macrophages. The c-fms proto-oncogene encodes for a transmembrane glycoprotein probably identical to the M-CSF receptor. We therefore examined c-fms expression in TAM. TAM showed levels of c-fms mRNA higher than peritoneal exudate macrophages (PEM). Having established that TAM express c-fms at levels higher than PEM, it was of interest to investigate M-CSF expression in TAM and sarcoma cells. TAM did not express appreciable levels of M-CSF mRNA while tumor cells from both sarcomas used in this study showed high levels of M-CSF transcripts. Moreover, supernatants from 2 fibrosarcomas have M-CSF activity on bone marrow cells and induced proliferation of peritoneal exudate and bone marrow-derived macrophages. These activities were blocked by anti-M-CSF antibody.

These observations outline the existence of a paracrine circuit in the regulation of TAM survival and proliferation, involving M-CSF, secreted by sarcoma cells and acting on c-fms expressing TAM.

TABLE 1

Metastatic capacity of melanoma cells after MCP-1 gene transfer[a]

Exp.	Clone	MCP-1	Mice with met.	Lung colonies (total number)	Weight (mg ± SE)	Extrapulmonary lesions[b]
1	V14	-	7/8	20	210 ± 21	0/8
	L12	+	5/5	<300	862 ± 156	1/5
2	V14	-	7/10	16	138 ± 66	1/10
	V16	-	9/9	23	76 ± 17	0/9
	L12	+	8/8	14	296 ± 116	8/8
	L4	+	7/7	15	174 ± 80	0/7

a) The human MCP-1 gene under the control of a retroviral promoter was transfered in the B78/H subline of the B16 melanoma. The obtainement and properties of MCP-1 expressing (L12-L4) and control (V14-V16) clones are described by Bottazzi et al (1992), 5×10^5 cells of in vitro cultured cells were injected in the tail vein and mice were autopsied on day 30 (experiment 1) or 34 (experiment 2).

b) Extrapulmonary metastases involved lymph nodes and liver

It is of interest that TAM from human Kaposi's sarcoma have been shown recently to have proliferative activity (C. Parravicini, unpublished).

ANTITUMOR POTENTIAL OF MACROPHAGES

Appropriately activated mononuclear phagocytes can kill tumor cells in vitro and elicit tumor-destructive reactions in vivo.

The latter involve vascular responses that are induced by cytokines (TNF and IL-1) released by monocytes (Mantovani et al 1992b). Macrophages can kill tumor cells through a variety of mediators, including soluble or membrane-associated cytokines (IL-1 and TNF), and reactive oxygen or nitrogen intermediates and probably other, as yet undefined, cytotoxic pathways. In most experimental systems, macrophage cytotoxicity involves a close interaction with tumor target cells. We have recently found that antibodies to leukocyte integrins (lymphocyte function-associated antigen (LFA)-1 in particular) inhibit human monocyte cytotoxicity including that exerted on targets that are sensitive to TNF (Bernasconi et al 1991, Jonjic et al 1992). These findings are compatible with a model in which contact between monocyte surface integrins and undefined ligands on tumor target cells allows local delivery of cytotoxic molecules.

Further evidence for the importance of the CD18-dependent adhesion pathway was recently obtained by a gene transfer approach. Transfer of the ICAM-1 gene in a "low ICAM-1" melanoma clone (2/21) relatively resistant to monocyte cytotoxicity resulted in augmented levels of killing (Jonjic et al, unpublished).

IMMUNOTHERAPY IN OVARIAN CARCINOMA

While the results obtained in rodent tumors and in vitro suggest that activated macrophages indeed have the potential to eliminate at least small numbers of tumor cells surviving after cytoreductive therapy, evidence for antitumor activity of macrophage activators in humans is limited. In the context of a long standing interest in exploring i.p. immunotherapy in ovarian cancer (e.g. Allavena et al 1990) attention was recently focused on IFNγ, a prototypic macrophage activating cytokine. In a large cooperative study with 98 patients, i.p. IFNγ showed definite antitumor activity in subjects with minimal residual disease resistant to chemotherapy (Allavena et al 1992, Pujade-Lauraine et al 1990). It is of interest that when IFNγ was administered systematically, no modulation of in situ effector cells and no clinical response were observed (Colombo et al., unpublished).

CONCLUDING REMARKS

Phagocytes infiltrating neoplastic tissues have peculiar membrane phenotype and functional properties. TAM play a complex, ambiguous role in the regulation of primary tumor growth and metastasis (a "macrophage balance", see Mantovani et al 1992a). Yet these cells are strategically located at the very interface between tumor and host and represent a potential target for immunomodulation. A better understanding of the regulation and function of TAM may provide a less empirical basis for rational design of therapeutic approaches, as vividly illustrated by the antitumor activity of i.p. interferon γ in ovarian cancer patients with minimal residual disease resistant to chemotherapy (Allavena et al, 1992).

ACKNOWLEDGEMENTS

This work was supported by finalized project ACRO. The generous contribution of the Italian Association for Cancer Research, Milan, Italy, is gratefully acknowledged.

REFERENCES

Allavena, P., Grandi, M., D'Incalci, M., Geri, O., Giuliani, F.C., and Mantovani, A., 1987, Human tumor cell lines with pleiotropic drug resistance are efficiently killed by Interleukin-2 activated killer cells and by activated monocytes. Int. J. Cancer, 40:104.

Allavena, P., Peccatori, F., Maggioni, D., Sironi, M., Colombo, N., Lissoni, A., Galazka, A., Meiers, W., Mangioni, C., and Mantovani A., 1990, Intraperitoneal recombinant g-interferon in patients with recurrent ascitic ovarian carcinoma: modulation of cytotoxicity and cytokine production in tumor-associated effectors and major histocompatibility antigen expression on tumor cells. Cancer Res., 50:7318.

Bernasconi, S., Peri G., Sironi, M., and Mantovani, A., 1991, Involvement of leukocyte (B2) integrins (CD18/CD11) in human monocyte tumoricidal activity. Int. J. Cancer, 49:267.

Bottazzi, B., Polentarutti, N., Acero, R., Balsari, A., Boraschi, D., Ghezzi, P., Salmona, M., and Mantovani, A., 1983, Regulation of the macrophage content of neoplasms by chemoattractants. Science, 220:210.

Bottazzi, B., Colotta, F., Sica, A., Nobili, N. and Mantovani, A., 1990a, A chemoattractant expressed in human sarcoma cells (Tumor-derived chemotactic factor, TCDF) is identical to monocyte chemoattractant protein-1/monocyte chemotactic and activating factor (MCP-1/MCAF). Int. J. Cancer, 45:795.

Bottazzi, B., Erba, E., Nobili, N., Fazioli, F., Rambaldi, A. and Mantovani, A., 1990b, A paracrine circuit in the regulation of the proliferation of macrophages infiltrating murine sarcomas. J. Immunol., 144:2409.

Bottazzi, B., Walter, S., Govoni, D., Colotta F., and Mantovani, A., 1992, Monocyte chemotactic cytokine gene transfer modulates macrophage infiltration, growth and susceptibility to IL-2 therapy of a murine melanoma. J. Immunol., 148:1280.

Colombo, N., Peccatori, F., Paganin, C., Bini, S., Brandely, M., Mangioni, C., Mantovani, A., and Allavena, P., 1992, Anti-tumor and immunomodulatory activity of intraperitoneal administration of IFN g in ovarian carcinoma patients with minimal residual tumor after chemotherapy, Int. J. Cancer, *in press*.

Evans, R., and Cullen, R.T., 1984, In situ proliferation of intratumor macrophages. Journal Leukocyte Biology, 35:561.

Furutani, Y., Nomura, H., Notake, M., Oyamada, Y., Fukui, T., Yamada, M., Larsen, C.G., Oppenheim, J.J., and Matsushima, K., 1989, Cloning and sequencing of the cDNA for human monocyte chemotactic and activating factor (MCAF). Biochem. biophys. Res. Commun., 159:248.

Jonjic, N., Jilek, P., Bernasconi, S., Peri, G., Martin-Padura, I., Cenzuales, S., Dejana, E., and Mantovani, A., 1992, Molecules involved in the adhesion and cytotoxicity of activated monocytes on endothelial cells. J. Immunol., 148:2080.

Mahoney, K.H., and Heppner, G.H., 1987, FACS analysis of tumor associated macrophage replication: Differences between metastatic and nonmetastatic murine mammary tumors. Journal Leukocyte Biology, 41:205.

Mantovani, A., Bottazzi, B., Colotta, F., Sozzani, S., and Ruco, L., 1992a, Origin and function of tumor-associated macrophages. Immunology Today, *in press*.

Mantovani, A., Bussolino, F., and Dejana, E., 1992b, Cytokine regulation of endothelial cell function. Faseb J., *in press*.

Matsushima, K., Larsen, C.G., DuBois, G.C., and Oppenheim, J.J., 1989, Purification and characterization of a novel monocyte chemotactic and activating factor produced by a human myelomonocytic cell line. J. Exp. Med., 169:1485.

Oppenheim, J.J., Zachariae, C.O.C., Mukaida, N., and Matsushima, K., 1991, Properties of the novel proinfammatoty supergene "Intercrine" cytokine family. Annual Review of Immunol., 9:617.

Pujade-Lauraine, E., Colombo, N., Namer, N., Fumoleau, P., Monnier, A., Nooy, M.A., Falkson, G., Mignot, L., Bugat, R., Oliveira, C.M.D., Mousseau, M., Netter, G., Oberling, F.,Coiffier, B., and Brandely, M., 1990, Intraperitoneal human r-IFN gamma in patients with residual ovarian carcinoma (OC) at second look laparotomy (SLL). ASCO, 9:156 abs., 111.

Sica, A., Wang, J.M., Colotta, F., Dejana, E., Mantovani, A., Oppenheim, J.J., Larsen, C.G., Zachariae, C.O., and Matsushima, K., 1990, Monocyte chemotactic factor gene expression induced in endothelial cells by IL-1 and tumor necrosis factor. J. Immunol., 144:3034.

Snyderman, R., and Cianciolo, G.J., 1984, Immunosuppressive activity of the retroviral envelope protein P15E and its possible relationship to neoplasia. Immunology Today, 5:240.

Valente, A.J., Fowler, S.R., Sprague, E.A., Kelley, J.L., Suenram, A.C. and Schwartz, C.J., 1984, Initial characterization of a peripheral blood mononuclear cell chemoattractant derived from cultured arterial smooth muscle cells. Am. J. Pathol., 117:479.

Van Damme, J., Decock, B., Lenaerts, J.P., Conings, R., Bertini R., Mantovani, A. and Billiau, A., 1989, Identification by sequence analysis of chemotactic factors for monocytes produced by normal and transformed cells stimulated with virus, double stranded RNA or IL-1. Europ. J. Immunol., 19:2367.

Walter, S., Bottazzi, B., Govoni, D., Colotta, F., and Mantovani, A., 1991, Macrophage infiltration and growth of sarcoma clones expressing different amounts of monocyte chemotactic protein/JE. Int. J. Cancer, 49:431.

Wang, J.M., Cianciolo, G.J., Snyderman, R., and Mantovani, A., 1986, Coexistence of a chemotactic factor and a retroviral P15E-related chemotaxis inhibitor in human tumor cell culture supernatants. J. Immunol., 137:2726.

Yoshimura, T., Yuhki, N., Moore, S.K., Appella, E., Lerman, M.I., and Leonard, E.J., 1989, Human monocyte chemoattractant protein-1 (MCP-1). Full-lenght cDNA cloning, expression in mitogen-stimulation blood mononuclear leukocytes, and sequence similarity to mouse competence gene JE. FEBS Letters, 244:487.

Zachariae, C.O.C., Anderson, A.O., Thompson, H.L., Appella, E., Mantovani, A., Oppenheim, J.J. and Matsushima, K., 1990, Properties of monocyte chemotactic and activating factor (MCAF) purified from a human fibrosarcoma cell line. J. Exp. Med., 171:2177.

SEPTIC SHOCK PATHOPHYSIOLOGY:
FOCUS ON THERAPEUTIC APPROACH

Giancarlo Palmieri*, Giuseppe Nicoletti, Silvia Cantoni*, and Lucio Bucci*

*Divisione Medica II Brera, Ospedale Niguarda Ca'Granda, Milano
Istituto di Microbiologia, Università di Catania, Catania, Italy

Over the last 30 years, the prevalence of sepsis, and its sequelae, namely sepsis syndrome and septic shock has increased among hospitalized patients mostly due to improvements in medical care and technology.

In the United States the incidence of septicemia has increased from 73.6 to 175.9 cases per 100,000 persons between 1979 and 1987 (MMWR reported data). The frequency with which septic shock ensues in patients with septicemia is more difficult to establish, mainly due to differences in definitions from one study to another. Overall estimates (Kreger *et al.*) suggest that it develops in about 40% of patients and that it is always associated with a poor prognosis with mortality ranging from about 77% up to 90% according to different study populations (Parker *et al.*)

Clinical definitions of sepsis syndrome and septic shock have recently been proposed by Bone.

A number of factors have contributed to the increased prevalence of the clinical spectrum of disorders associated with sepsis and several efforts have been made in recent years to elucidate the pathophysiology of these conditions and to develop new therapeutical approaches.

Gram-negative bacteria are a major component of humans' native microbial flora. Thus it is not surprising that they are the most commonly isolated microorganisms in patients with sepsis due to emerging microbial opportunism in the face of significant depression of host defenses secondary to the underlying disease process or to the widespread use of antimicrobial agents. However, septic shock can develop also during the course of infections caused by Gram-positive bacteria, fungi and probably also by viruses; frequently, the causative agent can not be isolated.

Bacterial products - such as lipid A (the toxic moiety of G- bacteria endotoxin); certain wall antigens from G+ bacteria (such as hemolytic group A streptococci which have an M protein that exerts toxic effects similar to those of endotoxin) (Ginsberg, 1972); exotoxin A produced by P. aeruginosa; exotoxin produced by certain G+ bacteria- as well as fungal and viral antigens have been shown to be potent activators of a number of humoral pathways along with macrophages and other cell types involved in inflammatory and immune reactions against infectious agents. Host sensitivity to the infecting microorganisms can be greatly enhanced by the concommitant presence of more than one bacterial product: levels of circulating endotoxin otherwise harmless may be rendered toxic by simultaneous release of cell wall components, including endotoxin itself, and exotoxins of G+ strains (Galanos *et al.*, 1990).

Bacterial products have been shown to activate the complement cascade both via the classic and alternative pathways. The former is mainly activated by complexes of cell wall components and antibody, while the latter can be activated experimentally by lipopo lysaccharide from the cell wall of G- bacteria and by G+ cell wall components (Glauser *et al.*, 1991). The alternative pathway appears to have an important function in providing non-specific opsonic support before specific antibodies become available; however, not all microorganisms seem capable of equally well activating this pathway (Guckian *et al.*, 1978) and thus have a requirement for type-specific antibodies for efficient opsonization. Both IgM and IgG antibodies have opsonic and bactericidal activities, particularly in the presence of complement, and also play a role in neutralizing toxins. There is evidence from immunization studies in humans that the protective antibody against endotoxin core is IgM rather than IgG (McCabe *et al.*, 1988).

Complement appears to play a major role in promoting blood stream clearance of microorganisms by enhancing phagocytosis and lysis of serum-sensitive bacteria. The inflammatory reaction it triggers is certainly beneficial to the host, but excessive complement activation, possibly resulting from a large bacterial challenge, may well turn out to be deleterious to the host himself. It has been demonstrated that increased concentrations of activated complement are associated with fatal outcome in septic shock due to G+ and G- bacteria (Hack *et al.*, 1989).

Endotoxin and peptidoglycan residues and teichic acid from the cell wall of G+ organisms, along with other bacterial products, have also been shown to activate factor XII (FXIIa), which in turn directly promotes the activation of the complement, coagulatin, fibrinolytic and bradykinin systems. Complement mediated in inflammatory reaction may thus be potentiated. Uncontrolled activation of coagulation will result in thrombosis and platelet clotting factor consumption leading to the clinical picture of acute disseminated intravascular coagulation, a coagulation disorder which frequently complicates septic shock.

Bacterial products may initiate the clotting cascade through at least two additional mechanisms. Procoagulant activity may be produced by leukocyte interaction with bacterial antigen-antibody complexes (Rothberger *et al.*, 1977), upon stimulation of macrophages and endothelial cell by LPS (Glauser *et al.*, 1991) and finally after endotoxin-mediated vascular injury, in all instances leading to activation of the extrisic coagulation pathway. Secondly, bacterial products also induce the release of tumor necrosis factor (TNF) which is also an activator of the extrinsic coagulation pathway through the expressing of tissue factor (van der Poll *et al.*, 1990). It also inhibits the fibrinolytic response by suppressing the release of tissue-type plasminogen activator (t-PA) and inducing the release of plasminogen activator inhibitor type I (PAI-I). Moreover, down-regulation of thrombomodulin brought about by TNF impairs activation of the anticoagulant protein C (van der Poll, 1990).

At the same time as clotting appears to be initiated, activation of the fibrinolytic system by FXIIa also occurs through the conversion of plasminogen proactivator to plasminogen activator and the subsequent conversion of plasminogen to plasmin. Along with the consumption of platelets and clotting factors, this may also lead to the bleeding tendency observed during septic shock. Worth remembering is the fact that plasmin itself can also initiate the complement cascade.

Finally, bradykinin production is also a consequence of FXII activation. This vasoactive peptide induces vasodilatation and increased vascular permeability: decreased peripheral vascular resistance along with leakage of fluid into the interstitial space will result in hypotension and hypoperfusion of critical organs.

Haemodynamic derangements also result from the vasoactive properties of other humoral mediators (e.g. complement, arachidonic acid metabolites) and from the release of myocardial depressant substance.

Since the great majority of microorganisms that are responsible for the clinical spectrum of sepsis displays resistance to the bactericidal activity of fresh human serum, the role of circulating neutrophils and monocytes and of the fixed phagocytes of the reticuloendothelial system is of paramount importance in clearing microorganisms from the blood stream. As already mentioned, phagocytosis in enhanced by both complement products and specific antibodies.

Moreover, phagocytic and immune-system cells also play an important role in the phatogenesis of sepsis by releasing a number of mediator molecules. Derivatives of arachidonic acid metabolism, free radical oxygen species and lysosomal enzymes are released upon activation of neutrophils with subsequent vasoactive effects on the microvasculature and endothelial cell cytotoxicity, thus exacerbating hypotension.

Macrophages and endothelial cells challenged with endotoxin also generate another potent vasodilator, endothelial-derived relaxing factor, recently identified as nitric oxide (Palmer *et al.*, 1987).

Under the stimulus of bacterial products, monocytes, lymphocytes, endothelial cells and other cell types are induced to synthesize and release several cytokines, such as tumor necrosis factor alpha, interleukin-1, 6 and 8, platelet activating factor. IL-1 and IL-6 in turn stimulate T lymphocytes to produce interferon gamma, IL-2, IL-4 and GM-CSF (Jacobs *et al.*, Dinarello *et al.*) Elevated levels of IL-1 are found in septic shock and it has been demonstrated that administration of low doses of IL-1 can induce clinical effects closely resembling shock (Bone, 1991).

Much attention has focussed on TNF which is currently considered to be one of the central mediators of sepsis, responsible for much of the pathophysiological changes associated with release of endotoxin and probably also with release of bacterial products other than endotoxin. Several cell types involved in the pathogenesis of sepsis are able to produce TNF: monocytes, lymphocytes, natural killer, Kupffer and endothelial cells. Its role is sepsis has been suggested by several experimental observations. Worth mentioning is that mice genetically unresponsive to endotoxin also lack the capacity to produce murine TNF (Beutler *et al.*, 1986). Moreover, administration of recombinant TNF to humans mimics most of the clinical, hystopathologic and laboratory findings commonly observed in Gram negative sepsis (Michie *et al.*, 1988; Beutler *et al.*, 1986; Blick *et al.*, 1987). TNF can trigger the coagulation cascade and the complement system; it promotes arachidonate metabolism and increases endothelial permeability (Bone, 1991). It has been suggested that high circulating TNF levels may portend a poor prognosis in patients with sepsis and its sequelae (Bone, 1991).

Under "normal" conditions, the immune and inflammatory reactions so far described are self-limited and highly efficient at cleaning the infection that has triggered them: bacteremia is transient and results in only mild fever with little if any hemodynamic changes. However, activation of these same defensive systems by a substantial inoculum of microorganisms in a seriously ill patient appears to be both disregulated, due to derangements of the regulatory mechanisms of the immune and inflammatory responses, and unable to control the infection. If the initial nidus of infection or mild bacteremia are not properly brought under control, release of endotoxin and esotoxins will trigger a systemic response to infection and the signs and simytoms of sepsis will ensue. Endothelial damage, resulting from persistence of activated mediators in the circulation, will then lead to organ failure, with a clinical picture of sepsis syndrome. Widespread endothelial damage coupled with sustained activation of inflammatory and immune system cells will result in the metabolic and hemodynamic derangements characteristic of septic shock.

In this view, sepsis, sepsis syndrome and septic shock should not be seen as separate, discrete entities but rather as a continuum clinical spectrum of increasingly severe stages of the same basic pathophysiologic processes.

In order to understand the rational behind the different therapeutical approaches proposed and the reasons why none of them seems curative in all patients presented with sepsis and its sequelae, it should be remembered that the development of this patholoigical entity does not require the persistent or massive release of bacterial products into the blood stream: all the different mediators secreted can interact with one another resulting in further amplification of the host response, even in the absence of significant amounts of circulating bacterial products.

On the basis of our present understanding of sepsis and its sequelae, there appears to be three specific points where therapy can be applied in order to effectively conteract the pathogenic sequence leading to irreversible septic shock.

First, the causative microorganism can be eradicated with specific antimicrobial therapy or by means of surgical drainage when appropriate.

Second, carefull monitoring and correction of metabolic and hemodynamic derangements should always be sought in the appropriate hospital environment, the intensive care unit.

Third, the recently developed specific inhibitors of the endogenous and exogenous mediators of sepsis will hopefully soon find a place in the management of septic patients.

ANTIMICROBIAL THERAPY

Surgical or pharmacologic measures aimed at eradicating the invading microorganism have been the mainstay of therapy in septic patients. Whenever possible, the most specific antibiotic should be chosen on the basis of biological fluid colture results; however, very often the causative agent can not be isolated before broad-spectrum antimicrobial therapy, effective against all the likely microorganisms involved, is indicated.

Large clinical studies have demonstrated that early, specific antimicrobial therapy is associated with significant improvement in survival, even in the most severely ill patients (Kreger et al., 1980; Bryan et al., 1983). However, once the clinical picture of advancing septic shock is developing, antibiotics alone can not reverse it (Parillo, 1991) and more aggressive interventions are required.

METABOLIC AND CARDIOVASCULAR SUPPORT

Sepsis syndrome and septic shock are complex and rapidly changing conditions that require continuous monitoring and rapid institution of intensive cardiovascular support. It has been shown that the use of therapy guided by invasive monitoring results in a significant decrease of mortality (Li et al., 1984; Reynolds et al., 1988). Moreover, experimental data support the hypothesis that intensive cardiovascular support may prolong survival sufficiently to allow antibiotics to eradicate the infecting microorganism (Natanson et al., 1990).

Adequate oxygenation should be ensured. Administration of fluids, inotropic agents and vaso-pressor should be taylored to the needs of each patient based upon invasive hemodynamic measurements. Metabolic abnormalities, such as hypoxaemia and acidosis, should be promptly corrected.

Septic shock is characterized by arteriolar vasodilatation which leads to a hyperdynamic state with low systemic vascular resistence, high cardiac output, hypotension and inadequate tissue perfusion.

Hypotension appears to be largely mediated by nitric oxide. Since it is produced by the endotoxin-cytokine-inducible NO synthase, specific inhibitors of ths enzyme have been developed and recently tried in patients with refactory hypotension. Two inhibitors, N- monomethyl-L-arginine (L-NMMA) and N-nitro-L-arginine methyl ester (L-NAME), have been tested and results are encouraging: rapid, dose-dependent increase in systolic, diastolic and mean arterial blood pressure associated with increased systemic vascular resistance have been recorded in the patients treated (Petros et al., 1991; Nava et al., 1991).

This approach, which prevents excessive vasodilation, seems a promising alternative to the use of vasoconstrictors which might lead to poor tissue perfusion. However, complete inhibition of NO synthesis could be harmful to the patient since NO has antimicrobial properties (Nathan et al., 1991), it inhibits platelet aggregation (Durante et al., 1991) and has been shown to play a protective role in patients with ARDS (Adult Respiratory Distress Syndrome) (Faule et al., 1991). Moreover, under certain experimental conditions, inhibition of NO synthesis potentiates endotoxin produced intestinal vasocinstriction inducing hemorrhages in the bowel wall (Hutcheson et al., 1990). This might give bacteria and their toxic products an access into the circulation, possibly exacerbating the septic condition.

At present, NO synthase inhibitors are still investigating drugs and clinical trials are needed in order to establish both the optimal therapeutical dose and the most appropriate mode of administration (bolus vs continuous infusion).

AGENTS EFFECTIVE AGAINST EXOGENOUS AND ENDOGENOUS HUMORAL MEDIATORS OF SEPSIS

Although aggressive antibiotic therapy and cardiovascular support have certainly improved survival rates among patients with severe, established septic shock, mortality is still high, remaining at 50% to 60% (Parillo et al., 1990). This has stimulated considerable interest in trying to improve survival developing new therapeutical approaches able to conteract the various mediators involved in the pathogenesis of this condition.

Glucocorticoids (GC) are known to be potent antiinflammatory and immunosuppressive agents and their administration has profound effects on many of the mediator systems involved in the pathogenesis of shock. Based upon experimental data, (GC) have long been thought to have a beneficial role in the reversal of septic shock.

However, large clinical studies (Sprung et al., 1984; Hinshaw et al., 1987; Bone et al., 1987) did not find any evidence of benefit from high-dose steroid administration. Conversely, it appeared that steroid recipients had significantly more secondary infections.

Some insight into the apparent failure of (GC) to reverse septic shock is provided by studies on the regulation of TNF. It has been shown that dexamethasone prevented TNF release when given before or during macrophage stimulation with endotoxin, but not if given afterward (Beutler et al., 1986). Put in practice, this means that it will seldom be possible to administor GC early enough to influence TNF - and probably other mediators also- production. Moreover, at least initially, the mediators released in response to the infectious agent are useful in clearing the infection and it is conceivable that blunting with high-dose GC this useful defensive reaction might be harmful to the host.

ANTIBODIES AGAINST ENDOTOXIN have been developed with the aim of blocking the adverse systemic reaction due to Gram negative bacteria endotoxin.

The first clinical trials have employed human polyclonal antiserum from volunteers immunized with a mutant strain of Escherichia coli (O111:B4), which induces an immune response to the core region of endotoxin containing lipid A. In clinical trials, the use of this antiserum proved to be of benefit in patients with Gram negative bacteremia resulting in significant reductlion in mortality rate (Ziegler et al., 1982) and to protect surgical patients at high risk of infection from septic shock (Baumgartner et al., 1985).

However, several reasons make this polyclonal antiserum of limited availability and value. First, vaccination is associated with mild toxicity and since there is no booster response, a person can donate only once; many volunteers need to be vacccinated in order to obtain enough antiserum; the antibody content of the antiserum is variable, so that its efficacy cannot be standadized. Moreover, there is the potential for transmitting infections via blood products.

The use of monoclonal antibodies (mAb) circumvents these problems. The first mAb to be used was the E5, a murine IgM antibody against lipid A. In a prospective. randomized; placebo-controlled trial (Gorelick et al., 1990) on 486 patients it was shown that among the 137 patients not in shock at entry to the study, those treated with E5 had a significantly lower mortality. However, mortality among E5 and placebo recipients who were in shock at enrollment or who did not have Gram negative shock did not differ.

A second mAb tried is HA-1A, a human IgM antibody that binds specifically to the endotoxins of a broad range of clinical isolates of Gram-negative bacteria. This antibody was used in a study group of 543 patients with sepsis or suspected Gram-negative infection (Ziegler et al., 1991). The study focussed on the 200 patients with documented Gram-negative bacteremia and showed that HA-1A use significantly reduced mortality, from 49% in the placebo group to 30% in the HA-1A group. Both patients with and without shock benefitted from treatment. However, in patients without proven Gram-negative bacteremia, no difference in outcome was demonstrated with the use of either HA-1A or plabebo.

Administration of both EJ5 and HA-1A was not associated with serious adverse reactions. In about half the patients treated with E5, a rise of antibody to murine immunoglobulin was noted, but this was of no clinical importance. None of the patients who received HA-1A had detectable anti-HA-1A antibodies.

The fact that one can not clinically differentiate patients with Gram-negative sepsis, the only benefit from this therapeutical approach, at the very onset of shock is the main limit to the widespread use of the monoclonal antibodies. Identification of the causative mocroorganism relies upon bacteriological cultures which not always are positive and become available some 20 hours after patient admission. At the present it is not known whether antibodies given at this time would still be effective. Additionally, in both studies only specific subgroups of patients had improved outcome after therapy with monoclonal antibodies (non- shocked vs shocked patients and Gram-negative infection vs other causative agents). We still do not know whether adjunctive therapy with antibodies would be most effective when used prophylactically or therapeutically, or whether late treatment would be equally effective as early administration and whether repeated doses of the antibody would be a more suitable way of therapy rather than a single bolus injection.

Thus, the inability to identify accurately those patients most suitable for treatment, uncertainties regarding specificity and mode of actions of the developed antibodies and the fact that only patients with documented Gram-negative sepsis are elegible for treatment, are clear indicators of the need for not only further clinical trails of anti-endotoxin antibodies, but also for alternative ways of treating patients with sepsis caused by microorganisms other than Gram-negative bacteria.

Considerable experimental evidence suggests that TUMOR NECROSIS FACTOR ALPHA (TNF-alfa) is an important mediator of septic shock and blocking or neutralising the TNF response by means of passive immunotherapy may have therapeutical potential. Contrary to initial experimental results, it is now clear that TNF concentrations remain high for many days, up to 120 days in one reported study (Cohen, 1991); Calandra et al., 1990), making therapy with specific antagonists feasible also later after the development of shock. Another potentially important advantage in making TNF, rather than endotoxin, a target for intervention is the possibility that TNF might play a part in the pathogenesis of shock due to agents other than Gram-negative bacteria.

A recent study (Silva et al., 1990) has shown that a single injection of a monoclonal antibody against recombinant murine TNF was effective in preventing death of mice injected experimentally with E. coli when given prophylactically or within 0.5 hour after challenge. This protection was significantly diminished if the injection was delayed until 2.5 hours after challenge and it was not due to enhanced bacterial clearance rates in the treated animals, nor to bactericidal properties of the mAb itself, but rather to neutralization of circulating TNF.

The good results obtained in the E. coli model of sepsis where not confirmed with the use of Pseudomonas aeruginosa as infecting agent. A protective effect was evident only during the first 24 hours; thereafter mortality in the treated group approached that of controls. TNF levels were effectively suppressed in the animals treated, suggesting that the protective effect of the mAb was bypassed by induction of a different host-derived mediator.

Similar negative results were obtained in neutropenic mice challenged with Klebsiella pneumonie, indicating that neutrophils play a central role in host defense. Again, TNF response was successfully suppressed by the antibody, but his was not sufficient to prevent death, thus emphasizing that, despite its central role, TNF is not the sole determinant of outcome, at least in this experimental model.

Human studies are only very preliminary. In a phase-1 study of 14 patients with severe, unresponsive shock, a single dose of murine mAb against TNF brought about only temporary improvement of clinical conditions (Exley et al., 1990). Favorable changes in temperature, pulse rate and blood pressure seemed to coincide with administration of the antibody, but overall survival did not differ from actual estimates of survival in septic shock patients receiving conventional therapy.

Very preliminary experience with intravenous infusion of high/dose purified C1-ESTERASE INHIBITOR is being carried out (Hack et al., 1992). Increased degradation of C1-esterase inhibitor occurs during septic shock and it is well known that activation of inflammatory pathways plays a major role in the pathogenesis of this condition. C1jk-esterase inhibitor administration was safe and devoid of untoward effects in a pilot study including 5 patients. Four of these patients responded to treatment with attenuation of complement and contact factor activation and with decreased demand for vasopressor medications. This therapeutical approach is still very preliminary and it is not possible yet to establish whether C1-esterase inhibitors do have a role in the treatment of septic shock.

Increased synthesis of IL-1 occurs during sepsis. However, recent studies (Granowitz et al. 1991) have demonstrated that concentrations of the IL-1-receptor antagonist, a naturally occurring antagonist of IL-1 which binds to the same receptor but does not stimulate the cell, are also elevated during challenge of human volunteers with E. coli endotoxin. The increased production of the antagonist suggests that substantial blockage of IL-1 receptors occurs physiologically during sepsis. Recombinant IL-1 receptor antagonist might have a place in the future treatment of septic shock since, even in the presence of physiological levels of the naturally occurring antagonist, a biological response can be induced by occupancy of less than 5% of IL-1 receptors and after binding of ILk-1 to its receptor, the complexes are internalized and receptors can recycle to the cell surface.

CONCLUSION

New therapeutical approaches are being developed for more effective treatment or prevention of sepsis syndrome and septic shock. They are aimed at supressing the key mediators responsible for the haemodynamic, inflammatory and immune derangements that result in severe shock. Clinical results are encouraging, but a deeper understanding of the pathophysiology of sepsis and its sequelae is probably needed in order to more effectively counteract the effects of the involved mediators.

The syndrome most probably results from complex interactions of many humoral mediators and cell populations. Moreover, most of the mediators can induce release of the others, making it difficult to ascribe a given effect to a specific mediator and, on the other hand, triggering a cascade of events that amplifies the original response. For these reasons blocking by means of antagonist molecules or specific antibodies only one mediator might not be sufficient to bring under control all the complex interactions leading to shock. To reverse the condition, pharmacological cocktails seem more indicated.

When considering the use and timing of anti-mediator therapies, the role of these same mediator in host defense against infection should also be taken into account. It follows the early, effective block of cell functions and cytokine actions in patients with sepsis with the purpose of counteracting potentially harmful levels of these mediators, may also impair the ability of the host to control the infection. This might result in worsening of the very infection that triggered the development of septic shock.

REFERENCES

- Baumgartner JD, Glauser MP, McCutchan JA, et al. Prevention of Gram negative shock and death in surgical patients by antibody to endotoxin core glycolipid. Lancet, 1985; ii: 59-63.
- Beutler B, Krochin N, Milsark IW, et al. Control of cachectin (Tumor Necrosis Factor) synthesis: mechanisms of endotoxin resi stance. Science, 1986; 232: 977-80.
- Blick M, Sherwin SA, Rosenbaum M, et al. Phase-1 study of recombinant Tumor Necrosis Factor in cancer patients. Cancer Res, 1987; 47: 2986-9.
- Bone RC. The pathogenesis of sepsis. Ann Intern Med, 1991; 115: 457-69.
- Bone RC, Fisher CJ Jr, Clemmer TP, et al. A controlled clinical trial of high-dose methylpred-nisolone in the treatment of severe sepsis and septic shock. N Engl J Med, 1987; 317: 653-58.
- Bryan CS, Reynolds KL, Brenner ER. Analysis of 1,186 episodes of Gram-negative bacteremia in non-university hospitals: the effects of antimicrobial therapy. Rev Infect Dis, 1983; 5: 629-38.
- Calandra T, Baumgartner JD, Grav GE, et al. Prognosis values of Tumor Necrosis Factor/ca-chectin, interleukin-1, alpha-interferon and gamma-interferon in the serum of patients with septic shock. J Infect Dis, 1990; 161: 982-87.
- Cohen J. Clinical role of tumor necrosis factor in septic shock. Update Intensive Care Emergency Med, 1991; 14: 262-68.

- Dinarello CA, Mier JW. Lymphokines. N Engl J Med, 1987; 317: 940-45.
- Durante W, Schini VB, Scott-Burden T, et al. Platelet inhibition by an L-arginine derived substance released by IL- 1beta-treated vascular smooth muscle cells. Am J Physiol, 1991; 261: H 2024-30.
- Exley AR, Cohen J, Buurman WA et al. Monoclonal antibody to Tu mor Necrosis Factor in severe septic shock. Lancet, 1990; 335: 1275-77.
- Faule KJ,Rossaint R, Keitel M et al. Successful treatment of severe adult respiratory distress syndrome with nitric oxide: the first three patients. Presented at Second International Meeting on the Biology of Nitric Oxide. London, october, 1991).
- Galanos C, Freudenberg MA, Matsuura M. Mechanisms of the lethal action of endotoxin and endotoxin hypersensitivity. In: Friedman H, Klein TW, Nokano M, Nowotny A, eds. Endotoxin, advances in ex perimental medicine and biology. New York: Plenum Press, 1990; 603-19.
- Ginsberg I. Mechanisms of cell and tissue injury induced by group A streptococci: relation to poststreptococcal sequelae. J Infect Dis, 1972; 126: 294-7.
- Glauser MP, Zanetti G, Baumgartner JD et al. Septic shock: pat hogenesis. Lancet, 1991; 338: 732-6.
- Gorelick K, Scannon PJ, Hannigan J et al. Randomized placebo- controlled study of E5 monoclonal antiendotoxin antibody. In: Borrebaeck CA, Larrick JW, eds. Therapeutic mono-clonal antibo dies. New York: Stockton Press, 1990: 253-61.
- Granowitz EV, Santos AA, Poutsiaka DD et al. Production of IL-1-receptor antagonist during experimental endotoxaemia. Lancet, 1991; 338: 1423-4.
- Guckian JC, Christensen WP, Fine DP. Evidence for quantitative variability of bacterial opsonic requirements. Infect Immun, 1978; 19: 882-5.
- Hinshaw LB, Peduzzi P, Young E et al. Effect of high-dose glucocorticoid therapy on mortality in patients with clinical signs of systemic sepsis. N Engl J Med, 1987; 317: 659-65.
- Hutcheson IR, Whittle B Jr, Boughton-Smith NK. Role of nitric oxide in maintaining vascular integrity in endotoxin-induced in testinal damage in the rat. Br J Pharmacol, 1990; 101: 815-20.
- Jacobs RF, Tabor DR. Immune cellular interactions during sepsis and septic injury. Crit Care Clin, 1989; 5: 9-26.
- Kreger BE, Craven DE, McCabe WR. Gram negative bacteriemia. IV Re-evaluation of clinical features and treatment in 612 patients. Am J Med, 1980; 68: 344-55.
- Kuhweide R, Van Damme J, Ceuppens JL. Tumor necrosis factor- alpha and interleukin 6 synergistically induce T cell growth. Eur J Immunol, 1990; 20: 1019-25.
- Li TC, Phillips MC, Shaw L et al. On-site physician staffing in a community hospital intensive care unit. Impact on test and pro cedure use and on patient outcome. JAMA, 1984; 252: 2023-7.
- McCabe WR, DeMaria A Jr, Berberich H et al. Immunization with rough mutants of Salmonella minnesota: protective activity of IgM and IgG antibody to the R595 (Re chemotype) mutant. J Infect Dis, 1988; 158: 29-30.
- Michie MR, Manogue KR, Springs DR et al.Detection of circulating tumor necrosis factor after endotoxin administration. N Engl J Med, 1988; 318: 1481-6.
- MMWR. Increase in national hospital discharge rates for septicemia. United States, 1979-1987, MMWR, 39: 31-4.
- Nathanson C, Danner RL, Reilly JM et al. Antibiotics versus car diovascular support in a canine model of human septic shock. Am J Physiol, 1990; 259 (5pt2) H 1440-7.
- Nathan CF, Hibbs JB. Role of nitric oxide synthesis in macrophage antimicrobial activity. Curr Opin Immunol, 1991; 3: 65-70.
- Nva E, Palmer RMJ, Moncada S. Inhibition of nitric oxide synthesis in septic shock: how much is beneficial? Lancet, 1991; 338: 1555-57.
- Palmer RMJ, Ferrige AG, Moncada S. Nitric oxide release accounts for the biological activity of endothelium-derived relaxing factor. Nature, 1987; 327: 524-26.
- Parker MM, Parrillo JE. Septic shock: hemodynamics and pathoge nesis. JAMA, 1983; 250: 3324-7.
- Parrillo JE. Management of septic shock: present and future. Ann Intern Med, 1991; 115: 491-93.
- Parrillo JE, Parker MM, Natanson C et al. NIH Conference. Septic shock in humans: advances in the understanding of pathogenesis, cardiovascular dysfunction and therapy. Ann Intern Med, 1990; 113: 227-42.

- Petros A, Bennett D, Vallance P. Effect of nitric oxide synthase inhibitors on hypotension in patients with septic shock. Lancet, 1991; 338: 1557-58.
- Reynolds HN, Haupt MT, Thill-Baharozian MC et al. Impact of critical care physician staffing on patients with septic shock in a university hospital medical intensive care unit. JAMA, 1988; 260: 3446-50.
- Rothberger H, Zimmerman TS, Spiegelberg HL et al. Leukocyte procoagulant activity: enhancement of production in vitro by IgG and antigen-antibody complexes. J Clin Invest, 1977; 59: 549-61.
- Silva AT, Bayston KF, Cohen J. Prophylactic and therapeutic ef fects of a monoclonal antibody to tumor necrosis factor-alpha in experimental Gram-negative shock. J Infect Dis, 1990; 162: 421- 27.
- Sprung CL, Caralis PV, Marcial E et al. The effect of high-dose corticosteroids in patients with septic shock. A prospective, controlled study. N Engl J Med, 1984; 311; 1137-43.
- Ziegler EJ, Fisher CJ, Sprung CL et al. Treatment of Gram nega tive bacteremia and septic shock with HA-1A human monoclonal an tibody against endotoxin. N Engl J Med, 1991; 324: 429-36.
- Ziegler Ej, McCutchan JA, Fierer J et al. Treatment of Gram ne gative bacteremia and shock with human antiserum to a mutant E scherichia coli. N Engl J Med, 1982; 307: 1225-30.

DIFFERENTIATING AGENTS AND CANCER THERAPY. ROLE OF CELLULAR LIPID PEROXIDATION AND ITS PRODUCT 4-HYDROXYNONENAL IN THE CONTROL OF CELL PROLIFERATION AND DIFFERENTIATION.

Vito M. Fazio,[1] Giuseppina Barrera,[2] Roberto Muraca,[2] Monica Rinaldi,[1] Silvia A. Ciafrè,[3] Marzia Lazzari,[4] Mario U. Dianzani[2] and Maria Giulia Farace.[1,3]

[1] Institute of Experimental Medicine, CNR, Rome, Italy
[2] Dept. of Experimental Medicine and Oncology, University of Torino, Italy
[3] Dept. of Exp. Medicine and Biochemical Sciences, "Tor Vergata" University, Rome
[4] Dept. of Surgery, "Tor Vergata" University, Rome, Italy

INTRODUCTION

Numerous experimental observations provide evidences that malignancy can be reversed by causing cancerous cells to differentiate and stop growing (1-5). This statement implies that transformation does not inevitably destroy the inherent potential for expression, under appropriate environmental conditions, of differentiated characteristics.

This is also demonstrated by the fact that tumors are generally heterogeneous with regard to the apparent state of differentiation of their cells. They are commonly composed of a mixture of malignant stem cells, which have a marked capacity for proliferation and a limited capacity for differentiation under normal homeostatic conditions, and of the possibly benign progeny of these malignant cells, at different degree of differentiation (5, 6).

In the cancer many more malignant cells are produced than differentiate. The cells of the neoplastic mass do not cycle faster than normal cells, but the tumor grows more rapidly because of the larger number of undifferentiated, proliferating malignant cells.

The restoration of the correspondent differentiated phenotype could be experimentally induced in cancer cells by culture in embryonic environment (5), by treatment with specific naturally occurring substances (5) or with some chemical compounds (5, 7). It is reasonable that the biochemical pathway for differentiation can be modified by a variety of molecules at various points in the pathway thereby enhancing or inhibiting the process. Several experimental data suggest that arresting multiplication by inducing differentiation bypasses many of the genetic abnormalities that originally disrupted the normal pattern of growth and differentiation (6). However, little is known about the nature of cancer-derived differentiated normal cells.

In this review we will briefly discuss the suggested mechanisms that lead to the induction of re-differentiation of tumor cells and we will compare these data with recent results which correlate cellular lipid peroxidation products to the control of cell proliferation and differentiation. We will also critically analyze the possibilities for a clinical use of differentiation inducer agents.

MECHANISMS OF MALIGNANT PROCESS REVERSAL

Models of Inducer-Mediated Differentiation. These studies are mainly performed *in vitro* on tumor cell lines of different embryonic derivation. Two models of induction to cell differentiation are generally accepted, according to the nature of the inducer and the cell lineage.

The first is cell cycle dependent (8) and relies on a specific sensitivity of the cells to the inducer only during a particular phase of the cell division. In this model, synchronized cells can be induced to differentiated with a single pulse of the inducer in the appropriate step of the cell cycle. Non-synchronized cells need at least one complete cell cycle (approximately 12 hours) to be induced the majority of them.

The second is a stochastic model (9, 10) in which the proportion of committed cells is directly related to the length of exposure to the inducer, without any connection to the cell cycle. Cells can be induced even in the absence of DNA synthesis and cell proliferation.
The molecular processes involved in the induction of cell differentiation in each of these models are not obviously so distant. It is possible that different inducers trigger the differentiation acting on the same biochemical pathway at different steps. Anyway, the precise mechanisms involved in the regulation of differentiation still remain relatively obscure.

Phases During Inducer-Mediated Differentiation. Generally speaking, the course of induced differentiation follows three progressive periods (7). Upon addition of the inducer, there results a **latent period**, whose lenght varies with the inducer used, but corresponds approximately to one cell cycle. After this period, cells undergo **commitment** to terminal differentiation and start to develop the differentiated phenotype. Commitment is defined as the capacity of cells to express the differentiated phenotype, despite removal of the inducer (11). Finally, upon continued exposure to the inducer, the following step is a progressive recruitment to **terminal differentiation**. Cell division ceases without affecting the viability, and the cells express the biochemical and morphogenetic markers of the normal nontransformed counterpart. Cell death is reached in few days following terminal differentiation according to the normal lifetime *in vitro* or *in vivo* of that particular terminally differentiated cell type.

Molecular Mechanisms. The molecular events involved in the process of differentiation are still relatively obscure and they may change with the different inducers and cell lineages. Obviously, the expression of genes related to cell proliferation is progressively decreased, while the expression of the gene/s involved in the constitution of the differentiated phenotype is greatly enhanced (12).

In some cases, as in retinoic acid induced differentiation, specific **cellular binding proteins/receptors** were found. Nuclear receptors (in humans: RAR a, ß andχ) (13-16) act like ligand-inducible, transcription enhancer factors and belong to the nuclear receptor superfamily which includes both thyroid and steroid hormone receptors (17-19). Moreover, a cytoplasmic binding protein (CRABP) was also found in different retinoic acid-responsive cells but not in others (20, 21). This protein seems to be indirectly involved in the induction of differentiation and to probably act through the nuclear receptors.

During the latent period, the inducer initiates a number of changes that lead to the establishment of the commitment. In myeloid and erythroid inducer-mediated differentiation the expression of nuclear proto-oncogenes, c-myc, c-myb, c-fos, and of **p53** gene is peculiarly modulated (22, 23). **C-myc** expression follows a characteristic early biphasic down-modulation accompanied by inhibition of **c-myb** and **c-fos** expression. The control of the expression of these genes acts both at transcriptional and post-transcriptional levels (24). A dis-regulated over-expression of c-myc during this period, blocks the induction of differentiation but not commitment (25, 26). The rapid early decline of c-myc expression following inducer treatment is not a prerequisite for the induction of differentiation (27) but the late definitive decline of c-myc mRNA is essential for the commitment process. On the contrary, the constitutive over-expression of c-myb completely inhibits erythroid differentiation (28).

One of the earliest events during the induction of differentiation is a **protein kinase-C-phosphoinositol-system-** mediated step. In myeloid and erythroblastoid cells protein kinase-C activity rapidly translocates from the cytoplasma to the plasma membrane (29, 30), with the combined production by proteolysis of a soluble protein kinase activity (31). In this process the ß-isophorm of protein kinase-C plays the most valuable role, since an exogenous form introduced into the cells accelerates the differentiation pattern (32).

Other inducer-mediated changes in the latent period include altered membrane fluidity, modifications in Ca, K, and Na flux (7).

In the inducer-mediated erythroid differentiation, following the latent period, the most salient biochemical changes, during the periods of commitment and terminal differentiation, are the accumulation of both the **globin** mRNA and protein, and assembling of complete hemoglobin (33). The main regulatory mechanism in this transition is at the level of globin gene transcription (12). Of course, similar changes develop also during the differentiation of other cell lineages, with the expression of the **specific differentiative marker/s** (10, 34). Several inducers can modulate differentiation in cell lineages of completely different embryonal derivation (5).

Other modifications in the biochemistry of inducer-mediated differentiating cells are a rapid increase in intracellular **cAMP**, followed by a gradual decrease (35). Interestingly, a marked increase in both basal and stimulated **adenylate cyclase** activity, regardless of the differentiation inducer utilized, appears only later.

It has been also demonstrated the inhibition of **ornithine decarboxylase** activity (a protein closely related to cell proliferation and indirectly to cell differentiation) (36) and the enhanced expression of the **epidermal growth factor receptor** (37), **TGF-ß receptor** (38) and **fibroblast growth factor-related proteins** (39) by retinoic acid.

It is worth noting that, at least in part, the anti-tumor actions of retinoids *in vivo* may be mediated through effects on the **immune-system**. These effects directly involve an intact T-cell response (40) and include increased macrophage or polymorphonuclear leukocyte functions (41, 42) and enhanced cell-mediated cytotoxicity (43).

MEMBRANE LIPID PEROXIDATION IN NORMAL AND TUMOR CELLS

Membrane lipid peroxidation is thought to be involved with a number of normal and abnormal physiological processes. Normal conditions include prostaglandin synthesis and aging while abnormal events include liver acute toxicity by several compounds, damage by cigarette smoke and atherogenesis (44 46). Lipid peroxidation largely results from free radical reactions in biological membranes which are rich in polyunsaturated fatty acids. Their unsaturated bonds undergo the autocatalytic process of peroxidation which yields a variety of intermediate and final products. Depending on the complexity of the system the unstable lipid hydroperoxydes LOOH, which are formed during the first step of lipid catalytic decomposition, may be converted in consecutive scission, fission, rearrangement and oxidation reactions into a great diversity of products (44). These derived molecules contain functional groups such as the aldehydo-, keto-, hydroxy-, epoxi-, carboxy-, and peroxi-.

Lipid peroxidation, and consequently its products, is notably decreased in regenerating rat liver in correlation with the maximum of DNA synthesis (47). Other rapidly growing tissues such as testis, bone marrow and intestinal epithelium were demonstrated to be resistant to lipid peroxidation to a certain extent (for rev. 48).

A striking relationship between proliferation rate, differentiation degree and lipid peroxidation was mainly demonstrated in tumor cells. A negative correlation exists between proliferative activity and/or anaplasia grade, and the ability of neoplastic cells to undergo lipid peroxidation (48). Lipid peroxidation is inversely related to the growth rate of the tumor, regardless of the prooxidant stimuli employed (49). Interestingly, preneoplastic nodules, slightly deviated and highly proliferating tumor cells have a progressive decrease in basal lipid peroxidation and peroxidizability (66). Highly undifferentiated anaplastic cell lines show undetectable levels of both basal or inducible lipid peroxidation (50, 51).

Several peculiar characteristics of neoplastic cells can account for an aberration in the oxy-radical metabolism and membrane lipid peroxidation (52). These cells lack the complex enzyme system of oxy-radical scavenging in a fashion which is inversely related to growth rate (48, 52). It must be pointed out that the decrease or lost in protective enzymes seems to be a peculiar characteristic of transformation and not simply a property related to the rapid proliferating activity of cancer cells (53). The most relevant rate-limiting factor in the decrease of peroxidation is the low poly-unsaturated fatty-acid availability in tumor cell membranes (for review: 48, 52) Concomitantly, the molecular order of the lipid bilayer increases while its fluidity decreases in correlation with the increase in tumor growth rate (48, 52).

4-HYDROXYNONENAL

Synthesis, Metabolism and Reactivity. The breakdown products of membrane lipid peroxidation found in the main quantitative proportion are malondialdehyde, 4-hydroxyalkenals, n-alkanals, 2-alkenals and cyclic peroxides (for review: 44). The hydroxyalkenal 4-hydroxy-2,3-trans-nonenal (HNE) is one of the major aldehydes formed during the peroxidation of linoleic, gamma-linoleic and arachidonic acid (44). Hydroxyalkenals are strong electrophilic reagents which react with nucleophiles, as the sulphydryl anion RS of low molecular weight thiols or -SH enzymes and proteins. 4-hydroxynonenal formed in biological system reacts at micromolar concentrations (1-100 μM) with -SH group. At higher concentrations HNE can react also with amino-groups in proteins and in other molecules. In contrast with other peroxidation products 4-hydroxyalkenals show a reaction rate much faster and a stability of reaction products much higher (60). According to numerous experimental data HNE is the lipid peroxidation product which shows the highest reactivity towards important biomolecules and cellular processes (54, 55).

The physiological level of HNE in several types of tissues ranges from 0.2 to 2.8 μM, while in normal cells induced to peroxidate increases to 7 μM (56). This level represents a steady state amount of HNE since it is continously produced and rapidly catabolized by normal cells (57). It was demonstrated that the capacity to metabolize HNE changes in various tissues and does not imply oxidative process (58).

Biological Activity of HNE and Cancer Cells. All the effects exerted by other products of lipid peroxidation on enzyme activities, proteins, nucleic acids and cellular processes, can be exhibited also by HNE, in some cases in a more specific and more pronounced way (44, 54-56). In agreement with a direct effect of 4-hydroxyalkenals on cell proliferation and transformation, many reports clearly show that these aldehydes posses carcinostatic activity in experimental animal tumors (54, 56, 59). It must be pointed out that the majority of the toxic effects described with HNE were obtained in experiments with concentrations often much higher than 10 μM (10, 54, 56). Since the physiological concentration in normal cells is in the 1 μM range, these results do not reproduce physiological conditions. At low micromolar concentrations HNE does not show toxic effects but modulates cellular functions. It stimulates polymorphonuclear leukocyte chemotactic activity by the activation of phosphoinositide-specific phospholipase-C cascade and increases basal adenylate cyclase activity (60, 61).

In an attempt to demonstrate a possible physiological role of HNE, we have conducted experiments at concentrations of HNE ranging from 10 nM to 100 μM. We have first demonstrated that human anaplastic cell lines (K562, HL60, etc.) have undetectable levels of both basal and induced lipid peroxidation, and consequently of its products (10, 51). This observation excluded alterations in HNE concentration due to endogenous production during the course of cell treatment and more precisely confirmed previous observations by other laboratories.

100 μM HNE was clearly toxic also after a single treatment for 1 hour and markedly decreased cell viability, RNA, DNA and protein synthesis (51, 62). On the contrary, specifically 1 μM HNE showed a marked general stimulatory effect on cell metabolism, and modulated the expression of specific genes (51). C-myc expression underwent a rapid biphasic down-modulation. Interestingly, the expression of genes related to erythroid cell differentiation (globins) was in parallel increased, while housekeeping gene expression (ß-actin) was unmodified. The regulation of c-myc expression was acted indifferently on messenger RNA from both the two major transcription start sites and mainly at post-transcriptional level, with only a very rapid transcriptional attenuation at 20 minutes after inducer treatment. All of these data are coincident with the gene modulation occurring in the course of chemically induced *in vitro* erythroid differentiation.

We also tested the activity of ornithine decarboxylase (ODC) which is directly related to cell proliferation and indirectly to differentiation (63). 1 μM HNE specifically inhibited ODC activity in whole K562 cells, but it was uneffective on cytosol preparation and it did not modify ODC half life. These observations are consistent with the induction of a cellular process which includes the inhibition of ODC activity (not a direct interaction of HNE with the enzyme), the modulation of the expression of c-myc and of genes related to cell differentiation, even if terminal differentiation was not yet achieved. The complex of these results was obtained with a single treatment for only one hour. Since all the accepted models of inducer-mediated differentiation imply a contact between the inducer and the cells for not less than 12 hours, HNE seems to be very effective in inducing differentiation. In order to test experimental conditions allowing a constant and stable concentration of HNE in culture medium, we analyzed by high pressure liquid chromatography (HPLC) the extinction rate of HNE in medium alone, in medium with 10% foetal calf serum, and in cell suspension in complete medium (10, 64). After 45 minutes from HNE (10 μM) addiction in neoplastic cell suspension (K562 and HL60) and complete medium, HNE was reduced to 2% of initial value. We therefore tested the possibility to maintain constant and stable concentrations by adding HNE every 45 minutes. In the course and following 10 and 12 repeated treatments with 1 μM HNE we tested by HPLC the concentration of 4-hydroxynonenal in the culture medium. No accumulation of HNE was detected and the concentration of the aldehyde was quite constant and stable. These results allowed us to demonstrate terminal differentiation of human promyelocytic HL60 cell line to granulocytic phenotype (10) by 12 repeated treatments with 1 μM HNE. HL60 cell proliferation was blocked without any change in cell viability until cell death following terminal differentiation. HNE induced chemiluminescence production, phagocytosing ability and enzymatic changes dealing with the differentiated phenotype. Even if this treatment was still below 12 hours, more than 50 % of cells were induced to terminal differentiation. Moreover, a striking correlation between the length of exposure to the inducer and the proportion of terminally differentiated cells was demonstrated.

Furthermore, recent preliminary results indicate also the involvement of protein-kinase C cascade in the mechanism of HNE action (A. Aquino and V.M. Fazio, unpublished results).

CONCLUSIVE CONSIDERATIONS

From the complex of the data discussed on the cellular lipid peroxidation in normal and cancer cells, the effects of 4-hydroxynonenal and the mechanism of inducer-mediated cancer cell re-differentiation, we believe to conclude that HNE can really have some role in the regulation of cell proliferation and differentiation. The typical modulation of c-myc expression, ODC activity, differentiation-related genes and proteins, adenylate cyclase, phosphoinositide-specific phospholipase C cascade, and protein kinase C, at concentrations close to the basal levels found in normal cells, are consistent with the mechanisms of inducer-mediated cell differentiation.

More studies are needed to better describe and specify the mechanism of HNE action in order to elucidate its role in cell proliferation and differentiation.

The establishment of effective cancer-specific differentiation therapy could solve many of the problems related to the toxicity of the chemotherapic protocols up to now performed in human cancer. HNE could combine several of the critical features for an effective differentiating agent. In fact, it specifically acts on cancer cells, its functional concentration in vitro is coincident with the basal level found in vivo in normal cells, induces differentiation after only 9-10 hour incubation, it is not accumulated, and at this concentration it is absolutely free of toxic effects.

In order to consider clinical experimental approaches to differentiation therapy, we will conclude briefly summarizing the characteristics and limits of differentiative anti-cancer chemotherapics.

Features and Limits of Differentiation Agents in Clinical Trials. As already discussed, the basic defect in neoplastic growth relies on an imbalance between the ability of cancer cells to proliferate and the initiation of their differentiation under normal homeostatic regulation. It seems that differentiating agents bypass the abnormal neoplastic pathway and act at different biochemical steps to re-induce the pattern of differentiation. This means that differentiation inducers suppress tumor growth not by killing cells but by inducing enhanced commitment to terminal differentiation, followed by normal cell death.

According to in vitro studies (5-7) and clinical trials (5, 7, 65, 66) there exist several problems in the interpretation of the results and in the treatment of tumors with differentiating agents:

- since these compounds do not kill the cells but the cells die only after several days following differentiation, it is not possible to observe a rapid cytoreduction of the tumor;

- not always specific, sensitive and feasible markers of differentiation are suitable in vivo to demonstrate the differentiation of neoplastic cells and to follow the efficacy of the treatment;

- these compounds are often toxic for normal cells because of the high effective concentration and/or the prolonged and continous minimum duration of treatment required to induce a substantial proportion of the population to differentiate;

- other pharmacological considerations, as the plasma half-life, high reactivity with blood and plasma components, and the pharmacokinetics.

If these are the disadvantages related to differentiating agents, is it warranted the development of differentiation therapy ? To answer it must be remembered that none of the cytotoxic antineoplastic drugs developed thus far have specificity for only the malignant cells. As a consequence, normal cells are killed during treatment, causing morbidity and at times death of the patient. A secoind point to be stressed is that many of the common cancers do not respond well or definitively to currently available chemotherapeutic agents.

The objectives for differentiation agents in the clinical trials could be:
- suppression of established tumors at various degrees of malignancy;
- treatment of preneoplastic, still benign, conditions;
- prevention of cancerous transformation.

It is over the purpose of this work to enumerate all the copious experimental data of clinical and pre-clinical trials with differentiating agents and to cite all the agents that gave interesting results (for more informations see reviews 5-8, 67, 68). However, it is worth remembering that at least the retinoic acid and its derivatives and the hybrid polar/apolar compounds and hexamethylene bisacetamide (HMBA) in particular, have proved to be very effective differentiation agents. For several pre-malignant lesions of the skin, head and neck, cervix, and bladder, and recently also most strikingly in promyelocytic leukemia, clinical activity of retinoids has been either established or strongly suggested (65, 66, 69-75). Polar/ apolar compounds, for which clinical studies began more recently, do not yet provided sufficient evidence for a sustained therapeutic benefit (65, 76). Interest in these compounds was recently enhanced with the demonstration that erythroleukemia cells, selected for a low level resistance to vincristine, show increased sensitivity to the action of polar/apolar inducers, including HMBA (77). Interestingly cells resistant to HMBA treatment become highly sensitive after they are selected for vincristine-resistance (78). Moreover, recent reports of increased induction of differentiation in primary AML blasts culture with the combinations of retinoic acid, HMBA and a cytotoxic agent as cytosine arabinoside or 6-thioguanine (79, 80), strongly suggest a potential role for combination therapy with differentiating agents (68).

Aknowledgments: This research was partly supported by CNR, Progetto Finalizzato BTBS to V.M.F. and by Progetto Finalizzato ACRO to M.G.F., and by Association for International Cancer Research (UK) to M.U.D.

REFERENCES

1. H. Beug, P.A. Blundell, T. Graff, Reversibility of differentiation and proliferative capacity in avian myelomonocytic cells transformed by E26 leukemia cells, Genes Devel. 1:277 (1987).
2. R.L. Brinster, The effects of cells transferred into the mouse blastocyst on subsequent development, J. Exp.. Med. 140:1049 (1974).
3. J.J. DeCosse, C.L. Gossens, J.F. Cuzma, Breast cancer: induction of differentiation by embryonic tissue, Science 181:1057 (1973).
4. E. Gootwine, C. Webb, L. Sachs, Participation of myeloid leukemia cells injected into embryos in hematopoietic differentiation in adult mice, Nature 299:63 (1982).
5. G.B. Pierce and W.C. Speers, Tumors as caricatures of the process of tissue renewal: prospects for therapy by directing differentiation, Cancer Res. 48:1966 (1988).
6. L. Sachs, Growth, differentiation and the reversal of malignancy, Sci. Am. 254:30 (1986).
7. E. Dmitrovsky, M. Markman and P.A. Marks, Clinical use of differentiating agents in cancer therapy, in: "Cancer Therapy; Cancer Chemotherapy and Biological Response Modifiers, Annual 11", H.M. Pinedo, B.A. Chabner and D.L. Longo, ed.s, Elsevier Science Publishers, Amsterdam-New York (1990).
8. A. Yen, L. Freeman and J. Fishbaugh, Leukemia Res. 11:63 (1987).
9. C. Tarella, D. Ferrero, E. Gallo, G.L. Pagliardi, and F.W. Ruscetti, Induction of differentiation of HL60 cells by dimethyl sulfoxide: evidence for a stochastic model not linked to the cell division cycle, Cancer Res. 42:445 (1982).
10. G. Barrera, C. Di Mauro, R. Muraca, D. Ferrero, G. Cavalli, V.M. Fazio, L. Paradisi, and M.U. Dianzani, Induction of differentiation in human HL60 cells by 4-hydroxynonenal, a product of lipid peroxidation, Exp. Cell Res. 197:148 (1991).
11. E. Fibach, R.C. Reuben, R.A. Rifkind, and P.A. Marks, Effect of hexamethylene bisacetamide on the commitment to differentiation of murine erythroleukemia cells, Cancer Res. 37:440 (1977).
12. P. Charnay, and T. Maniatis, Transcriptional regulation of globin expression in the human erythroid cell line K562, Science 220:1281 (1983).

13. V. Giguere, E.S. Ong, P. Segui, and R.M. Evans, Identification of a receptor for the morphogen retinoic acid, Nature 330:624 (1987).

14. H. DeThe, A. Marchio, P. Tiollais, and A. Dejean, A thyroid hormone receptor-related gene inappropriately expressed in human hepatocellular carcinoma, Nature 330:667 (1987).

15. M. Petkovich, N.J. Brand, A. Krust and P.A. Chambon, A human retinoic acid receptor which belongs to the family of nuclear receptors, Nature 330:440 (1987).

16. N. Brand, M. Petkovich, A. Krust, P.A. Chambon, H. DeThe, A. Marchio, P. Tiollais, and A. Dejean, Identification of a second human retinoic acid receptor, Nature 332:850 (1989).

17. R.M. Evans, The steroid and thyroid hormone receptor superfamily, Science 240:889 (1988).

18. C. Nervi, J.F. Grippo, N.I. Sherman, M.D. George, and A.M. Jetten, Identification and characterization of nuclear retinoic acid binding activity in human myeloblastic leukemia HL60 cells, Proc.Natl.Acad.Sci. USA 86:5854 (1989).

19. A. Krust, P. Kastner, M. Petkovich, A. Zelent, and P. Chambon, A third human retinoic receptor, hRAR-gamma, Proc. Natl. Acad. Sci. USA 86:5310 (1989).

20. C.M. Stoner, and L.J. Gudas, Mouse cellular retinoic acid binding proteins: cloning, molecular complementary DNA sequence, and messenger RNA expression during the retinoic acid induced differentiation of F9 wild type and RA-3-10 mutant teratocarcinoma, Cancer Res. 49:1497 (1989).

21. H.J. Lawrence, K. Conner, M. Kelly, M.R. Haussler, P. Wallace, and G.C. Bagby Jr., Cis-retinoic acid stimulates the clonal growth of myeloid leukemia cells in vitro, Blood 69:302 (1987).

22. H.M. Lachman, and A.I. Skoultchi, Expression of c-myc changes during differentiation of mouse erythroleukemia cell differentiation, Nature 310:592 (1984).

23. V. Richon, R.G. Ramsay, R.A. Rifkind, and P.A. Marks, Modulation of the c-myb, c-myc, and p53 mRNA and protein levels during induced murine erythroleukemia cell differentiation, Oncogene 4:165 (1989).

24. A. Nepveu, K.B. Marcu, A.I. Skoultchi, and M. Lachman, Contributions of transcriptional and post-transcriptional mechanisms to the regulation of c-myc expression in mouse erythroleukemia cells, Genes Develop. 1:938 (1987).

25. J.A. Coppola and M.D. Cole, Constitutive c-myc oncogene expression blocks mouse erythroleukemia cell differentiation but not commitment, Nature 320:760 (1986).

26. H.M. Lachman, G. Cheng, and M.A. Skoultchi, Transfection of mouse erythroleukemia cells with myc sequences changes the rate of induced commitment to differentiate, Proc. Natl. Acad. Sci. USA 83:6480 (1986).

27. T.U. Kume, S. Takada, and M. Obinata, Probability that the commitment of murine erythroleukemia cell differentiation is determined by the c-myc level, J. Mol. Biol. 202:779 (1988).

28. M.F. Clarke, J.F. Kukowska-Latallo, E. Westin, M. Smith, and E.V. Prochownik, Constitutive expression of a c-myb cDNA blocks Friend murine erythroleukemia cell differentiation, Mol. Cell. Biol. 8:884 (1988).

29. K.J. Balazovich, D. Potnow, L. Boxer, and E.V. Prochownik, Changes in protein kinase C activity are associated with differentiation of Friend erythroleukemia cells, Biochim. Biophys. Acta 927:247 (1987).

30. X.Wu, G. Shao, S. Chen, X. Wang, and Z.-Y. Wang, Studies on the relationship between protein kinase C and differentiation of human promyelocytic leukemia cells by retinoic acid, Leukemia Res. 15:869 (1989).

31. E. Melloni, S. Pontremoli, M. Michetti, O. Sacco, A.G. Cakiroglu, J.F. Jackson, R.A. Rifkind, and P.A. Marks, Protein kinase C activity and hexamethylene bisacetamide induced erythroleukemia cell differentiation, Proc. Natl. Acad. Sci. USA 84:5282 (1987).

32. E. Melloni, S. Pontremoli, B. Sparatore, M. Patrone, F. Grossi, P.A. Marks, and R.A. Rifkind, Introduction of the ß- isozyme protein kinase C accelerates induced differentiation of murine erythroleukemia cells, Proc. Natl. Acad. Sci. USA 87:4417 (1990).

33. P.A. Marks, M. Sheffrey, and R.A. Rifkind, Induction of transformed cells to terminal differentiation and the modulation of gene expression, Cancer Res. 47:659 (1987).

34. C. Thiele, C.P. Reynolds, and M. Israel, Decreased expression of N-myc precedes retinoic acid-induced morphological of human neuroblastoma cells, Nature 313:404 (1985).

35. J. Fontana, G. Miksis, and J. Durham, Elevation of adenylate cyclase activity during leukemic cell differentiation, Exp. Cell Res. 168:487 (1987).

36. K.F.F. Scott, F.L. Meyskens Jr, and D.H. Russel, Retinoids increase transglutaminase activity and inhibit ornithine decarboxylase activity in Chinese hamster ovary cells and in melanoma cells stimulated to differentiate, Proc. Natl. Acad. Sci. USA 79:4093 (1982).

37. A.R. Rees, E.D. Adamson, and C.F. Graham, Epidermal growth factor receptors increase during differentiation of embryonal carcinoma cells, Nature 281:309 (1979).

38. A. Rizzino, Appearance of high-affinity receptors for type -ß transforming growth factor during differentiation of murine embryonal carcinoma cells, Cancer Res. 47:4386 (1987).

39. A. Rizzino, C. Kuszynski, E. Ruff, and J. Tiesman, Production and utilization of growth factor related to fibroblast growth factor by embryonal carcinoma cells and their differentiated cells, Dev. Biol. 129:61 (1988).

40. S.A. Eccles, S.C. Barnett, and P. Alexander, Inhibition of growth and spontaneous metastasis of syngeneic transplantable tumors by an aromatic retinoic acid analogue.1. Relationship between tumor immunogenicity and responsiveness, Cancer Immunol. Immunother. 19:109 (1985).

41. J.A. Badwey, J.M. Robinson, J.T. Curnette, M.J. Karnowsky, and M.L. Karnowsky, Retinoids stimulate the release of superoxide by neutrophils and change their morphology, J. Cell Physiol. 127:223 (1986).

42. K. Tachibana, S. Sone, E. Tsubura, and Y. Kishino, Stimulatory effects of vitamin A on tumoricidal activity of rat alveolar macrophages, Br. J. Cancer 49:343 (1984).

43. R. Lotan, and G. Dennert, Stimulating effects of vitamin A analogs on induction of cell-mediated cytotoxicity in vivo, Cancer Res. 39:55 (1979).

44. H. Esterbauer, Aldehydic products of lipid peroxidation, in: Free Radicals, Lipid Peroxidation and Cancer, D.H.C. McBrien, and T.F. Slater, ed.s, Academic press, 101-125 (1982).

45. B. Frei, T.M. Forte, B.N. Ames, and C.E. Cross, Gas phase oxidants of cigarette smoke induce lipid peroxidation and changes in lipoprotein properties in human blood plasma. Protective effects of ascorbic acid, Biochem. J. 277:133 (1991).

46. H.F. Hoff, and J.A. O'Neil, Oxidation of LDL: role in atherogenesis, Klin.-Wochenschr. 69:1032 (1991).

47. K.H. Cheeseman, M. Collins, S. Maddix, A. Milia, K. Proud foot, T.F. Slater, G.W. Burton, A. Webb, and K.A. Ingold, Lipid peroxidation in regenerating rat liver, FEBS Lett. 209:191 (1986).

48. L. Masotti, E. Casali, and T. Galeotti, Lipid peroxidation in tumor cells, Free Radical Biol. Med. 4:377 (1988).

49. S. Borrello, G. Minotti, G. Palombini, A. Grattagliano, and T. Galeotti, Superoxide-dependent lipid peroxidation and vitamin E content of microsomes from hepatomas with different growth rate, Arch. Biochem. Biophys. 238:588 (1985).

50. M.U. Dianzani, G. Poli, R.A. Canuto, M.A. Rossi, M.E. Biocca, F. Biasi, G. Cecchini, G. Muzio, M. Ferro, and H. Esterbauer, New data on kinetics of lipid peroxidation in experimental hepatomas and preneoplastic nodules, Toxicol. Pathol. 14:404 (1986).

51. V.M. Fazio, G. Barrera, S. Martinotti, M.G. Farace, B. Giglioni, L. Frati, V. Manzari, and M.U. Dianzani, 4-hydroxy-nonenal, a product of cellular lipid peroxidation, which modulates c-myc and globin gene expression in K562 cells, Cancer Res. 52:4866 (1992).

52. T. Galeotti, L. Masotti, S. Borrello, and E. Casali, Oxy-radical metaboilsm and control of tumor growth, Xenobiotica 21:1041 (1991).

53. S. Borrello, A. Seccia, T. Galeotti, G.M. Bartoli, and F. Serri, Protective enzymes in human epidermal carcinomas and psoriasis, Arch. Dermatol. Res. 276:338 (1984).

54. H. Esterbauer, Lipid peroxidation products: formation, chemical properties and biological activities, in: Free Radicals in Liver Injury, G. Poli, K.H. Cheeseman, M.U. Dianzani, T.F. Slater, ed.s, IRL press, 29-47 (1985).

55. H. Esterbauer, H. Zollner, and R.J. Schaur, Hydroxyalkenals: cytotoxic products of lipid peroxidation, in: ISI Atlas of Science: Biochemistry (1988).

56. H. Esterbauer, R.J. Schauer, and H. Zollner, Chemistry and biochemistry of 4-hydroxynonenal, malonaldehyde and related aldehydes, Free Radic. Biol. Med. 11:81 (1991).

57. G. Poli, M.U. Dianzani, K. Cheeseman, T.F. Slater, J. Lang, and H. Esterbauer, Biochem. J. 227:629 (1985).

58. H. Esterbauer, H. Zollner, and J. Lang, Metabolism of the lipid peroxidation product 4-hydroxynonenal by isolated hepatocytes and by liver fractions, Biochem. J 228:363 (1985).

59. H.M. Tillian, H. Esterbauer, and E. Schauenstein, Improved cytostatic effect of 4-hydroxynonenal compared with 4-hydroxypentenal on Ehrlich ascites tumor cells (EATC) in vitro, Naunin Schmiedebergs Arch. Pharmacol. 321 9:20 (1982); S. Hauptlorenz, H. Esterbauer, W. Moll, R. Pumpel, E. Schauenstein, and B. Puschendorf, Effect of the lipid peroxidation product 4-hydroxynonenal and related aldehydes on proliferation and viability of cultured ascites tumor cells, Biochem. Pharmacol. 34: 3803 (1982); E. Schauenstein, Effects of low concentrations of aldehydes on tumor cells and tumor growth, in: Free Radicals, Lipid Peroxidation and Cancer, D.C.H. McBrien, T.F. Slater, ed.s, Academic press 159-171 (1982).

60. M.A. Rossi, M. Curzio, C. Di Mauro, F. Fidale, A. Garramone, H. Esterbauer, M. Torrielli, and M.U. Dianzani, Experimental studies on the mechanism of action of 4-hydroxy-2,3-trans-nonenal, a lipid peroxidation product di splaying chemotactic activity toward rat neutrophils, Cell Biochem. Funct. 9:163 (1991).

61. L. Paradisi, C. Panagini, M. Parola, G. Barrera, and M.U. Dianzani, Effect of 4-hydroxynonenal on adenylate cyclase and 5'-nucleotidase activities in rat liver plasma membranes, Chem. Biol. Interactions 53:209 (1985).

62. G. Barrera, S. Martinotti, V.M. Fazio, V. Manzari, L. Paradisi, M. Parola, L. Frati, and M.U. Dianzani, Effect

113

of 4-hydroxynonenal on c-myc expression, Toxicol. Pathol. 15:238 (1987).

63. G. Barrera, O. Brossa, V.M. Fazio, M.G. Farace, L. Paradisi, E. Gravela, and M.U. Dianzani, Effects of 4-hydroxynonenal, a product of lipid peroxidation, on cell proliferation and ornithine decarboxylase activity, Free Rad. Res. Comm. 14:81 (1991).

64. G. Barrera, F. Biasi, V.M. Fazio, L. Paradisi, and M.U. Dianzani, Repeated treatments with low HNE concentration affect K562 cell proliferation, in: Chemical Carcinogenesis 2, A. Columbano, et al, ed.s, Plenum press, 337-342 (1991).

65. C.W. Young, M.P. Falucchi, T.D. Walsh, L. Baltzer, S. Yaldaei, Y.-W. Stevens, C. Gordon, W. Tong, R.A. Rifkind, and P.A. Marks, Phase I trial and clinical pharmacological evaluation of examethylene bisacetamide administration by ten-day continous intravenous infusion of twenty-eight-day intervals, Cancer Res. 48:7304 (1988).

66. C. Chomienne, P. Ballerini, N. Balitrand, M. Amar, J.F. Bernard, P. Boivin, M.T. Daniel, R. Berger, S. Castaigne, and L. Degos, Retinoic acid therapy for promyelocytic leukemia, Lancet Sept. 23:746 (1989).

67. P.A. Marks, and R.A. Rifkind, Differentiating agents in cancer therapy, in: Cancer Therapy; Cancer Chemotherapy and Biological Response Modifiers, Annual 12, H.M. Pinedo, D.L. Longo, and B.A. Chabner, ed.s, Elsevier Science Publishers (1991).

68. G.E. Francis, and J.M. Cunningham, Growth and differentiation control, in: Cancer Therapy; Cancer Chemotherapy and Biological Response Modifiers, Annual 11, H.M. Pinedo, B.A. Chabner, and D.L. Longo, ed.s, Elsevier Science Publishers (1990).

69. S.M. Lippman, J.F. Kessler, and F.L. Meyskens Jr., Retinoids as preventive and therapeutic anticancer agents, Cancer Treat. Rep. 71:493 (1987).

70. W.K. Hong, J. Endicott, L.M. Itri, W. Doos, J.G. Batsaiis, ...and S. Strong, 13 cis-retinoic acid in the treatment of oral leukoplakia, N. Engl. J. Med. 315:1501 (1986).

71. U.E. Studer, C. Biedermann, D. Chollet, P. Karrer, R. Kraft, H. Toggenburg, and F. Vonbank, Prevention of recurrent superficial bladder tumor by oral etretinate: preliminary results of a randomized, double blind multicenter trial in Switzerland, J. Urol. 131:47 (1984).

72. J.L. Misset, G. Mathe, G. Santelli, J. Gouveia, J.P. Homasson, M.C. Sudre, and H. Gaget, Regression of bronchial epidermoid metaplasia in heavy smokers with etretinate, Cancer Detect. Prev. 9:167 (1986).

73. S.A. Weiner, E.A. Surwit, V.E. Graham, and F.L. Meyskens Jr., A phase 1 trial of topically applied trans retinoic acid in cervical dysplasia, Invest. New Drugs 4:241 (1986).

74. F.L. Meyskens Jr., L. Edwards, and N.S. Levine, Role of topical tretinoin in melanoma and dysplastic nevi, J. Am. Acad. Dermatol. 15:822 (1986).

75. M.E. Huang, Y.C. Ye, S. Chen, J.R. Chai, J.X. Lu, L. Zhoa, L.J. Gu, and Z.Y. Wang, Use of all-trans retinoic acid in the treatment of acute promyelocytic leukemia, Blood 72:567 (1988).

76. E.L. Rowinsky, D.S. Ettinger, W.P. McGuire, D.A. Noe, L.B. Grochow, and R.C. Donehower, Prolonged infusion of hexamethylene bisacetamide: a phase I and pharmacological study, Cancer Res. 47:5788 (1987).

77. E. Melloni, S. Pontremoli, G. Damiani, P. Viotti, N. Weich, R.A. Rifkind, and P.A. Marks, Vincristine-resistant erythroleukemia cells have marked increased sensitivity to hexamethylene bisacetamide induced differentiation, Proc. Natl. Acad. Sci. USA 85:3835 (1988).

78. V.M. Richon, N. Weich, L. Lens, H. Kiyokawa, L. Ngo, R.A. Rifkind, and P.A. Marks, Characteristics of erythroleukemia cells selected for vincristine resistance which have accelerated inducer mediated differentiation, Proc. Natl. Acad. Sci. USA (1991).

79. H.T. Hassan, and J.K.H. Rees, Triple combination of retinoic acid + low concentration of cytosine arabinoside + hexamethylene bisacetamide induce differentiation of human AML blasts in primary culture, Hematol. Oncol. 7:429 (1989).

80. H.T. Hassan, and J.K.H. Rees, Triple combination of retinoic acid + 6-thyoguanine + hexamethylene bisacetamide induces differentiation of human AML blasts in primary culture, Leukemia Res. 14:109 (1990).

INHIBITION OF HIV REPLICATION AND ENHANCEMENT OF IMMUNE FUNCTIONS BY THE ACYCLIC NUCLEOSIDE PHOSPHONATE 9-(2-PHOSPHONYL-METHOXYETHYL)ADENINE (PMEA)

CF. Perno[1], V. Del Gobbo[1], J. Balzarini[2], E. Balestra[1], G. Milanese[3], S. Aquaro[1], F. Sesa[1], A. Holy[4], E. De Clercq[2], N. Villani[1], R. Caliò[1]

[1]Dept. Exp. Medicine, and [3]Dept. of Public Health, University of Rome "Tor Vergata", Italy; [2]Rega Inst. for Med. Res, K.U. Leuven, Belgium and [4]Inst. of Organic Chem. and Biochem., Czech. Acad. Sci., Prague, Czechoslovakia

SUMMARY

9-(2-phosphonyl-methoxyethyl)adenine (PMEA) is an acyclic nucleoside phosphonate analogue with potent activity against DNA viruses (i.e. herpesviruses) and retroviruses, including human immunodeficiency virus (HIV). To assess the clinical potential advantages of this drug, we evaluated the anti-HIV activity of PMEA in monocyte-macrophages (M/M) (cells of crucial importance in the pathogenesis of HIV-related disease). We also assessed the capacity of this nucleoside analogue to modulate some functions of the natural immunity, such as natural killer (NK) activity and interferon production. We found that PMEA inhibits HIV replication in M/M and in lymphocytes at nanomolar and micromolar concentrations respectively. In addition, PMEA was also found to enhance NK activity and to stimulate interferon production. PMEA has unique capability of being both an antiviral agent, effective against retroviruses as well as herpesviruses, and an immunomodulating agent. Its therapeutic potential should be further assessed in patients with HIV-related disease.

INTRODUCTION

Since human immunodeficiency virus (HIV) is the cause of acquired immunodeficiency syndrome (AIDS), efforts have been made to develop an efficient therapy to inhibit the replication of the virus and thus indirectly reverse the profound immunosuppression associated with this disease. Clinical studies have revealed the ability of several nucleoside analogues, such as 3'-azido-2',3'-dideoxythymidine (AZT) and 2',3'-dideoxyinosine (DDI), to inhibit HIV replication, to increase the number of circulating CD4 lymphocytes, and to improve some immune functions, (i.e. lymphocyte proliferation upon antigen stimulus, skin tests) (1-3). However, improvement is transient, and progression of the disease was often seen in spite of treatment (4). Immunosuppression in patients with AIDS can also be of iatrogenic origin, since AZT, akin to most nucleoside analogues commonly used in anticancer therapy, is able per se to

Combination Therapies 2, Edited by A.L. Goldstein and E. Garaci Plenum Press, New York, 1993

decrease the number of CD4-lymphocytes and to suppress some functions of the immune system (5,6).

It is conceivable that drugs with potent anti-HIV activity and non-immunosuppressive potential or, even better, with immunostimulating activity, could be of benefit for patients with AIDS.

In the search of antiviral compounds with these characteristics, we studied a series of acyclic nucleoside phosphonates (7.8). They inhibit the replication of various DNA viruses (i.e. herpesviruses) and retroviruses, including HIV (9). In particular, 9-(2-phosphonyl-methoxyethyl)adenine (PMEA) has been shown to be a potent inhibitor of both herpes viruses (i.e. herpes simplex virus, cytomegalovirus) and HIV (10). In view of the clinical interest in this compound, we investigated some additional aspects of its antiviral activity and immunomodulating potential of PMEA. In particular, we assessed the antiviral effect of PMEA in cells of the monocyte/macrophage lineage (M/M), a prominent reservoir for HIV in tissues (11,12). We also monitored the effects of PMEA on some immune responses, such as natural killer (NK) activity and interferon production.

MATERIALS AND METHODS

Compound. PMEA was dissolved in phosphate-buffered saline, and stored at 4°C until used. For in vivo experiments, PMEA was prepared freshly for each intraperitoneal inoculation of mice.

Antiviral assay. Purified M/M were obtained from peripheral blood of healthy HIV-negative volunteers by enrichment with Ficoll followed by further purification by 5-day adherence. Details about this procedure are described elsewhere (12-14). M/M were exposed to different concentrations of PMEA 30 minutes before challenge with HIV-1/HTLV-III$_{Ba-L}$ (called HIV-BaL) strain. Virus production was assessed by measurement of HIV-p24 production (using a commercially available enzyme linked immunosorbent assay) in the supernatants, and syncytium formation. Suppression of virus production by PMEA in M/M was then compared to that achieved in normal peripheral blood lymphocytes exposed to a lymphocytotropic strain of HIV (HTLV-III$_B$). Details about these techniques are described in other papers of our group (12-16).

Immunological assay. For the assessment of natural killer (NK) activity, 6-week old male C57Bl/6 mice were treated with various concentrations of PMEA, and then sacrificed at different time points. NK activity of spleen cells was evaluated by the 4-hour incubation assay described by Herberman and Ortaldo (17), in which Yac-1 lymphoma cells were used as target. Results are expressed as percent of cell cytotoxicity based on 51-Cr release in the supernatants of labeled target cells.

Interferon production assay was based on the inhibition of the cytopathic effect of vescicular stomatitis virus (VSV) in L929 fibroblastoid cells exposed to appropriate dilutions of the sera of PMEA-treated mice (6).

RESULTS

The structure of PMEA is reported in Fig. 1. In preliminary experiments, we assessed the ability of PMEA to inhibit HIV replication in M/M and T-lymphocyates (Table 1).

Complete suppression of HIV antigen expression in the M/M culture supernatants was achieved at 0.3 uM PMEA: this concentration is about 30 fold lower than that required to completely block HIV antigen expression in T-lymphocytes (data not shown). The EC$_{50}$ of PMEA in M/M was 0.02 uM (Table 1), while in T-lymphocytes the EC50 was about 4 uM. PMEA was not toxic for M/M at concentrations up to 100 uM, while for (proliferating) T-lymphocytes PMEA was toxic at concentrations of 50 uM. Thus, the therapeutic index (ratio of CCso to EC50) is substantially higher in M/M than in

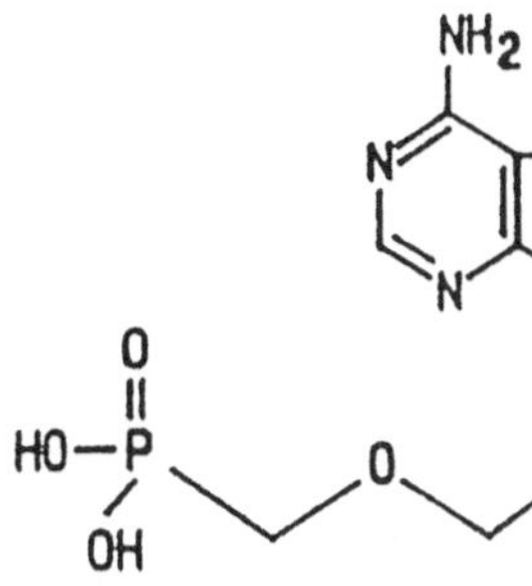

PMEA

FIG. 1

Table 1. Anti HIV activity of PMEA in M/M and lymphocytes

CELLS	EC_{50}*	CC_{50}*	T.I.*
M/M	0.02 μM	>100 μM	>5,000
Lymphocytes (MT-4)	3.7 μM	50	14

*EC_{50}: Effective concentration; CC_{50}: 50% cytotoxic concentration; T.I.: therapeutic index (ratio of CC_{50} to EC_{50}).

T-lymphocytes. These data also suggests that cytotoxicity of these nucleoside analogues may be related to the cell cycle, as already reported for other compounds, including 2',3'-dideoxynucleosides (11,15).

The effect of PMEA on NK activity is shown in Fig. 2a. At a dose of 25 mg/kg/day, PMEA induced a substantial enhancement of NK-mediated cytotoxicity in mice. This enhancement exceeded by more than 100% that of the control NK activity

Kinetics of NK cell cytotoxic activity in mice treated with PMEA

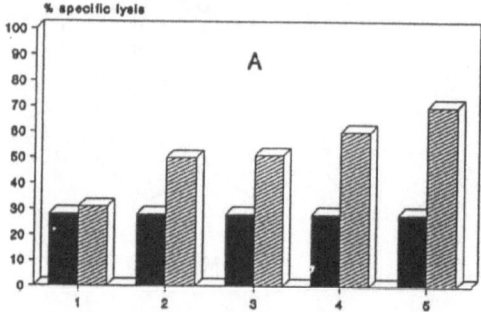

IFN titration in mice during PMEA treatment

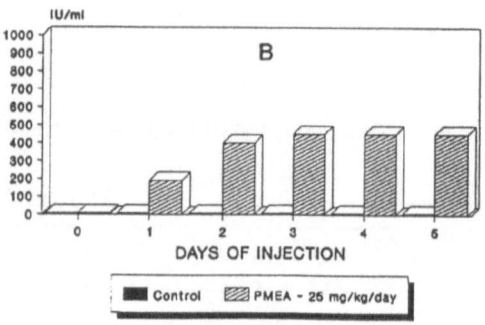

FIG. 2

Mice were inoculated daily with PMEA for five consecutive days. NK activity and IFN production were assessed daily up to the fifth day of PMEA administration.
(control mice), and was in the range of that achieved by poly I:C, a well-known enhancer of NK activity.

Since the increase of NK activity is often mediated by interferon (IFN), we also determined the IFN levels in the sera of PMEA-treated mice. The results, reported in Fig. 2b, clearly indicate that substantial IFN was produced in PMEA-treated mice, while, as expected, no IFN was detected in control animals. Thus, PMEA is able to induce IFN production and to stimulate NK activity in mice. The two phenomena seem to be related to one another.

Based on the data obtained upon acute (5 days) treatment (Fig. 2), we then assessed the ability of PMEA to enhance NK function and IFN production following chronic treatment.

As shown in Fig 3a, PMEA-induced NK activation was maintained, even though sligthly decreased overtime, upon long-term (20 days) treatment with the drug (25 mg/kg/day).

NK cell activity

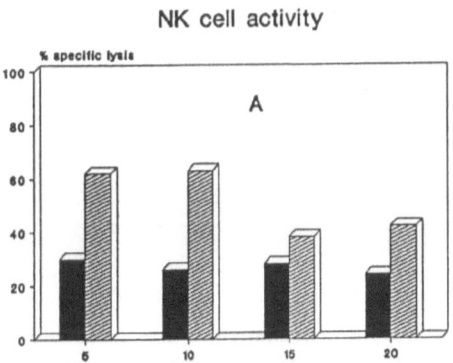

IFN titration

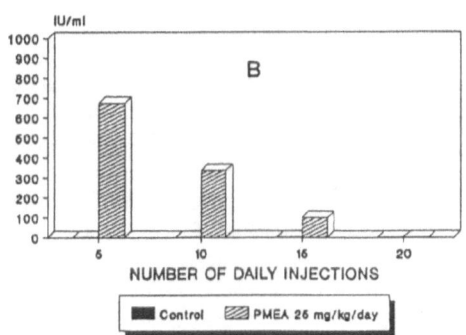

FIG. 3

NK ACTIVITY AND IFN PRODUCTION IN MICE CHRONICALLY TREATED WITH PMEA

Conversely, IFN production decreased with time, and by the twentieth consecutive day of PMEA administration, it was annihilated (Fig. 3b). These data are in agreement with the general phenomenon that repeated administration of IFN inducers (like Poly I:C) leads to hyporesponsiveness, and finally, abrogation of IFN production. We then treated mice with lower doses of PMEA (5 mg/kg/day) for 20 consecutive days. As shown in Fig.4, this drug dosage induced a less pronounced, but more sustained NK enhancement, as compared to the 25 mg/kg/day dosage regimen. However, interferon production could not be detected in mice treated with PMEA at 5 mg/kg/day (data not shown).

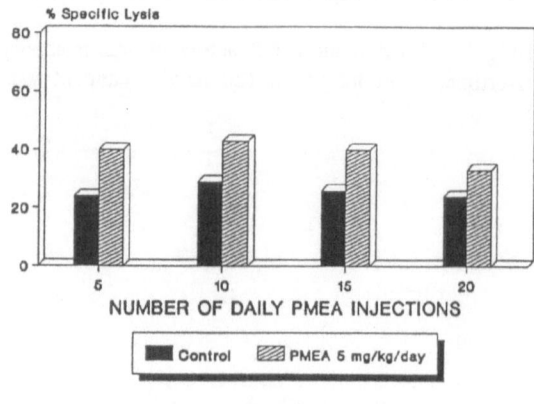

NK cell activity

% Specific Lysis

NUMBER OF DAILY PMEA INJECTIONS

■ Control   ▧ PMEA 5 mg/kg/day

FIG.4

Thus, long-term treatment of mice with low doses of PMEA still leads to NK enhancement, but this effect is apparently not accompanied with detectable IFN production.

DISCUSSION

The results reported in this paper indicate that the acyclic nucleoside phosphonate PMEA is a potent inhibitor of HIV replication in T-lymphocytes and M/M, and can upregulate some natural immune functions such as NK activity and interferon production. Since HIV infection results in a potent immunosuppression, antiviral drugs (often immunosuppressive per se, like in the case of AZT) should be associated with immunomodulators able to enhance immune functions. This may also counteract the drug-induced potentiation of the immunosuppressive effect caused by the virus itself (5).

We have previously shown that acyclic nucleoside phosphonates not only inhibit the replication of DNA viruses and retroviruses, but are also able to activate natural defense functions (6). The biochemical explanation underlying the latter phenomenon is still unclear. From the data presented here and in our previous papers (6), it appears that NK enhancement by PMEA may be mediated through a mechanism involving, at least in part, IFN production. However, NK activation is sustained for at least 20 days following treatment with PMEA at 25 mg/kg/day when IFN is no longer detectable. Furthermore, when administered at 5 mg/kg/day for 20 days, PMEA induces NK enhancement in the absence of IFN production. Thus, the sustained NK enhancement achieved under these conditions may be related to production of various cytokines other than IFN. In this context, it should be mentioned that preliminary evidence suggest that PMEA per se is able to activate some functions of peritoneal M/M (data not shown). It is conceivable that M/M (which are able to produce various cytokines) may be involved in the maintenance of NK activation. This issue is now under investigation.

The overall data suggest that PMEA is an interesting candidate for further evaluation in the clinic, in patients with AIDS or, in general, HIV infections. As both an antiviral agents, active against HIV as well as herpesviruses, and an immunomodulatory agent, PMEA distinguishes itself from all other candidate drugs currently considered for clinical trials in patients infected with HIV.

ACKNOWLEDGEMENTS

Authors deeply acknowledge the help of Mrs. Franca Serra and Mrs. Patrizia Saccomandi for the skilled technical help in performing the experiments, and Mr. Vincenzo Serra and Mrs. Christiane Callebaut for their dedicated editorial help in the preparation of the manuscript.
This work has been supported by a grant from the Project AIDS of the Ministry of Health (Italy), and a grant from the Project FATMA of the National Research Council of Italy.

REFERENCES

1   Yarchoan R, Klecker RW, Weinhold KJ, Markham PD, Lyerly Hk, Durack DT, Gelmann E, Nusinoff Lehrmann S, Blum RM, Barry Dw, Shearer GM, Fischl MA, Mitsuya H, Gallo RC, Collins JM, Bolognesi DP, Myers CE and Broder S. *Lancet* **i**, 575-582, 1986

2   Fischl MA, Richman DD, Grieco MH, Gottlieb MS, Volberding PA, Laskin OS, Leedom JM, Groopman JE, Mildvan D, Schooley RT, Jackson GG, Durack DT, King D. *New Engl. J. Med.* **317**, 185-190, 1987.

3   Yarchoan R, Mitsuya H, Thomas RV, Pluda JM, Hartman NR, Perno CF, Marczyk KS, Allain JP, Johns DG, and Broder S. *Science* **245**, 412-417, 1989.

4   Reiss P, Lange JMA, Boucher CA, Danner SA, Goudsmit J.*Lancet i*, 421-423, 1988.

5   Yarchoan R, Pluda JM, Perno CF, Mitsuya H and Broder S. *Blood* **78**, 859-884, 1991.

6   Del Gobbo V, Foli A, Balzarini J, De Clercq E, Balestra E, Villani N, Marini S, Perno CF and Caliò R. *Antiviral Res.* **16**, 65-75, 1991.

7   De Clercq E, Holy A, Rosenberg I, Sakuma T, Balzarini J and Maudgal PC. *Nature* **323**, 464-467, 1986.

8   Balzarini J, Naesens L, Herdewijn P, Rosenberg I, Holy A, Pauwels R, Baba M, Johns DG and De Clercq E. *Proc. Natl. Acad. Sci.* USA **86**, 332-336, 1989.

9   Balzarini J, Naesens L, Slachmuylders J, Niphuis , Rosenberg I, Holy A, Shellekens H, and De Clercq E. *AIDS 5*, 21-28, 1991.

10   De Clercq E, Sakuma T, Baba M, Pauwels R, Balzarini J, Rosenberg I and Holy A. *Antiviral* Res. **8**, 261-272, 1987.

11   Perno CF, Yarchoan R, Cooney DA, Hartman NR, Gartner S, Popovic M, Hao Z, Gerrard TL, Wilson YA, Johns DG and Broder S. *J. Exp. Med.* **168**, 1111-1125, 1988.

12   Gartner S, Markovitz P, Markovits DM, Kaplan MH, Gallo RC and Popovic M. *Science* **233**, 215-219, 1986.

13   Perno CF, Yarchoan R, Cooney DA, Hartman NR, Webb DSA, Hao Z, Mitsuya H, Johns DG and Broder S. J. *Exp. Med.* **169**, 933-951, 1989.

14   Perno CF, Baseler MW, Broder S and Yarchoan R. J. *Exp. Med.* **171**, 1043-1056, 1990.

15   Perno CF, Yarchoan R, Balzarini J, Bergamini A, Milanese G, Pauwels R, De Clercq E, Rocchi G and Caliò R. *Antiviral Res.* **17**, 289-304, 1992.

16   Balzarini J, Perno CF, Schols D and De Clercq E. *Biochem. Biophys. Res. Comm.* **178**, 329-335, 1991.

17   Herberman RB and Ortaldo JR. *Science* 214, 24-30, 1981.

MODULATION OF INFLAMMATORY CYTOKINES BY A RECEPTOR ANTAGONIST, AUTOANTIBODIES, AND FEVER.

Klaus Bendtzen,[1] Morten B. Hansen,[2] and Morten Svenson[1,2]

[1]Department of Medicine TTA
[2]Department of Infectious Diseases M
Rigshospitalet University Hospital
DK-2200 Copenhagen N, Denmark

INTRODUCTION

The inflammatory reactions that follow infections and traumatic injuries are initiated and controlled by proteins and glycoproteins produced by cells engaged in these reactions, including cells of the immune system. These mediators, cytokines, form a complex network of molecules that act at extremely low concentrations (10^{-14} to 10^{-10} M) through specific and often dynamically expressed receptors on many different target cells [1]. Most cytokines act regionally near the production site, but some cytokines act systemically as pleiotropic hormones with overlapping and potentially harmful effects (immunoinflammatory hormones). The most important cytokines in this regard, interleukin (IL)-1α, IL-1β, IL-6, and tumor necrosis factor (TNF)α are centrally involved in complications to severe infections and trauma such as disseminated intravascular coagulation DIC, adult respiratory distress syndrome (ARDS), multiorgan failure (MOF), non-hemorrhagic shock and the development of cachexia in chronic infections such as AIDS [1-8] (Table 1).

Since cytokines are being increasingly used as biological response modifiers (BRM), and because treatment of many infections and inflammatory disorders is aimed at modifying endogenously produced cytokines, detailed knowledge of the regulation of the complex cytokine network becomes increasingly important. The awareness of the presence of highly specific naturally occurring modulators of inflammatory cytokines should help to develop BRMs that may improve the management of many infectious and immunoinflammatory reactions.

CLINICAL SIGNIFICANCE OF INFLAMMATORY CYTOKINES

IL-1α and -1β, IL-6 and TNFα produce a number of symptoms characteristic of infectious and inflammatory diseases (Table 1). These symptoms are usually part of the acute-phase reaction which in some situations, may lead to DIC, ARDS, MOF, shock and death.

Combination Therapies 2, Edited by A.L. Goldstein
and E. Garaci   Plenum Press, New York, 1993

Table 1. Inflammatory cytokines known to be pathogenetically important in systemic complications to infections and trauma.

Functions	IL-1α/β	IL-6	TNFα
Coactivators of			
T- and B-lymphocytes	+	+	+
hepatocytes (acute-phase protein production)	+	+	+
hemopoietic stem cells (neutrophilia)	+	+	
endothelial cells	+		+
fibroblasts	+		+
neuronal cells		+	
keratinocytes		+	
synovial cells	+		+
Fever	+	+	+
Slow-wave sleep	+		+
Nonspecific resistance to infection	+	+	+
Radioprotection	+		+
Muscle protein degradation[1]	+		+
Loss of fat depots[1]	+		+
Non-hemorrhagic shock syndrome	+	(+)	+

[1] If prolonged and inappropriately controlled production occurs, these effects lead to cachexia. Hence, the acronym *cachectin* was previously used for TNFα [9].

Fever

Fever as a clinical symptom has been known for thousands of years, from the Old Testament and Hippocrates to Wunderlich who invented the thermometer only a century ago.

It is now clear that IL-1α, IL-1β, IL-6 and TNFα are identical with the leukocytic factors responsible for fever in experimental animals, and originally described as *endogenous* or *leukocytic pyrogen*. It is noteworthy that prostaglandin E$_2$ is a second mediator of the cytokine-induced activation of the thermoregulatory center in the brain [1,10]. Therefore, cyclooxygenase inhibitors such as aspirin ameliorate the pyrogenic action of the IL-1s, IL-6 and TNFα, even though the cytokines may still circulate in the blood. Other functions of IL-1α/β, TNFα and IL-6 that do not require prostaglandins as second messengers are intact. This explains why aspirin lowers the temperature of a febrile patient without reducing the tendency to sleep or jeopardizing the defense against infection.

The Acute-Phase Reaction

Fever is often part of an acute-phase reaction, and administration of IL-1α, IL-1β, IL-6 or TNFα reproduces this reaction [2,9-11]. The reaction is usually seen during acute and chronic infectious and inflammatory diseases, in cancer, and during posttraumatic syndromes. IL-6 and, to a lesser extent, the IL-1s and TNFα induce hepatocytes to synthesize acute-phase proteins and, at the same time, reduce the blood level of albumin. Associated manifestations are drowsiness, leukocytosis and altered levels of trace metals in the blood. An elevated level of fibrinogen, especially if accompanied by anemia, causes an increased sedimentation rate of the blood; still a commonly used clinical parameter of *inflammation*.

DIC, ARDS, MOF and Shock

In some situations, the acute-phase reaction may progress to life-threatening syndromes. It was previously thought that microbial products, particularly endotoxins, were directly responsible for these syndromes, for example during infections with gram-negative bacteria or, indirectly, through release of endotoxins from the gut flora during severe hypotensive conditions. This, however, is in all likelihood incorrect. First, coagulation abnormalities and non-hemorrhagic shock may develop without detectable circulating levels of endotoxins. Second, endotoxins, along with many other bacterial and nonbacterial products, are potent inducers of IL-1α/β, IL-6 and TNFα in macrophages, and all patho-physiological processes associated with the above mentioned life-threatening conditions can be reproduced in experimental animals by injection of TNFα and, to a lesser extent, by IL-1 [2,12]. Third, neutralizing antibodies to TNFα or IL-6, and a selective inhibitor of IL-1α/β (see below), prevent these serious complications in infected animals or in animals given otherwise lethal doses of endotoxin [13-15]. Finally, endotoxins do not induce shock in the endotoxin-resistant C3H/HeJ mouse. In these animals, a mutation decreases transcription of the endotoxin-inducible TNFα gene and thus prevents the production of this particular cytokine [9]. TNFα and IL-1α/β, therefore, appear to be central mediators of many manifestations of severe inflammation, including metabolic acidosis, DIC, ARDS, MOF and shock.

NATURAL REGULATORS OF INFLAMMATORY CYTOKINES

Apart from being involved in systemic complications to infections and trauma, the inflammatory cytokines are now known to play a crucial role in the pathogenesis of many autoimmune diseases, including rheumatic and autoimmune connective tissue diseases, and autoimmune endocrine diseases such as insulin-dependent diabetes mellitus [16]. Consequently, naturally occurring regulators of the functions of these hormones are of potential clinical importance [1]. Table 2 lists some of the natural inhibitors of production and function of the inflammatory cytokines.

Table 2. Natural inhibitors of inflammatory cytokines (CK).

Inhibitors of production/secretion of
    CK and CK-receptor gene activation: glucocorticoids, vitamin D3, PGE, cAMP
    CK secretion: glucocorticoids

CK- and CK-receptor binding proteins:
    soluble CK receptors
    autoantibodies to CK
    serum factors: α2-macroglobulin, lipoproteins
    CK receptor-binding proteins: IL-1ra

Destruction of CK:
    temperature-induced polymerization/transformation: IL-1β, (IL-1ra)
    proteases (nonspecific, specific?)

Target cell regulation:
    functionally counteracting CK: IL-10, transforming growth factor β
    miscellaneous: PGE, cAMP, glucocorticoids, vitamin D3

This paper deals briefly with three recently recognized means of natural inhibition of IL-1α/β, IL-6 and TNFα:

1. The IL-1 receptor antagonist protein (IRAP or IL-1ra).
2. Autoantibodies to IL-1α and IL-6.
3. Temperature-induced denaturation of IL-1β and IL-1ra.

1. The IL-1 Receptor Antagonist (IL-1ra)

IL-1ra is a naturally occurring peptide which is structurally related to IL-1β and, to a lesser extent, IL-1α [18,19]. IL-1ra is produced by the same cells that produce IL-1α and IL-1β. The molecule is biologically unique, because it is the only known hormone that selectively interferes with the receptor binding of other hormones to prevent their biological functions. Hence, IL-1ra binds to the two known types of membrane IL-1 receptors without causing internalization of the receptor or activation of the target (Figure 1). IL-1ra thereby blocks the biological activities of both IL-1α and IL-1β, apparently on all targets known to respond to IL-1α/β [20].

As shown in Figure 1, both IL-1 receptors may be found in soluble forms for instance in biological fluids. Interestingly, soluble IL-1 type I receptors (sIL-1RI) preferentially bind to IL-1ra, whereas soluble IL-1 type II receptors (sIL-1RII) almost exclusively bind IL-1β [17]. IL-1α has little affinity for the soluble forms of the IL-1 receptors; the main serum factor that binds to IL-1α is high-affinity autoantibodies to this particular IL-1 species. These antibodies are detectable in the majority of normal individuals (see below).

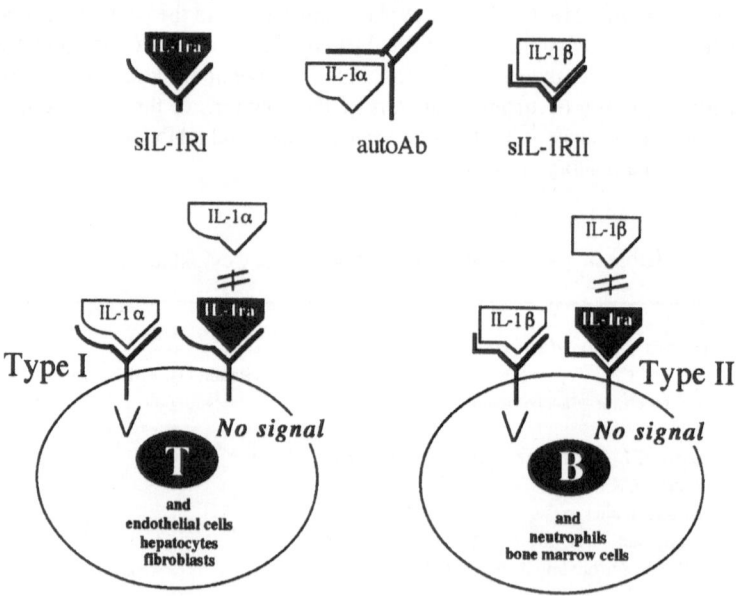

Figure 1. Type I and type II IL-1 receptors on T-lymphocytes, B-lymphocytes and other cell types, competitive inhibition of IL-1 receptor antagonist (IL-1ra), and selective binding of IL-1α, IL-1β and IL-1ra to soluble serum factors.

Although cross-binding exists, IL-1α and IL-1β preferentially bind to the type I and type II receptors on T- and B-lymphocytes, respectively. IL-1ra binds equally well to both types of membrane receptors. In contrast, each member of the IL-1 family of molecules binds to selective molecules in serum. IL-1ra binds strongly to the soluble IL-1 type I receptor (sIL-1RI) with little or no binding to sIL-1RII. The latter binds preferentially to IL-1β, and the predominant IL-1α-binding serum factor is IgG autoantibody (autoAb) [17].

Table 3. IL-1ra-induced reduction / prevention of disease in animal models. [1]

Endotoxin-induced:
  acute inflammation, hypoglycemia, shock, lethality

Interleukin 1-induced:
  acute inflammation, fever, sleep, synovitis and cartilage erosion

E. coli-induced:
  shock, lethality

Miscellaneous:
  arthritis, inflammatory bowel disease, graft-versus-host disease, cerebral malaria

---

[1] see 10,14,20-27.

Clinical Significance of IL-1ra. IL-1ra is produced and found at elevated levels in the circulation in several diseases, and it inhibits many symptoms of disease in animal models (Table 3). IL-1ra therefore appears to be an important natural and, possibly, therapeutic modulator of many infectious and inflammatory conditions. Positive, preliminary findings have been obtained in the treatment of patients with septic shock [14].

2. Autoantibodies to Human IL-1α and IL-6

Specific antibodies to IL-1α and IL-6 in sera of normal as well as diseased individuals have been reported recently [28-32]. The characteristics of these autoantibodies are summarized in Table 4.

Table 4. Autoantibodies to IL-1α and IL-6 in healthy adults.

	anti-IL-1α Ab	anti-IL-6 Ab
Frequency	30-75%	15%
increased with age	yes	no
increased in males	yes	no
Block cytokine binding to receptor	yes	yes
Block bioactivity	yes	yes
Recognize native cytokines	yes	yes
Immunoglobulin class	$IgG_{4,2,1}$	IgG_1
Found in pharmaceutical IgG preparations	yes	yes
Ligand binding:		
K_d	$< 10^{-11}$ M	$< 10^{-10}$ M
maximum binding	30 ng/ml serum	300 ng/ml serum
bind with Fab fragments	yes	yes
association *in vitro* at 37°C (t/2)	< 3 min	< 5 min
dissociation *in vitro* at 37°C (t/2)	2 h < t/2 < 60 h	1.5 h < t/2 < 60 h

Up to 50% of the autoantibodies to IL-1α, isolated from normal sera, are of the IgG4 subtype (normally only 1% of total IgG) [33,34]. These, and the antibodies to IL-6, are polyclonally derived, and their Fab parts bind IL-1α or IL-6 with exquisite specificity and with high affinities [33,35]. It is therefore not surprising that these antibodies inhibit receptor binding and thus the bioactivities of the cytokines to which they are specifically aimed.

Circulating anti-IL-1α and anti-IL-6 autoantibodies are often detectable in apparently healthy individuals of both sexes (Table 4). They occur at different concentrations and, possibly, in different forms in certain inflammatory disorders [35,36].

Antibodies Binding to Other Cytokines. Recently, antibodies binding TNFα, TNFβ and the interferons (IFN) have been detected in sera of apparently healthy humans [37-40]. Antibodies to IL-2 have also been reported, particularly after therapeutic use of the cytokine [41]. In addition, IgE antibodies to TNFα, TNFβ, IFNγ and IL-4 may be responsible for triggering histamine release from basophils of AIDS patients [42]. IL-1β also binds to serum factors, but specific anti-IL-1β antibodies have not yet been reported.

It is important to realize that naturally occurring antibodies to cytokines, apart from those against IL-1α and IL-6, not always bind the cytokines in a specific manner or, indeed, with any appreciable affinity. For example, Western blotting techniques may show some degree of specificity even though the binding between antibody and ligand is weak and topographically unassociated with the specific binding sites of the antibodies. Also, antibody-induced neutralization of the bioactivity of a cytokine may to a large degree depend upon the target cell; for discussion, see Hansen et al. [43].

Clinical Significance of Autoantibodies to Cytokines. The (patho) physiological role of autoantibodies to IL-1α and IL-6 is unknown but almost certain considering the force by which these antibodies bind the ligands (as strong as, or stronger than, the corresponding receptors and most antibodies raised by immunization of animals). In case of IL-1α, the antibodies may function as selective suppressors of both the membrane-associated and the soluble forms of the cytokine [33,34]. Since IL-1α associated with the cytoplasmic membrane of antigen-presenting cells appears to be particularly important in the triggering of T-lymphocytes, the presence of neutralizing antibodies to this form of IL-1α may contribute to immunosuppression. Also, IgG1 and IgG2 antibodies to IL-1α may trigger cytotoxic processes directed against both IL-1α-producing and IL-1α-responding cells.

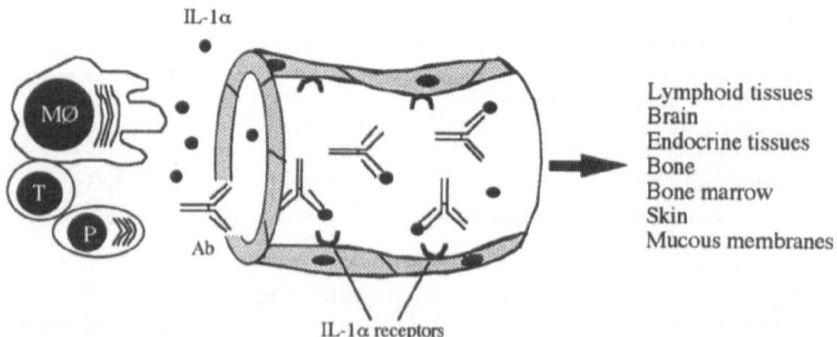

Figure 2. Function of IgG4 autoantibodies as specific carriers of IL-1α.

The antibodies (Ab) prevent IL-1α from binding / activating endothelial cells. This may block systemic vascular effects of the cytokine(s). The antibodies may target IL-1α to high-affinity receptors in other organs (see also Figure 3).

MØ: macrophage.   T: T-lymphocyte.   P: Ab-producing plasma cell.

The predominance of IgG4 antibodies to IL-1α indicates that this type of antibody may provide another level of regulation [34]. IgG4 does not activate complement, and lattice formation is limited with these antibodies. Hence, precipitation of cytokine/anti-cytokine IgG4 is unlikely to occur to any significant degree *in vivo*. IgG4 anti-cytokine antibodies may therefore function as specific neutralizers of cytokines in the circulation. This might explain why some cytokines, if tested by bioassay, 'disappear' within minutes after injection in the circulation. At the same time, these immunoglobulins may act as highly specific carriers which protect the cytokines against proteolytic degradation, removal by filtration in the kidneys and consumption by absorption to endothelial cell receptor molecules. This would enable cytokines to circulate to distant sites in the organism despite the presence of medium-affinity receptors in the vascular bed (Figure 2). Experimental support for this hypothesis has recently been published [32].

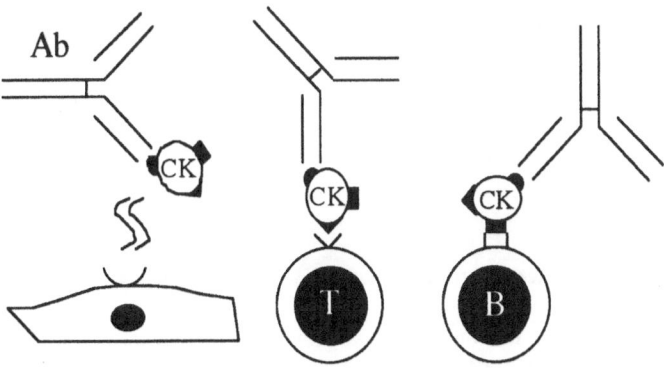

Figure 3. Model for antibody-mediated site-direction of a pleiotropic cytokine .

The cytokine (CK) binds to different targets with topographically distinct binding sites. The part of the molecule (●) that binds to endothelial cells is directly or indirectly blocked by antibody (Ab). This blockade, however, does not apply when the cytokine binds to other targets, such as T-lymphocytes or B-lymphocytes (T and B).

Although the epitope specificities of the antibodies to IL-1α and IL-6 are unknown, and even though antibodies from individual sera appear to recognize more than one epitope, it is tempting to speculate that these autoantibodies might serve to direct IL-1α or IL-6 to specific high-affinity receptor combinations for these pleiotropic cytokines (Figure 3) [1,34]. In this case, autoantibodies to cytokines become important regulatory components of the cytokine network. Such a site-directed function of antibodies to classical hormones has been suggested recently by Aston et al. [44,45].

In any event, it is likely that inappropriate production or function of antibodies to inflammatory cytokines may be pathogenetically involved in many inflammatory diseases and, possibly, in systemic complications to infections and trauma. Therapeutic application of these antibodies is of obvious clinical interest. In fact, the presence of these antibodies in pharmaceutically prepared preparations of human immunoglobulin (see Table 4) may, at least in part, explain the often dramatic modifications of immunologic reactions that accompany intravenous administration of large amounts of human immunoglobulin [46].

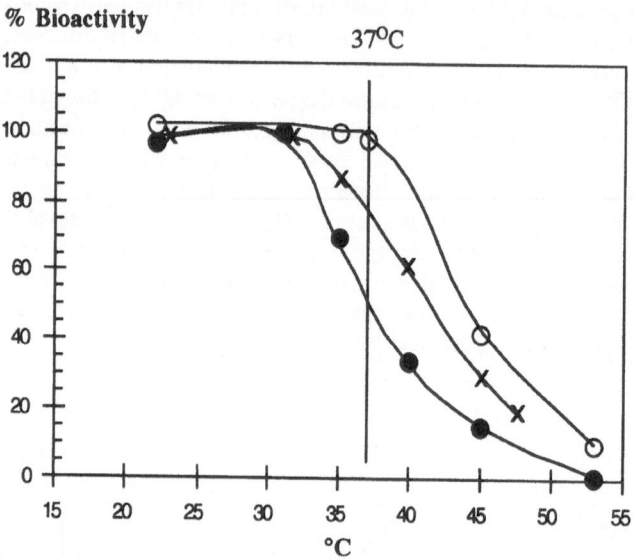

Figure 4. Thermoinactivation (4 h) of the three human IL-1 species in the absence of serum. Bioactivities were tested on murine T-lymphocytes [47].

● - ●: IL-1β.   x - x : IL-1ra.   o - o: IL-1α.

4. Temperature-Induced Denaturation of IL-1β and IL-1ra

Endogenous pyrogen was one of several previously used synonyms for the IL-1s, IL-6, TNFα, TNFβ and the IFNs [1,2,10]. Although these mediators are considered centrally involved in the generation of fever in man and experimental animals, little attention has been devoted to a possible thermal modulation of the structures and functions of these pyrogens.

We have obtained evidence that human recombinant- and native IL-1β, but not IL-1α, is thermally denatured even at physiological temperature (Figure 4) [48,49]. Indeed, IL-1β and IL-1ra lose significant activity at temperatures which may be reached during fever in man and, particularly, in experimental animals, whose core temperatures often reach higher levels than those of humans. Interestingly, the presence of serum more than double the rate by which IL-1β is inactivated at 37°C. When incubated at 40°C in the presence of serum, IL-1β loses 50% of its bioactivity and immunoreactivity within 60 min, most likely because serum factors such as albumin, α2-macroglobulin and lipoproteins bind to the denatured form(s) of IL-1β [48,49]. The other endogenous pyrogens IL-1α (see Figure 4), IL-6 and TNFα are relatively heat-stable [49].

Clinical Significance of IL-1β and IL-1ra Thermoinactivation. The clinical significance of these findings is unclear, but the fact that IL-1β, probably the most important endogenous pyrogen, is transformed into an inactive form even at normal temperatures makes a physical means of IL-1β regulation *in vivo* an attractive hypothesis [49].

The thermoinstability of IL-1β and perhaps other pyrogenic or nonpyrogenic cytokines is of significant practical importance. The clinical use of pyrogenic cytokines, or BRMs that induce the production of pyrogenic cytokines, would benefit from detailed knowledge of the fate in the organism of exogenous or endogenous cytokines at normal and elevated body temperatures. Perhaps more importantly, cytokines and cytokine inhibitors such as IL-1ra may function poorly if produced, or injected, in already febrile individuals. These considerations may be even more relevant in studies using experimental animals, whose physiological temperatures are often above that of humans.

Cytokine thermoinstability may also affect the development of reagents used to monitor these cytokines. We have obtained evidence that some antibodies used for immunometric assays and histological detection of IL-1β preferentially or exclusively recognize the thermo-inactivated form of IL-1β [50]. As shown in Figure 5, radioimmunoassay of native and heat-denatured mature IL-1β gave surprisingly variable results when different preparations of polyclonal rabbit antibodies to mature IL-1β were used.

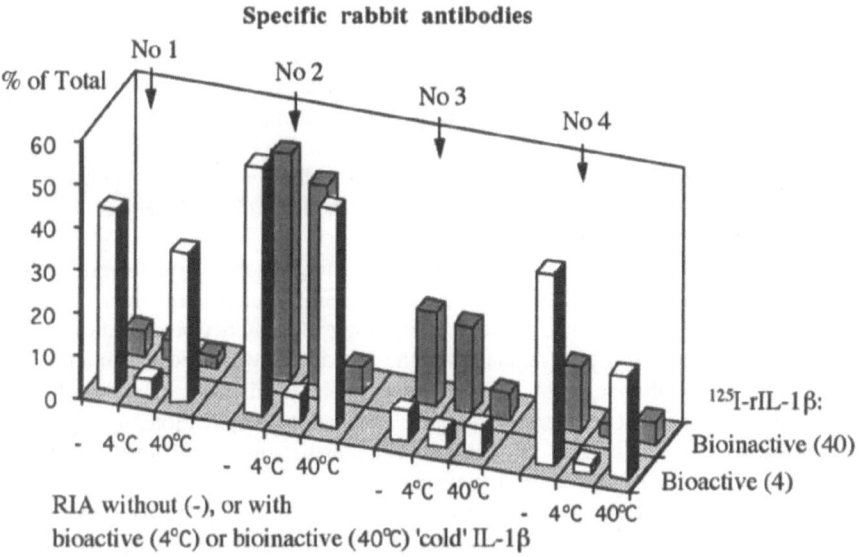

Figure 5. Radioimmunoassay (RIA) of bioactive ^{125}I-IL-1β (kept at 4°C) and bioinactive ^{125}I-IL-1β (preheated at 40°C) using four different polyclonal antibodies.

Antibodies were prepared by immunization of rabbits with:

No 1: mature IL-1β coupled to diphtheria toxoid and absorbed to Al(OH)₃,

No 2: mature IL-1β preheated at 39-40°C for 18 h, and

No 3: untreated mature IL-1β (a kind gift from H. Worsaae; Novo-Nordisk, Gentofte, Denmark) [52].

No 4: rabbit antibody against mature IL-1β (provided with an IL-1β RIA kit; Amersham).

Interestingly, antibody reactivity seemed to depend upon whether IL-1β had been immobilized to a carrier before immunization. If this precaution was not taken, the resulting antibodies almost completely failed to react with the native bioactive form of the cytokine (Figure 5, No 3). Somewhat similar data were recently reported by Hogquist et al. [51], using antibodies to mature murine IL-1β. Cross-over, competitive analyses indicated that each antiserum contained specific antibodies to either the native or the denatured form of mature recombinant IL-1β (Figure 5). Cross-reactive antibodies were however present in one of the antisera (No 4).

The most likely explanation of the above findings is that untreated IL-1β, unlike carrier-immobilized IL-1β, may undergo complete or partial heat-denaturation after injection into animals. This exposes new epitopes not accessible on the native form of the cytokine. The resulting antibodies, therefore, recognize structures on denatured IL-1β not necessarily present on the native cytokine. In some situations, the generated antibodies may not bind to any epitope on the native molecule (Figure 5, No 3). Failure to realize this would lead to erroneous interpretations, particularly if such antibodies are used to localize and/or quantify IL-1β in tissues or biological fluids originating from febrile individuals.

CONCLUSION

At low levels, inflammatory cytokines are essential for optimal functioning of our defense and repair systems. The same cytokines, however, are potentially harmful mediators of infectious and immunoinflammatory reactions. Many cytokines induce the production of other cytokines, and some cytokines augment production and secretion of themselves. Some cytokines, particularly the evolutionary old *endogenous pyrogens*, function systemically as pleiotropic hormones with overlapping effects on many cell types. They appear to engage in a complex network of mediators with both agonistic and antagonistic effects.

Considering the potency by which these mediators exert their many different local and systemic functions, it comes as no surprise that a number of different regulatory mechanisms have emerged during evolution. Regulation takes place at the gene activation stage, during protein synthesis and -secretion, in circulation, and at the level of cytokine-receptor interactions and target cell responses.

Since BRMs of the inflammatory cytokines, including the mediators themselves, are being increasingly used for therapeutic purposes, and because treatment of many immunoinflammatory disorders is aimed at modifying endogenously produced cytokines, detailed knowledge of the natural regulation of the cytokine network becomes increasingly important. Knowing the means by which *Nature* regulates this network should help to improve the management of many potentially dangerous complications to infections, autoimmune diseases and surgical and nonsurgical traumatic conditions. Finally, structural changes to cytokines at physiological or elevated temperatures, though usually overlooked, is decisive for accurate determinations of some cytokines. This is probably of great clinical importance for monitoring cytokine-modulating BRMs, including therapeutic use of cytokines themselves.

REFERENCES

1. K. Bendtzen, Clinical significance of cytokines. Natural and therapeutic regulation, *Sem.Clin.Immunol.* 3:5 (1991).
2. K. Bendtzen, Interleukin 1, interleukin 6 and tumor necrosis factor in infection, inflammation and immunity, *Immunol.Lett.* 19:183 (1988).
3. H. Wada, S. Tamaki, M. Tanigawa, M. Takagi, Y. Mori, A. Deguchi, N. Katayama, T. Yamamoto, K. Deguchi, and S. Shirakawa, Plasma level of IL-1β in disseminated intravascular coagulation, *Thromb. Haemost.* 65:364 (1991).
4. S.K. Leeper-Woodford, P.D. Carey, K. Byrne, J.K. Jenkins, B.J. Fisher, C. Blocher, H.J. Sugerman, and A.A. Fowler III, Tumor necrosis factor. Alpha and beta subtypes appear in circulation during onset of sepsis-induced lung injury, *Am.Rev.Respir.Dis.* 143:1076 (1991).
5. T.M. Hyers, S.M. Tricomi, P.A. Dettenmeier, and A.A. Fowler, Tumor necrosis factor levels in serum and bronchoalveolar lavage fluid of patients with the adult respiratory distress syndrome, *Am.Rev. Respir.Dis.* 144:268 (1991).
6. A.S. Fauci, Cytokine regulation of HIV expression, *Lymphokine Res.* 9:527 (1990).
7. M. Odeh, The role of tumour necrosis factor-α in acquired immunodeficiency syndrome, *J.Int.Med.* 228: 549 (1990).
8. C. Bernard and A. Tedgui, Cytokine network and the vessel wall. Insights into septic shock pathogenesis, *Eur.Cytokine Net.* 3:19 (1992).
9. B. Beutler and A. Cerami, Cachectin (tumor necrosis factor) and lymphotoxin as primary mediators of tissue catabolism, inflammation, and shock, *in:* "Lymphokines and the Immune Response," S. Cohen, ed., CRC Press, (1990), p. 199.
10. C.A. Dinarello, Interleukin-1 and interleukin-1 antagonism, *Blood* 77:1627 (1991).

11. T. Hirano, S. Akira, T. Taga, and T. Kishimoto, Biological and clinical aspects of interleukin 6, *Immunol.Today* 11:443 (1990).

12. V. Lehmann, M.A. Freudenberg, and C. Galanos, Lethal toxicity of lipopolysaccharide and tumor necrosis factor, *J.Exp.Med.* 165:657 (1987).

13. A. Fomsgaard, M.A. Freudenberg, K. Bendtzen, and C. Galanos, Quantitation and biological activities of native tumour necrosis factor from LPS-stimulated human monocytes, *APMIS* 98:529 (1990).

14. K. Ohlsson, P. Björk, M. Bergenfeldt, R. Hageman, and R.C. Thompson, Interleukin-1 receptor antagonist reduces mortality from endotoxin shock, *Nature* 348:550 (1990).

15. H.F. Starnes,Jr., M.K. Pearce, A. Tewari, J.H. Yim, J.C. Zou, and J.S. Abrams, Anti-IL-6 monoclonal antibodies protect against lethal *Escherichia coli* infection and lethal tumor necrosis factor-α challenge in mice, *J.Immunol.* 145:4185 (1990).

16. K. Bendtzen, Immune hormones (cytokines); pathogenic role in autoimmune rheumatic diseases and endocrine diseases, *Autoimmunity* 2:177 (1989).

17. M. Svenson, M.B. Hansen, P. Heegaard, K. Abell, and K. Bendtzen, Purification of a high-affinity IL-1ra binding serum factor using specific antibodies to the human IL-1 type I receptor (sIL-1RI). Unpublished.

18. S.P. Eisenberg, R.J. Evans, W.P. Arend, E. Verderber, M.T. Brewer, C.H. Hannum, and R.C. Thompson, Primary structure and functional expression from complementary DNA of a human interleukin-1 receptor antagonist, *Nature* 343:341 (1990).

19. D.B. Carter, M.R. Deibel, C.J. Dunn, C.S.C. Tomich, A.L. Laborde, J.L. Slightom, A.E. Berger, M.J. Bienkowski, and F.F. Sun, Purification, cloning, expression and biological characterization of an interleukin-1 receptor antagonist protein, *Nature* 344:633 (1990).

20. W.P. Arend, H.G. Welgus, R.C. Thompson, and S.P. Eisenberg, Biological properties of recombinant human monocyte-derived interleukin 1 receptor antagonist, *J.Clin.Invest.* 85:1694 (1990).

21. G.O. Wakabayashi, J.A. Gelfand, J.F. Burke, R.C. Thompson, and C.A. Dinarello, A specific receptor antagonist for interleukin 1 prevents *Escherichia coli*-induced shock in rabbits, *FASEB J.* 5:338 (1991).

22. T.R. Ulich, S.M. Yin, K.Z. Guo, J. Delcastillo, S.P. Eisenberg, and R.C. Thompson, The intratracheal administration of endotoxin and cytokines. 3. the interleukin-1 (IL-1) receptor antagonist inhibits endotoxin-induced and IL-1-induced acute inflammation, *Am.J.Pathol.* 138:521 (1991).

23. H.R. Alexander, G.M. Doherty, C.M. Buresh, D.J. Venzon, and J.A. Norton, A recombinant human receptor antagonist to interleukin-1 improves survival after lethal endotoxemia in mice, *J.Exp.Med.* 173:1029 (1991).

24. M.R. Opp and J.M. Krueger, Interleukin 1-receptor antagonist blocks interleukin 1-induced sleep and fever, *Am.J.Physiol.* 260:R453 (1991).

25. B. Henderson, R.C. Thompson, T. Hardingham, and J. Lewthwaite, Inhibition of interleukin-1-induced synovitis and articular cartilage proteoglycan loss in the rabbit knee by recombinant human interleukin-1 receptor antagonist, *Cytokine* 3:246 (1991).

26. R.J. Smith, J.E. Chin, L.M. Sam, and J.M. Justen, Biologic effects of an interleukin-1 receptor antagonist protein on interleukin-1-stimulated cartilage erosion and chondrocyte responsiveness, *Arthritis Rheum.* 34:78 (1991).

27. D.K. Podolsky, Inflammatory bowel disease I, *N.Engl.J.Med.* 325:928 (1991).

28. M. Svenson, L.K. Poulsen, A. Fomsgaard, and K. Bendtzen, IgG autoantibodies against interleukin 1α in sera of normal individuals, *Scand.J.Immunol.* 29:489 (1989).

29. H. Suzuki, T. Akama, M. Okane, I. Kono, Y. Matsui, K. Yamane, and H. Kashiwagi, Interleukin-1-inhibitory IgG in sera from some patients with rheumatoid arthritis, *Arthritis Rheum.* 32:1528 (1989).

30. M.B. Hansen, M. Svenson, M. Diamant, and K. Bendtzen, Anti-interleukin-6 antibodies in normal human serum, *Scand.J.Immunol.* 33:777 (1991).

31. H. Suzuki, T. Ayabe, J. Kamimura, and H. Kashiwagi, Anti-IL-1α autoantibodies in patients with rheumatic diseases and in healthy subjects, *Clin.Exp.Immunol.* 85:407 (1991).

32. J.-H. Saurat, J. Schifferli, G. Steiger, J.-M. Dayer, and L. Didierjean, Anti-interleukin-1α autoantibodies in humans: Characterization, isotype distribution, and receptor-binding inhibition--Higher frequency in Schnitzler's syndrome (urticaria and macroglobulinemia), *J.Allergy Clin.Immunol.* 88:244 (1991).

33. M. Svenson, M.B. Hansen, and K. Bendtzen, Distribution and characterization of autoantibodies to interleukin 1α in normal human sera, *Scand.J.Immunol.* 32:695 (1990).

34. K. Bendtzen, M. Svenson, V. Jønsson, and E. Hippe, Autoantibodies to cytokines friends or foes? *Immunol.Today* 11:167 (1990).

35. M.B. Hansen, M. Svenson, M. Diamant, and K. Bendtzen, High-affinity IgG autoantibodies to IL-6 in sera of normal individuals are competitive inhibitors of IL-6 *in vitro*, *Cytokine* (1992). Submitted

36. M.B. Hansen, M. Svenson, and K. Bendtzen, Human anti-interleukin 1α antibodies, *Immunol.Lett.* 30:133 (1991).

37. A. Fomsgaard, M. Svenson, and K. Bendtzen, Auto-antibodies to tumour necrosis factor α in healthy humans and patients with inflammatory diseases and Gram-negative bacterial infections, *Scand.J. Immunol.* 30:219 (1989).

38. E.W.B. Jeffes, E.K. Ininns, K.L. Schmitz, R.S. Yamamoto, C.A. Dett, and G.A. Granger, The presence of antibodies to lymphotoxin and tumor necrosis factor in normal serum, *Arthritis Rheum.* 32:1148 (1989).

39. C. Ross, M.B. Hansen, T. Schyberg, and K. Berg, Autoantibodies to crude human leucocyte interferon (IFN), native human IFN, recombinant human IFN-α2b and human IFN-γ in healthy blood donors, *Clin.Exp.Immunol.* 82:57 (1990).

40. A. Turano, A. Balsari, E. Viani, S. Landolfo, L. Zanoni, F. Gargiulo, and A. Caruso, Natural human antibodies to gamma interferon interfere with the immunomodulating activity of the lymphokine, *Proc.Natl.Acad.Sci.USA* 89:4447 (1992).

41. H. Kirchner, A. Körfer, P. Evers, M.M. Szamel, J. Knüver-Hopf, H. Mohr, C.R. Franks, U. Pohl, K. Resch, M. Hadam, H. Poliwoda, and J. Atzpodien, The development of neutralizing antibodies in a patient receiving subcutaneous recombinant and natural interleukin-2, *Cancer* 67:1862 (1991).

42. M. Pedersen, H. Permin, C. Bindslev-Jensen, K. Bendtzen, and S. Norn, Cytokine-induced histamine release from basophils of AIDS patients. Interaction between cytokines and specific IgE antibodies, *Allergy* 46:129 (1991).

43. M.B. Hansen, M. Svenson, and K. Bendtzen, Serum-induced suppression of interferon (IFN) activity. Lack of evidence for the presence of specific autoantibodies to IFN-α in normal human sera, *Clin. Exp.Immunol.* 88:559 (1992).

44. R. Aston, W.B. Cowden, and G.L. Ada, Antibody-mediated enhancement of hormone activity, *Mol. Immunol.* 26:435 (1989).

45. D.A. Rathjen, K. Cowan, L.J. Furphy, and R. Aston, Antigenic structure of human tumor necrosis factor: recognition of distinct regions of TNFα by different tumour cell receptors, *Mol.Immunol.* 28:79 (1991).

46. J.M. Dwyer, Manipulating the immune system with immune globulin, *N.Engl.J.Med.* 326:107 (1992).

47. M. Svenson, M.B. Hansen, L. Kayser, .K. Rasmussen, C.M. Reimert, and K. Bendtzen, Effects of human anti-IL-1α autoantibodies on receptor binding and biological activities of IL-1, *Cytokine* 4:125 (1992).

48. M. Svenson, M.B. Hansen, and K. Bendtzen, Specific and nonspecific binding of cytokines to human IgG, *J.Immunol.Methods* (1992). Submitted.

49. K. Bendtzen, M.B. Hansen, M. Diamant, P. Heegaard, and M. Svenson, Cytokine regulation during inflammation. Modulation by autoantibodies and fever, *in:* "The Wenner-Gren Center International Symposium: Neuro-immunology of fever," T. Bartfai, ed., Pergamon Press, New York (1992). In press.

50. M. Svenson, M.B. Hansen, and K. Bendtzen, Accuracy of immunometric methods for the detection of IL-1β. Commentary on antibody specificity, *J.Immunol.Methods* (1992). Submitted.

51. K.A. Hogquist, M.A. Nett, K.C.F. Sheehan, K.D. Pendleton, R.D. Schreiber, and D.D. Chaplin, Generation of monoclonal antibodies to murine IL-1β and demonstration of IL-1 in vivo, *J.Immunol.* 146:1534 (1991).

52. J. Mølvig, B. Sehested Hansen, H. Worsaae, K.R. Hejnæs, M. Helle, H. Dalbøge, and J. Nerup, Comparison of biological and immunological activities of human monocyte-derived interleukin 1β and human recombinant interleukin 1β, *Scand.J.Immunol.* 31:225 (1990).

CANCER IMMUNOCHEMOTHERAPY: PRELIMINARY STUDIES WITH TRIAZENE COMPOUNDS

Grazia Graziani[2], Stefania D'Atri[1], Anna Giuliani[1], Annibale Franchi[2], Daniela Piccioni[2], Giuseppe Papa[3], and Enzo Bonmassar[1]

[1]Institute of Experimental Medicine, National Council of Research (CNR), Via C.Marx 15, 00137 Rome, Italy
[2]Department of Experimental Medicine and Biochemical Sciences, University of Rome Tor Vergata, Via O. Raimondo, 00173 Rome, Italy
[3]Department of Internal Medicine, S. Eugenio Hospital, P.le dell'Umanesimo 10, 00144 Rome, Italy

INTRODUCTION

One of the most challenging problems of cancer immunotherapy in the clinic concerns the poor immune response of the host for the autochthonous tumor. This is, at least in part, due to the scarce immunogenicity of neoplastic cells, which are not recognized by host's natural or antigen-dependent immune apparatus. In order to overcome this difficulty, the immunopharmacological approach of "Chemical Xenogenization" (CX) has been introduced by our laboratory in 1970 (1). It has been found that in vivo treatment of leukemia-bearing mice with triazene compounds (TZC) leads to the appearance of novel transplantation antigens on the membrane of neoplastic cells (2-4). TZC-treated cells are rejected by syngeneic hosts and elicit specific cytotoxic T lymphocyte (CTL) responses (1-14). The principal features of CX in mouse leukemias are summarized in Table 1.

Large experimental evidence is now available on the crucial role played by the DNA repair enzyme ^{6}0-alkylguanine-DNA-alkyl-transferase (OGAT, 25) in the biochemical effects of TZC (21). This enzyme removes the ^{6}0-guanine alkyl adducts (Figure 1), including those produced by DNA methylating agents, such as TZC, nitrosoureas, MNNG, etc. High OGAT levels associated with neoplastic cells are expected to prevent either the antitumor and the CX-inducing activity of TZC (26).

Table 1. Main features concerning CX in murine leukemia models

---

Experimental design and results   References

---

a. CX generation in vivo.
 1.Treatment of leukemic mice with TZC for 2-6 transplant generations converts the entire leukemia cell population into highly immunogenic blasts.   1-4
 2.Similar results can be obtained with mouse melanoma.   5

b. CX generation in vitro.
 1.CX can be obtained with cultured mouse tumor cells exposed in vitro to active TZC (e.g. =N-N=N-monomethyl derivatives) or to TZC inactive in vitro (i.e. dimethyl-TZC) if the drug is activated (i.e. demethylated) with liver microsomes.   6-7

c. Antigenic properties of TZC-treated tumors (TZC/T)
 1.TZC/T retain their original tumor-associated transplantation antigen(s) (TATA) if present, and show novel "drug-mediated tumor antigens" (DMTA).   8-10
 2.TZC/T are rejected by histocompatible mice with rejection kinetics similar to those detectable for H-2 incompatible tumors.   11
 3.TZC/T elicit in vivo or in vitro specific CTL and specific humoral antibodies in syngeneic mice.   9,12-17

d. Molecular mechanisms involved in CX generation.All available data favour the hypothesis that CX is induced by somatic mutation mechanisms.
 1.CX is inhibited by an antimutagenic agent (Quinacrine).   18
 2.Highly immunogenic TUM- variant clones have been obtained by Boon,treating leukemia cells with the mutagenic DNA-methylating agent MNNG.   19
 This is due to point mutation (GC - AT transition) produced by GT mispairing generated by methyl adducts to ^{6}O-guanine of DNA.   20
 3.TZC produce methyl adducts to ^{6}O-guanine of DNA comparable to those induced by MNNG.   21
 4.The sequence containing point mutations, responsible of TZC-induced CX, has been identified.   22

e. Use of CX for therapeutic approaches.
 1.Use of TZC-induced CX for immunochemotherapy of murine leukemias.   23
 2.Use of immunogenic TZC/T to protect against scarcely immunogenic parental tumor cells.   8
 3.Immunochemotherapy of leukemias in the brain.   24

Since CX phenomenon and OGAT levels could be of great potential interest for innovative strategies in the treatment of human cancer, preliminary studies have been performed with blasts of patients with acute myelogenous leukemia (AML) exposed in vitro or in vivo to TZC (27). The results suggest that: (a) TZC-treated blasts immortalized with HTLV-I elicit autologous CTL responses, and (b) OGAT levels are inversely associated with blast sensitivity to TZC.

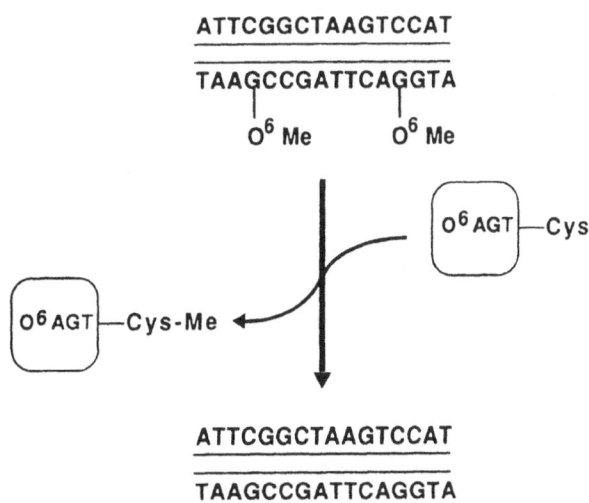

Figure 1. Repair of ^6O-methyl-guanine DNA adducts by OGAT.

MATERIALS AND METHODS

Drugs

5-(3,3'-dimethyl-1-triazeno)-imidazole-4-carboxamide(DTIC) (Deticene, marketed by Rhone-Poulenc Rorer, Milan, Italy), that requires metabolic demethylation for activation, was used for in vivo studies as described elsewhere (27).

Temozolomide, a cyclic TZC which decomposes spontaneously in vitro to monomethyl-triazene-imidazole-carboxamide (MTIC) (21), the active form of DTIC, was used in vitro to evaluate the chemosensitivity of blast cells to this drug.

4-(3-methyl-1-triazeno)benzoic acid potassium salt (MTBA), a TZC active in vitro (28), was used for in vitro treatment of human tumor cells.

Patients

26 leukemic patients, bearing acute myelogenous leukemia (AML) entered the study. 10 out of 26 underwent to treatment with DTIC as described (27).

Assay Of OGAT Activity

This method has been described in detail elsewhere (29). Briefly supernatants obtained after sonication of blast cells were assayed for OGAT activity by measuring the transfer of ^{3}H-labeled methyl groups from substrate DNA (29) to the OGAT protein (30). OGAT activity was expressed in terms of fentomoles of methyl group transferred per mg of protein (i.e. fmoles/mg).

Assay Of Sensitivity To Temozolomide

Blast cells were suspended in medium conditioned with 10% (vol/vol) supernatant of the 5637 cell line (31), plated in quadruplicate in 96-microplate well, and exposed to graded concentrations of Temozolomide for 48 h as previously described (27). 1µCi of (methyl-^{3}H)thymidine (Amersham U.K.) was then added to each well for additional 16 h. Chemosensitivity was expressed in terms of IC50, corresponding to the concentration of Temozolomide capable of producing a 50% inhibition of thymidine uptake by cultured blast cells, using linear regression analysis.

In Vitro Treatment Of Blast Cells With MTBA And Infection With HTLV-I

Blast cells of a patient with AML were washed and treated with MTBA (100 µg/ml) for 1h at 37°C in a Dubnoff metabolic shaker. Untreated or MTBA-treated cells were then washed, exposed to HTLV-I by coculture with HTLV-I donor, radiation-inactivated MT-2 cells (32) and maintained in continuous culture.

Detection Of HTLV-I Provirus DNA

Genomic DNA (1 µg) was amplified in 30 repetitive three-step cycles: 15s at 94°C, 30s at 53°C and 30s at 72°C (33). Amplifications were carried out in a Perkin-Elmer Cetus thermal cycler. All reaction products were assayed by liquid hybridization (LH) of the amplified DNA with a ^{32}P-end labelled oligonucleotide, followed by electrophoresis on 8% polyamylamide gel and then autoradiography (34). Primer pair and probe used respectively for Polymerase Chain Reaction

(PCR) (SK54/55) and LH (SK56) (35) are specific for HTLV-I pol region, which encodes the reverse transcriptase required for virus replication.

In Vitro Generation Of Human CTL

Peripheral blood mononuclear cells (MNC) were separated from heparinized blood obtained from a 52-year old female leukemic (AML) patient in complete remission, on a Ficoll-Hypaque gradient. Primary CTL were generated by incubating MNC at 37·C in a 5% CO_2 humidified atmosphere with irradiated (10.000 R) AML blasts obtained from the same patients, immortalized with HTLV-I, untreated (CL1) or MTBA treated (CL1-MTBA). After an incubation period of 6 days effector cells were collected and tested in a cytotoxicity assay against TZC-treated or untreated leukemic blasts and against the unrelated Burkitt lymphoma Daudi cell line. Primary CTL were further stimulated with the appropriate sensitizer cell line for additional 6 days, and then tested for cytotoxicity (secondary CTL generation).

Cytotoxicity Assay

Target (T) cells were labeled by incubation with 100 μCi of $Na^{51}CrO_4$ (Amersham) and added to effector cells (E) to give an E to T cell ratio ranging from 100:1 to 12.5:1. The percentage of specific lysis was calculated as follows:

$$\% \text{ specific cytotoxicity} = \frac{\text{test cpm} - \text{autologous cpm}}{\text{total cpm incorporated}} \times 100$$

where "test cpm" is the mean cpm released in the presence of effector cells, "autologous cpm" is the mean cpm released by target cells incubated with unlabeled autologous cells in place of effector cells, and "total cpm" is the total amount of ^{51}Cr incorporated in target cells.

RESULTS

Relationship Between OGAT Levels And Suceptibility Of AML Blasts To TZC

A total of 26 AML blast samples were collected from 10 patients which were then treated with DTIC (see Materials and Methods), and from additional 26 patients not scheduled for TZC treatment. Table 2 illustrates (a) relationship between OGAT levels of AML blasts and in vivo susceptibility to DTIC in terms of blast reduction in bone marrow or in peripheral blood; (b) relationship between enzyme levels and in vitro susceptibility to growth inhibition by Temozolomide. The results show a reasonably good inverse relationship between OGAT levels and chemosensitivity to TZC of AML blasts.

Table 2. Relationship between OGAT activity associated with AML blast cells and susceptibility to antitumor effects of TZC.

OGAT activity (fmoles/mg protein)	in vivo response[a]	in vitro chemosensitivity[b]
High (more than 200)	0/4	12/18 (>300)
		6/18 (200-300)
Medium (100-200)	0/1	1/3 (>300)
		2/3 (50-200)
Low (less than 100)	5/5	1/5 (>300)
		4/5 (50-200)

[a] evaluated in vivo in terms of number of cases over total, showing significant reduction or disappearance of AML blasts in bone marrow and/or peripheral blood of patients, on day 7 after treatment with DTIC (0.8mg/mq/day, day 1,2 and 3).

[b] evaluated in vitro in terms of number of samples over total showing the values of IC50 of Temozolomide (see Materials and Methods) indicated in parenthesis.

Attempts To Detect CX In AML Blasts Treated In Vitro With TZC

Bone marrow cells (99% AML blasts) of a 52-year old female patient were treated with MTBA and exposed to HTLV-I infection, as described in Methods section. Infected parental (CL1) or MTBA-treated (CL1/MTBA) cells were tested for (a) presence of HTLV-I viral genome by PCR followed by LH; (b) capability of generating autologous CTL, using normal, immunocompetent MNC obtained by the same patient after chemotherapy-induced complete remission, using Ara-C (1g/sqm/day, for 6 days) plus Mitoxantrone (6mg/sqm/day, for 6 days, 27).

The results of these studies show that (a) both control or MTBA-treated lines immortalized with HTLV-I, harbour HTLV-I retrovirus associated with genomic DNA (lanes B,C, Figure 2); (b) autologous primary or secondary CTL sensitized against CL1/MTBA line are cytotoxic for the TZC-treated line but show little or no cytolytic activity against parental or unrelated target cells (Figure 3). Conversely primary CTL immune against the parental CL1 line are preferentially lytic for the parental rather than the TZC-treated CL1/MTBA line (Figure 3).

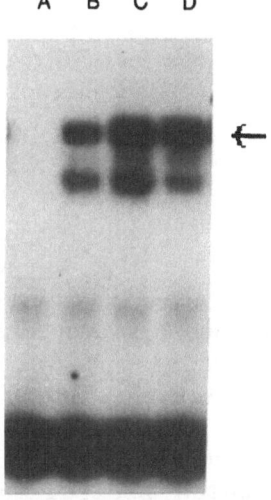

Figure 2. Presence of HTLV-I provirus, POL region, (indicated by the arrow), in infected CL1 or CL1/MTBA lines, but not in original non-infected bone marrow cells of origin.
A= untreated and uninfected AML blasts; B= HTLV-I infected AML blasts (CL1); C= HTLV-I infected and MTBA-treated AML blasts (CL1/MTBA); D= HTLV-I donor cell line (MT-2).

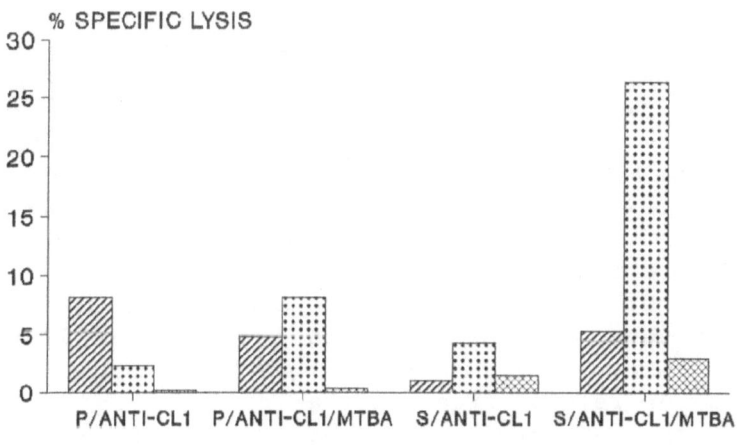

Figure 3. Cytotoxic activity of primary (P) or secondary (S) CTL against autologous parental (CL1) or MTBA-treated (CL1/MTBA) leukemic blasts and against the unrelated Daudi target cells. Lytic activity is expressed in terms of percentage of specific lysis at the E:T ratio of 25:1.

DISCUSSION

Preclinical studies in mouse leukemias and melanoma (1-5), a pilot study in patients with refractory AML (27) and the present preliminary investigation in human AML blast cells (Table 2) point out that (a) TZC could have a role in the treatment of acute leukemias in the clinic; (b) CX could provide a contribution to the antitumor effects of TZC, although further studies are required to support this point; (c) evaluation of OGAT activity in leukemic cells or in other cancer cells, including melanomas, could have a crucial role in determining the susceptibility of individual neoplasias to the antitumor and/or CX-inducing activity of TZC.

The inverse relationship between OGAT levels and chemosensitivity of a number of tumors or tumor lines to nitrosoureas or triazenes has been described by many authors (21,26,36). It is surprising however that little is known about in vivo relationship between OGAT activity and response of the patient to these agents.

Of particular interest appears to be the recent pilot clinical study in which pretreatment with high dose of Streptozotocin has been used to inhibit OGAT activity of tumor cells. The patients were then subjected to treatment with nitrosoureas, which appeared to be more active than in control subjects not pretreated with the OGAT inhibitor (37).

The possibility that TZC could induce CX in human cancer cells appears to be still an open question. The results described in Figure 2 point out that control or TZC-treated cells harbour HTLV-I provirus. Therefore the differential antigenic pattern of CL1 and CL1/MTBA cells recognized by specific CTL, as illustrated in Figure 3, does not seem to be conditioned by the presence of the retrovirus. However the nature of the antigen(s) recognized by autologous CTL on CL1/MTBA has not been identified and no data are available to support the hypothesis that these antigen(s) are generated by exposure to TZC. The present results therefore do not allow to draw any conclusion on the possible role played by CX in blast suppression afforded by TZC in AML patients.

Further studies are required to establish whether (a) T-cell dependent autoreactivity can be confirmed with TZC-treated blasts in a consistent number of cases, and (b) increase of relapse-free interval or possible number of "cures" can be obtained if TZC treatment is properly combined with biological response modifiers (Tentori L. et al, in preparation) capable of antagonizing the immunodepressive effects of TZC (38,39) and amplifying possible host's responses against TZC-induced DMTA.

SUMMARY

Induction of novel "drug-mediated transplantation antigens" (DMTA) by drug treatment of tumor-bearing mice (i.e. "chemical xenogenization", CX) has been obtained in our laboratory, using DTIC and other triazene compounds (TZC). The antitumor and the CX-inducing properties of TZC have been found to be negatively regulated by the DNA repair enzyme $6O$-alkyl-guanine-DNA-alkyl-transferase (OGAT), which removes the $6O$-methyl adducts at DNA guanine produced by TZC. These adducts are responsible of the cytotoxic activity of these drugs and of their CX-inducing effects, since $6O$-methyl-guanine mispairs with thymine, resulting in point mutation(s) (GC-AT transition) and DMTA appearance. The present preliminary study performed in patients bearing refractory acute myeloblastic leukemia (AML), shows that: (a) inverse relationship can be found between OGAT levels of leukemic blasts and their in vivo or in vitro chemosensitivity to TZC; (b) leukemic blasts exposed in vitro to TZC and immortalized with HTLV-I infection elicit autologous cytotoxic T lymphocytes in vitro, using responder cells of the donor patient after remission induction obtained with conventional chemotherapy. These results point out the potential therapeutic value of TZC in refractory AML, when low OGAT levels are associated with leukemic blasts. However further studies are required to establish the role that could be played by CX in TZC treatment of human leukemias or of other human neoplasias.

AKNOWLEDGMENTS

The present work has been supported in part by a grant of the "Istituto Superiore di Sanita'"(Rome),Italy-USA program on therapy of Neoplasias (Legge 531, 29/12/1987), and in part by a grant of the Italian Association for Cancer Research (AIRC), Milan, Italy.

The authors are grateful to Dr G.P.Margison (Department of Carcinogenesis, Paterson Institute for Cancer Research, Christie Hospital and Holt Radium Institute, Manchester, UK) who generously provided the $3H$-labeled methylated DNA substrate, and to Dr M. Stevens (Department of Pharmaceutical Sciences, Aston University, Birmingham, UK) who kindly furnished Temozolomide.

The authors are also grateful to "ENEA" (Rome, Italy), for having supported the PhD fellowship of Dr. Daniela Piccioni.

The authors are also grateful to Ms Barbara Bulgarini and to Ms Alessia De Vincenzi for their excellent technical assistance.

REFERENCES

1. E.Bonmassar, A.Bonmassar, S.Vadlamudi, and A.Goldin, Immunological alteration of leukemic cells in vivo after treatment with an antitumor agent, Proc.Natl.Acad.Sci. (USA) 66:1089 (1970).

2. E.Bonmassar, A.Bonmassar, S.Vadlamudi, and A.Goldin, Antigenic changes of L1210 leukemia in mice treated with 5-(3-3'-dimethyl-1-triazeno)-imidazole-4-carboxamide, Cancer Res. 32:1446 (1972).

3. A.Nicolin, F.Spreafico, E.Bonmassar, and A.Goldin, Antigenic changes of L5178Y lymphoma after treatment with 5-(3-3'-dimethyl-1-triazeno)-imidazole-4-carboxamide in vivo, J.Natl.Cancer Inst. 56:89 (1976).

4. P.Puccetti, L.Romani, and M.C.Fioretti, Chemical xenogenization of experimental tumors, Cancer Metast. Reviews 6:93 (1987).

5. M.Allegrucci, P.Fuschiotti, P.Puccetti, L.Romani, and M.C.Fioretti, Changes in the tumorigenic and metastatic properties of murine melanoma cells treated with a triazene derivative, Clin.Expl.Metastasis 7:329 (1989).

6. B.Nardelli, A.R.Contessa, L.Romani, G.Sava, C.Nisi, and M.C.Fioretti, Immunogenic changes of murine lymphoma cells following in vitro treatment with aryl-triazene-derivatives, Cancer Immunol. Immunother. 16:157 (1984).

7. A.R.Contessa, A. Bonmassar, A.Giampietri, A.Circolo, A.Goldin, and M.C.Fioretti, In vitro generation of a highly immunogenic subline of L1210 leukemia following exposure to 5-(3-3'-dimethyl-1-triazeno)-imidazole-4-carboxamide, Cancer Res. 41:2476 (1981).

8. D.P.Houchens, E.Bonmassar, M.R.Gaston, M.Kende, and A.Goldin, Drug-mediated immunogenic changes of virus-induced leukemia in vivo, Cancer Res. 36:1347 (1976).

9. O.Marelli, P.Franco, G.Canti, L.Ricci, N.Prandoni, A.Nicolin, H.Festenstein, DTIC xenogenized lines obtained from an L1210 clone: clonal analysis of cytotoxic T lymphocyte reactivity, Br.J.Cancer 58:171 (1988).

10. M.C.Fioretti, R.Bianchi, L.Romani, and E.Bonmassar, Drug-induced immunogenic changes of murine leukemic cells: dissociation of onset of resistance and emergence of novel immunogenicity, J.Nat.Cancer Inst. 71:1247 (1983).

11. C.Riccardi, M.C.Fioretti, A.Giampietri, P.Puccetti, and A.Goldin, Growth and rejection patterns of murine lymphoma cells antigenically altered following drug treatment in vivo, Transplantation 25:63 (1978).

12. A.Nicolin, A.Bini, E.Coronetti, and A.Goldin, Cellular immune response to a drug treated L5178Y lymphoma subline, Nature 251:654 (1974).

13. A.Santoni, Y.Kinney, A.Goldin, Secondary cytotoxic response in vitro against Moloney lymphoma cells antigenically altered by drug-treatment in vivo, J.Natn.Cancer Inst. 60:109 (1978).

14. L.Romani, M.C.Fioretti, and E.Bonmassar, In vitro generation of primary cytotoxic lymphocytes against L5178Y leukemia antigenically altered by 5-(3,3'-dimethyl-1-triazeno)-imidazole-4-carboxamide in vivo, Transplantation 28:218 (1979).

15. L.Romani, P.Puccetti, M.C.Fioretti, and M.G. Mage, Humoral response against murine lymphoma cells xenogenized by drug treatment in vivo. Int.J. Cancer 36:225 (1985).

16. C.Testorelli, Y.I.Archetti, P.Aresca, and L.Del Vecchio, Monoclonal antibodies to the L1210 murine leukemia cell line and to a drug-altered subline. Cancer Res. 45:5299 (1985).

17. L.Romani, U.Grohmann, F.Fazioli, P.Puccetti, M.G.Mage, and M.C.Fioretti, Cell-mediated immunity to chemically xenogenized tumors. I. Inhibition by specific antisera and H-2 association of the novel antigens, Cancer Immunol. Immunother. 26:48 (1988).

18. A.Giampietri, M.C.Fioretti, A.Goldin, and E.Bonmassar, Drug-mediated antigenic changes in murine leukemia cells: antagonistic effects of Quinacrine, an antimutagenic compound, J.Natl. Cancer Inst. 64:297 (1980).

19. T.Boon, Antigenic tumor cell variants obtained with mutagens, Adv.Cancer Res. 39:121 (1983).

20. E.De Plaen, C.Lurquin, A.Van Pel, B.Mariame', J.P.Szikora, T.Wolfel, C.Sibille, P.Chomez, and T.Boon, Immunogenic (tum) variants of mouse tumor P815: cloning of the gene of tum antigen P91A and identification of the tum mutation. Proc.Natl.Acad.Sci.(USA) 85:2274 (1988).

21. C.V.Catapano, M.Broggini, E.Erba, M.Ponti, L.Mariani, L.Citti, and M.D'Incalci, In vitro and in vivo methazolastone induced DNA damage and repair in L1210 leukemia sensitive and resistant to chloroethylnitrosoureas, Cancer Res. 47:4884 (1987).

22. U.Grohmann, L.Binaglia, P.Puccetti, and M.C.Fioretti, Murine leukemia virus gp70 antisense oligonucleotides inhibit CTL-mediated lysis of a drug-treated lymphoma, 8th Int. Congr. of Immunology, Budapest, Hungary August 23-28, 1992.

23. A.Giampietri, A.Bonmassar, P.Puccetti, A.Circolo, A.Goldin, and E.Bonmassar, Drug-mediated increase of tumor immunogenicity in vivo for a new approach to experimental cancer immunotherapy, Cancer Res. 41:681 (1981).

24. L.Romani, M.C.Fioretti, R.Bianchi, B.Nardelli, and E.Bonmassar, Intracerebral adoptive immunotherapy of a murine lymphoma antigenically altered by drug treatment in vivo, JNCI 68:817 (1982).

25. A.E.Pegg, L.Wiest, R.S.Foote, S.Mitra, and W.Perry, Purification and properties of O6-methylguanine-DNA-transmethylase from rat liver, J.Biol.Chem.258:2327(1983)

26. J.Domoradzki, A.E.Pegg, M.E.Dolan, V.M.Maher, and J.J.McCormick, Correlation between O6-methylguanine-DNA-methyltransferase activity and resistance of human cells to the cytotoxic and mutagenic effect of N-methyl-N'-nitro-N-nitrosoguanidine, Carcinogenesis 5:1641 (1984).

27. A.Franchi, G.Papa, S.D'Atri, D.Piccioni, M.Masi, E.Bonmassar, Cytotoxic effects of Dacarbazine in patients with acute myelogenous leukemia: a pilot study, Haematologica 77:146 (1992).

28. M.C.Fioretti, L.Romani, E.Bonmassar, Antigenic changes related to drug-action, in: "Biology of Cancer" (13th Int. Cancer Congress, Part B), E.A.Mirand, W.B.Hutchinson, and E.Mihich eds., Alan R.Liss Inc., New York (1983).

29. G.P.Margison, D.P.Cooper, J.Brennan, Cloning of the E.Coli O^6 methylguanine and methylphosphotriester methyl transferase gene using a functional DNA repair assay, Nucleic Acid Res. 13:1939 (1985).

30. G.N.Major, E.F.Gardner, A.F.Carne, P.D.Lawley, Purification to homogeneity and partial amino acid sequence of a fragment which includes the methyl acceptor site of the human DNA repair protein for O^6-methylguanine, Nucleid Acid Res. 18:1351 (1990).

31. K.Welte, E.Platzer, L.Lu et al, Purification and biochemical characterization of human pluripotent hematopoietic colony-stimulating factor, Proc. Natl. Acad. Sci. (USA) 82:1526 (1985).

32. G.Graziani, D.Pasqualetti, M.Lopez, C.D'Onofrio, A.M.Testi, F.Mandelli, R.C.Gallo and E.Bonmassar, Increased susceptibility of peripheral mononuclear cells of leukemic patients to HTLV-I infection in vitro. Blood 69:1175 (1987).

33. G.D.Ehrlich, S.Greenberg and M.Abbot, Detection of human T-cell lymphoma/leukemia viruses, in: "PCR protocol. A guide to methods and applications", M.A.Innis, D.H.Gelfand, J.J. Sninsky, and T.J.White eds., Academic Press Inc. (1990).

34. M.A.Abbot, B.J.Poiesz, B.C.Byrne, S.Kwok, J,J.Sninsky and G.D.Ehrlich, Enzimatic gene amplification: qualitative and quantitative methods for detecting proviral DNA amplification in vitro, J.Infect.Dis. 158:1158 (1988).

35. S.Knok, G.Ehrlich, B.Poiesz. R. Kalish and J.J.Sninsky, Enzymatic amplification of HTLV-I viral sequences from peripheral blood mononuclear cells and infected tissues, Blood 72:1117 (1988).

36. P.Robins, A.L.Harris, L.Goldsmith, and T.Lindahl, Cross-linking of DNA, produced by chloroethylnitrosourea is prevented by O^6-methylguanine-DNA-methyltransferase, Nucleic Acid Res. 11:7743 (1983).

37. T.J.Panella, D.C.Smith, S.C.Schold, M.P.Rogers, E.P.Winer, R.L.Fine, J.Crawford, J.E.Herndon II, and D.L.Trump, Modulation of O^6-alkylguanine-DNA-alkyltransferase-mediated Carnmustine resistance using Streptozotocin: a phase I trial, Cancer Res. 52:2456 (1992).

38. B.Nardelli, P.Puccetti, L.Romani, G.Sava, E.Bonmassar, and M.C.Fioretti, Chemical xenogenization of murine lymphoma cells with triazene derivatives: immunotoxicological studies, Cancer Immunol.Immunother. 17:213 (1984).

39. S.D'Atri, L.Tentori, M.Tricarico, and E.Bonmassar, Effects of triazenes on immune responses, in: "Triazenes. Chemical, Biological and Clinical aspects", T.Giraldi, T.A.Connors, and G.Cartei eds., Plenum Press, New York-London (1990).

THYMOSIN α1 AND α-INTEFERON WITH CISPLATIN AND ETOPOSIDE IN

ADVANCED NON-SMALL-CELL LUNG CANCER: A PHASE II STUDY

Massimo Lopez,[1] Giovanni Bonsignore,[2] Modesto D'Aprile,[3] Cartesio Favalli,[4] Marina Della Giulia,[1] Luigi Di Lauro[1], Patrizia Vici[1] and Enrico Garaci[4]

[1]Istituto Regina Elena
V.le Regina Elena, 291
00161 - Roma
[2]Istituto di Pneumologia
Università di Palermo
Via Trabucco, 180
90146 - Palermo
[3]Centro Oncologico "G.Porfiri"
Ospedale S.M. Goretti
Via Canova
04100 - Latina
[4]Cattedra di Microbiologia
Università di Roma "Tor Vergata"
Via Orazio Raimondo, 8
00173 - Roma

INTRODUCTION

In recent years, biological response modifiers (BRMs) have emerged as an important new class of agents for treating cancer. Agents such as interferon (IFN) and interleukin 2 (IL-2) have been reported to induce significant tumor regression in various types of cancer usually resistant to chemotherapy (1,12), but their use in non-small-cell lung cancer (NSCLC) has received little attention.

IFN is known to stimulate natural killer (NK) activity, and patients with lung cancer have been reported to have decreased NK activity (2). There is an increasing body of evidence that thymic hormones (TH) may have a role in enhancing the host immune response against tumors. TH have been shown to increase IFN and IL-2 production in vitro (14) and to modulate the expression of high affinity IL-2 receptors in normal human lynphocytes stimulated by PHA (9). Enhancement of NK activity by TH has been reported both in vitro and in vivo (13). In a series of experiments (3,4), thymosin α1 (TA1), a synthetic polipeptide of thimic origin, and IFN, singly or in combination with cytotoxic agents, were injected into normal and immunosuppressed mice. While IFN, as expected, significantly increased NK activity in normal mice, neither TA1 or IFN were effective in restoring NK activity in both cyclophosphamide (CTX)-treated and tumor-bearing immunosuppressed mice. Furthermore, treatment with CTX and TA1 plus IFN was significantly more effective than CTX alone or in combination with TA1 or IFN against Lewis lung carcinoma in mice.

In 1989, we undertook a phase II study in patients with advanced NSCLC to

Combination Therapies 2, Edited by A.L. Goldstein
and E. Garaci Plenum Press, New York, 1993

verify wether TA1 and low dose IFNα could potentiate the activity of cytotoxic chemotherapy in this disease.

PATIENTS AND METHODS

Between April 1989 and August 1991, 60 patients with histologically or cytologically proven advanced NSCLC were enrolled into the study. All patients had had no prior chemotherapy, and were 75 years of age or younger. All patients had measurable disease, World Health Organization (WHO) performance status (PS) ≤ 2, adequate renal (serum creatinine < 1.5 mg/dl), hepatic (serum bilirubin ≤ 1.5 mg/dl, SGOT ≤ 4 times normal limit) and bone marrow (WBC ≥ 4,000/mm^3 and platelets ≥ 100,000/mm^3) functions, no serious cardiac or pulmonary disease, and no other concomitant malignant disease. Informed consent was obtained from all patients.

The treatment consisted of cisplatin 100 mg/m^2 on day 1, etoposide 120 mg/m^2 I.V. on days 1-3, TA1 1 mg subcutaneously (s.c.) on days 8-11 and 15-18 and recombinant IFNα2a 3x10^6 IU s.c. on days 11 and 18, 1h after the injection of TA1.

Cisplatin was given by i.v. bolus with adequate prehydration and posthydration and forced diuresis. No specific antiemetic treatment was recommended in the protocol. Paracetamol 500 mg t.i.d. was given orally to prevent and control IFN-related flu-like symptoms. Doses of ciplatin and etoposide were reduced by 25% if the WBC nadir was ≤ 1,000/mm^3 and/or platelet nadir ≤ 25,000/mm^3. Cisplatin was withheld if the serum creatinine rose to ≥ 2 mg/dl and did not recover. No dose reduction was planned for TA1 and IFN.

Treatment was repeated every 3 weeks and continued to a maximum of six courses or until progression or major toxicity.

Before treatment, patients underwent staging evaluation including medical history, phisical examination, fiberoptic bronchoscopy with biopsy (optional), chest x-rays, computed tomography of the brain, chest and abdomen, and bone scan. Complete blood cell count was performed weekly; blood chemistries and urinalysis were determined before each course and on day 8. Changes in different immunologic parameters were evaluated in blood samples obtained on days 1, 4, 8, 12, 15 and 19 of each course.

Response and toxicity were evaluated according to WHO criteria (11). Survival from the first day of treatment to death was calculated by the method of Kaplan and Meier (6).

RESULTS

Characteristics of the 60 patients are summarized in Table 1. The majority of patients were male, were ambulatory (PS = 0-1), and had experienced weight loss of less than 10% of usual body weight. The predominant histologic types were squamous cell carcinoma (43%) or adenocarcinoma (33%). The median follow-up time for all patients was 12.3 months and the median follow-up in surviving patient was 18.8 months. At the time of this analysis 75% of patients had died. Out of 55 evaluable patients, 2 achieved a complete response (CR) and 22 a partial response (PR) for an overall response rate of 43.6 (95% confidence interval 30.5% to 56.7%). No statistical difference in response rate was found with regards to the stage of disease (stage III vs stage IV), the performance status (PS 0-1 vs PS 2) or the cell type (squamous cell carcinoma vs adenocarcinoma). Twenty-four patients experienced stable disease, whereas disease progression was observed in 7 patients.

The median duration of response was 7.9 months. Median duration of stable disease was 6.6 months. These findings are not statistically different.

The median survival for all patients was 12.6 months. It was 15.7 months in responding, and 10 months in non responding patients.

NK activity and lymphocyte subpopulations were evaluated in 20 patients who received the combined treatment, and were compared with that observed in 7 patients treated with cisplatin and etoposide alone. NK activity was depressed by chemotherapy in both groups. However, while this effect persisted for several days in the chemothe-

TABLE 1. PATIENT CHARACTERISTICS

ENTERED/EVALUABLE	60/55
SEX: M/F	54/6
AGE: MEDIAN (RANGE)	60 (36-75)
PS (WHO)	
0	4
1	50
2	6
WEIGHT LOSS	
< 10%	53
≥ 10%	7
HISTOLOGY	
SQUAMOUS CELL CARCINOMA	26
ADENOCARCINOMA	20
OTHER NON SMALL CELL	14
STAGE	
III A	6
III B	27
IV	27
PRIOR TREATMENT	
NONE	46
PRIOR SURGERY	12
PRIOR IRRADIATION	5

rapy group, recovery was significantly shortened in the chemoimmunotherapy group.

Furthermore this latter group benefited of an increase in NK activity from basal value. In both groups, NK activity reached the basal values by day 21.

CD4+ and CD8+ cells were also depressed by chemotherapy. Values sloped down until the 19th day in the chemotherapy group, whereas in the chemoimmunoterapy group there was an increase in CD4+ cells concomitantly with the administration of TA1 and IFN, and complete recovery was observed by day 15.

The incidence of toxic effects observed during the combined treatment is listed in Table 2.

TABLE 2. TREATMENT TOXICITY IN 60 PATIENTS

	N° OF PATIENTS WITH TOXIC EFFECT OF WHO GRADE			
TOXIC EFFECT	1	2	3	4
NAUSEA AND VOMITING	5	37	16	0
MUCOSITIS	3	1	0	0
ALOPECIA	0	10	49	0
LEUKOPENIA	11	13	15	7
THROMBOCYTOPENIA	13	3	4	3
ANEMIA	22	20	6	0
CREATININE	12	3	3	1
TRANSAMINASES	5	0	1	0
PERIPHERAL NEUROPATHY	7	1	0	0

Myelosuppression was recorded in the mayority of the patients, and was substantial. Most patients were distressed by nausea and vomiting, but this was tolerable in almost all patients. Alopecia occurred often, whereas infrequent side effects were mild stomatitis, slight neuropathy, and SGOT elevation. Transient serum creatinine elevation was recorded in 30% of the patients. Apart from moderate fever and minimal flu-like symphtoms, no other toxic reactions were related to o the administration of IFN.

Thymosin α1 is apparently devoid of toxicity. There were no treatment related deaths.

DISCUSSION

NSCLC is still a therapeutic challenge for the oncologist. Despite numerous attempts to maximising the activity of available chemotherapeutic agents, the impact of chemotherapy on the natural history of this disease has been, at best, marginal (5).

Treatment with various biological agents, including IFN, has been disappointing.

Theoretically, the combination of cytotoxic agents with BRMs should be synergistic for treating cancer, because these agents have different mechanisms of action. The observation that combined treatment with chemotherapy and IFN + TH was highly effective in experimental tumors (4), prompted us to test this new approach in the clinical setting.

In this study, the overall response rate of 44% is encouraging, and compares favorably with several randomized (7,8) and non randomized (5) studies using the combination of cisplatin and etoposide. As in other studies (8,10), there was no statistical difference in response rate between patients with locally advanced and those with metastatic disease, although a trend in favor of the former was observed. As is true in most cancers, NSCLC patients who achieved an objective response lived longer than those who do not. However, it is of interest the overall survival of 12.6 months, which appears to be longer than that reported in the literature (5). Patients with stable disease lived as long as responding patients. This could indicate that slowing tumor growth may result in patient benefit, and that objective response may not be the most appropriate criterion to evaluate treatment outcome when we are dealing with biological agents.

Tolerance was not a major problem. Although leukopenia was frequent, there were only two instances of infection episodes.

Although encouraging, the results of this study need to be confirmed in a randomized trial. This trial is now underway in our Institute, and results will be available next year.

REFERENCES

1. E.T. Creagan, D.L. Ahmann, S.J. Green, H.J. Long, S. Frytak, J.R. O'Fallon and L.M. Itri, Phase II study of low-dose recombinant leukocyte a interferon in disseminated malignant melanoma, J. Clin. Oncol. 9:1002 (1984).
2. W.K. Evans, D.W. Nixon, J.M. Daly, et al., A randomized study of oral nutritional support versus ad lib nutritional intake during chemotherapy for advanced colorectal and non-small-cell lung cancer, J. Clin. Oncol. 5:113 (1987).
3. C. Favalli, A. Mastino, T. Jezzi, S. Grelli, A.L. Goldstein, E. Garaci, Synergistic effect of thymosin α1 and α -interferon on NK activity in tumor-bearing mice, Int. J. Immunopharmac. 11:443 (1989).
4. E. Garaci, A. Mastino, F. Pica, C. Favalli, Combination treatment using thymosin α1 and interferon after cyclophosphamide is able to cure Lewis lung carcinoma in mice, Cancer Immunol. Immunother. 32:154 (1990).
5. D.C. Ihde, J.D. Minna, Non-small cell lung cancer Part II: Treatment, Curr. Probl. Cancer May/June (1991).

6. E.L. Kaplaplan, P. Meier, Nonparametric estimation from incomplete observations, J. Am. Stat. Assoc. 53:457 (1958).

7. J. Klastersky, J.P. Sculier, P. Ravez, P. Libert, J. Michel, G. Vandermoten, P. Rocmans, Y. Bonduelle, M. Mairesse, T. Michiels, J. Thiriaux, P. Mommen, O. Dalesio, A randomized study comparing a high and a standard dose of cisplatin in combination with etoposide in the treatment of advanced non-small-cell lung carcinoma, J. Clin. Oncol. 4:1780 (1986).

8. J. Klastersky, J.P. Sculier, G. Bureau, P. Libert, P. Ravez, G. Vandermoten, J. Thiriaux, J. Lecomte, R. Cordier, G. Dabouis, D. Brohee, L. Themelin, P. Mommen, Cisplatin versus cisplatin plus etoposide in the treatment of advanced non-small-cell lung cancer, J. Clin. Oncol. 7:1087 (1989).

9. K.D. Leichtling, S.A. Serrate and M.B. Sztein, Thymosin alpha 1 modulates the expression of high affinity interleukin-2 receptors on normal human lymphocytes, Int. J. Immunopharmac. 12:19 (1990).

10. E. Longeval and J. Klastersky, Combination chemotherapy with cisplatin and etoposide in bronchogenic squamous cell carcinoma and adenocarcinoma, Cancer 50:2751 (1982).

11. A.B. Miller, B. Hoogstraten, M. Staquet, A. Winkler, Reporting results of cancer treatment, Cancer 47:207 (1981).

12. S. Negrier, T. Philip, G. Stoter, S.D. Fossa, S. Janssen, A. Iacone, F.S. Cleton, O. Eremin, L. Israel, C. Jasmin, C. Rugarli, H.V.D. Masse, N. Thatcher, M. Symann, H.H. Bartsch, L. Bergmann, J.T. Bijman, P.A. Palmer and C.R. Franks, Interleukin-2 with or without LAK cells in metastatic renal cell carcinoma: a report of a European Multicentre Study, Eur. J. Cancer Clin. Oncol. 25:S21 (1989).

13. K.K. Oates and A.L. Goldstein, Thymosin, in: Biologic Therapy of Cancer, ed. V.T. De Vita, Jr. S. Hellman, S.A. Rosenberg, Publisher   J.B. Lippincott Company, Philadelphia (1991).

14. S.A. Serrate, R.S. Schulof, L. Leonidaridis, A.L. Goldstein, M.B. Sztein, Modulation of human natural killer cell cytotoxic activity. Lymphokine production, and interleukin 2 receptor expression by thymic hormones, J. Immunol. 7:2338 (1987).

COMBINATION OF CHRONIC INDOMETHACIN AND INTERMITTENT IL-2 THERAPY IN THE TREATMENT OF DISSEMINATED CANCER

Peeyush K. Lala[1,3], Nahla Al-Mutter[1], Ranjit Parhar[1], Mary Nel Saarloos[1], Diponkar Banerjee[2], Vivien Bramwell[3] and William C. Mertens[3]

Departments of [1]Anatomy, [2]Pathology and [3]Oncology
The University of Western Ontario
London, Ontario, Canada N6A 5C1

INTRODUCTION

Numerous effector cells of the immune system are capable of killing tumor cells *in vitro* as well as *in vivo* when properly activated. Antigen-specific T lymphocytes when exposed to certain tumor-specific antigens (TSA) in association with self MHC antigen can be triggered to produce tumor-specific cytotoxic cells in the presence of a second signal derived from T helper cells, now recognized as interleukin-2 (IL-2). However, only a small minority of spontaneously-derived tumors express TSA[1]. Secondly, T lymphocytes infiltrating tumor sites often remain inactive *in situ* because of host or tumor-related suppressor mechanisms, so that immunotherapy employing IL-2 alone may not be fully effective. However, the findings that tumor-infiltrating lymphocytes (TIL), when adoptively transferred, can selectively migrate to the tumor site, have led to promising therapeutic strategies employing IL-2 therapy in combination with TIL, or therapy with genetically modified TIL designed to deliver tumoricidal molecules at the tumor site[2]. Other anti-tumor effector cells do not require antigen-specific priming. These are natural killer (NK) lymphocytes and macrophages. When appropriately activated, e.g. with IL-2 or IL-2 in combination with other cytokines, these cells can kill a large spectrum of tumor cells *in vitro* as well as *in vivo*, and thus constitute a major effector arm of IL-2 therapy. Both these cell classes, NK cells in particular, represent a major component of the tumor-infiltrating mononuclear cells[3-6]. However, these cells also remain inactive *in situ*[5,6] and may resist adequate activation with IL-2 therapy alone. Our aims have been to elucidate the mechanisms underlying this inactivation and exploit this information to achieve maximal *in situ* activation of all killer cell lineages for eradication of the metastatic disease.

Combination Therapies 2, Edited by A.L. Goldstein
and E. Garaci Plenum Press, New York, 1993

In the present paper we show that host-derived or tumor-derived prostaglandin E_2 (PGE_2) presents a universal immunosuppressor molecule in the tumor-bearing host, responsible for inactivation of all IL-2-dependent killer cell lineages inclusive of T cells, NK cells and macrophages, because of its ability to down-regulate IL-2 receptors on effector cells and also to block IL-2 production. We also show that chronic indomethacin therapy (CIT), designed to block PGE_2 production, when initiated early, can reactivate NK cells *in situ*, halt primary tumor growth and prevent metastasis of certain murine tumors. CIT when combined with IL-2 therapy is then shown to eradicate established metastasis in a variety of murine tumor models and human tumors grown in nude mice, by activating all IL-2 dependent killer cell lineages *in situ*. Finally, we have recently tested this combination therapy in a phase 2 human trial for treating advanced renal cell carcinoma and melanoma patients with promising results. These results also raise the strong possibility that CIT (in combination with ranitidine therapy) without IL-2 therapy may offer an effective therapeutic modality for certain melanoma patients.

PGE$_2$-MEDIATED INACTIVATION OF HOST EFFECTOR CELLS

PGE_2 has long been recognized as a potential suppressor of a variety of immune responses[7]. Many tumors have been shown to produce high levels of PGE_2[8,9]. In addition, PGE_2 may also be host-derived. We have shown that tumor-bearing triggers host macrophages into PGE_2 production which increases with increasing tumor burden[10,11]. While the exact nature of this trigger remains to be identified, we observed that a loss of surface I-A antigen provides a phenotypic marker for this functional switch in host macrophages[12]. We believe that the maintenance of macrophage I-A expression requires the presence of IFN-γ in their micro-environment and that PGE_2 down-regulates the local production of IFN-γ by the immune cells[12]. Increased in situ levels of PGE_2, whether tumor-derived or host-derived, results in a functional inactivation of all potentially tumoricidal effector cells of the host. We found that in spite of an increased number of natural killer cells in the tumor-bearing host, they rapidly lose their killer function owing to this mechanism[5,6]. We have also noted that PGE_2 produced by macrophages isolated from tumor-bearing hosts can prevent *in vitro* activation of NK cells, LAK cells as well as tumoricidal macrophages[11]. At least two mechanisms have been identified for this pan-suppressor effect of PGE_2 on killer cells: down regulation of IL-2 receptors[13] and an inhibition of IL-2 production[13,14]. A down regulation of transferrin-receptors[14] as well as IFN-γ receptors[15] may represent additional mechanisms.

METASTASIS-PROMOTING ROLE OF PGE$_2$ BY ADDITIONAL TUMOR-RELATED MECHANISMS

While PGE_2 can promote metastasis owing to an inactivation of host natural effector cells such as NK cells and macrophages as described above, additional tumor-related mechanisms have also been proposed, such as promotion of tumor angiogenesis[10], and promotion of migrating ability of metastatic tumor cells[16].

PREVENTION OF SPONTANEOUS METASTASIS WITH CHRONIC INDOMETHACIN THERAPY

We tested the effects of CIT instituted early during the subcutaneous growth of spontaneously metastasizing (to the lungs) mammary adenocarcinomas in C3H/HeJ mice, some of which had been clonally derived in our laboratory from a spontaneous mammary tumor in the same mouse strain[17]. CIT given continuously at a dose of 14 μg indomethacin/ml of drinking water abrogated the NK-suppressor function of tumor-derived macrophages, revived the killer function of host NK cells and halted the growth of the primary tumors. More significantly, there was a complete prevention of spontaneous metastasis of metastasizable tumors. This therapy, when provided to C57BL/6 mice with established experimental lung metastasis of B16F10 melanomas, caused a reduction of the metastasis burden, but failed to eradicate the metastatic disease[18], apparently because the endogenous IL-2 production was still inadequate for an optimal activation and amplification of host killer cells *in situ*. These findings provided the rationale for combining CIT with IL-2 therapy for the treatment of well established metastases, as summarized below.

ERADICATION OF EXPERIMENTAL AND SPONTANEOUS METASTASES IN MICE BY THE COMBINATION OF CIT AND IL-2 THERAPY

We tested the therapeutic efficacy of this combination therapy in a variety of murine tumor models: experimental (following intravenous inoculation of tumor cells) lung metastasis of B16F10 melanoma in C57BL/6 mice[18,19], KHT35L1 fibrosarcoma in C3H/HeJ mice[20], experimental as well as spontaneous (following subcutaneous inoculation of tumor cells) lung metastasis of a highly metastatic C3L5 mammary adenocarcinoma (these cells had been selected *in vivo* for their strong lung-metastasizing ability) in C3H/HeJ mice[21,22]. In addition, we also tested this combination therapy in nude mice bearing experimental lung metastasis of human melanoma line P52[23], or multi-organ (lung, skin, lymph nodes and brain) metastasis of human melanoma line 70W[24]. CIT was started in each tumor model following the documented establishment of lung metastases, at a non-toxic dose of 14 μg indomethacin/ml of drinking water. IL-2 therapy was then added as multiple (2 or more) 5 day rounds of Cetus IL-2 given as 25,000 Cetus U (1.5 x 10^5 I.U.) i.p., every 8 h, starting 5 days after the onset of CIT and repeated after 5 days of IL-2 free intervals. This IL-2 regimen was based on our own experience as well as experience in the murine model reported by the Rosenberg group[25].

Results in all of the above tumor models were highly encouraging. CIT alone, or one or two rounds of IL-2 alone, although capable of a significant reduction in the metastasis burden, failed to result in a complete eradication of metastasis. CIT combined with one IL-2 round nearly completely abrogated the visible metastasis when examined shortly after the IL-2 round[18], but failed to result in lasting cure[19]. CIT combined with two or more rounds of IL-2 resulted in permanent cure in 30-80% of the hosts, depending on the tumor-model. Intermittent indomethacin therapy provided during the IL-2 rounds alone (as conventionally done in many human trials) showed no significant improvement in results as compared to IL-2 therapy alone[19]. CIT alone activated host killer cells with NK-like

(Asialo GM-1[+], Thy-1[-], Lyt-2[-]) phenotype and function, whereas the combination therapy generated highly active killer cells in the spleen as well as the metastasis site (lungs) inclusive of lymphoid cells with LAK-like phenotype (Asialo-GM-1[+], Thy-1[+], Lyt-2[-]) and cytolytic activity, as well as tumoricidal macrophages (Asialo-GM-1[+]). Simultaneous administration of anti-Asialo GM-1 antibody totally abrogated the therapeutic effects, indicating that the effects were largely due to Asialo GM-1[+] killer cells[19]. In the case of the spontaneous metastasis model, primary mammary adenocarcinomas as well as their metastases regressed completely in the majority of animals[21,22]. In this tumor model, which is moderately immunogenic, most of the tumor-free mice surviving after the immunotherapy exhibited a complete resistance to a second tumor challenge, indicating their acquisition of T cell immunity. Therapeutically activated host killer cells in this tumor model also exhibited additional ADCC-like activity in the presence of sera from treated mice, indicative of a beneficial B cell stimulation. The fact that this combination therapy was equally effective in nude mice bearing human melanomas[23,24] suggested that this regimen can work in the absence of functional T lymphocytes. Finally, we have shown that ibuprofen (another inhibitor of PGE_2 synthetase) can effectively replace indomethacin (if required because of low indomethacin tolerance in certain cases) in this immunotherapeutic protocol. C3H/HeN mice (which showed a lower indomethacin tolerance than C3H/HeJ mice) bearing C3L5 mammary adenocarcinoma metastases exhibited very good anti-tumor responses when ibuprofen was substituted for indomethacin[26].

We have further shown that this therapeutic protocol has no detrimental effect on host hemopoietic stem cells. Our results in the C3L5 mammary adenocarcinoma model in C3H/HeJ mice reveal that the total number of hemopoietic spleen colony forming units (CFU-S) in the body increases significantly in the tumor-bearing host in spite of the induction of certain CFU-S suppressor cells. The CIT + IL-2 therapy in these animals leads to a further amplification of the CFU-S numbers in the body[27].

APPLICATION OF THE COMBINATION THERAPY IN A PHASE 2 HUMAN TRIAL

Encouraged by the success of this combination therapy in the animal models, we applied this therapy to a Phase 2 human trial of 25 advanced renal cell carcinoma[28,29] and 21 advanced melanoma[30,31] patients (patient profile given in Table 1), as summarized below.

Treatment Regimen:

Patients were placed on oral indomethacin (50 mg thrice daily, escalated later to 75 mg/dose if patient tolerance permitted) and ranitidine (150 mg twice a day, to reduce indomethacin-induced dyspepsia), at least one week prior to IL-2 therapy, and continued until intolerance or disease progression. Continuous venous infusion of IL-2 was administered for at least one course, and three courses in most patients, each consisting of 5 days of treatment at 3×10^6 Cetus U (18×10^6 I.U.)/m²/day for the first course, with escalation during the subsequent courses (to

Table 1   Profile of treated patients

	Renal Cell Cancer	Melanoma
Number		
Total/male/female	25/17/8	21/9/12
Mean age (years)	50	48
WHO performance status (0/1/2)	11/11/3	10/9/2
Previous therapy		
Surgery	19/25	15/21
Chemo	1/25	3/21
Radiation	6/25	3/21
Other	2/25	-
Disease (metastasis) site		
Subcutaneous (nodes)	-	17/25
Lung	4/25	6/25
Bone	2/25	2/25
Liver	2/25	7/25
Other abdominal	17/25	3/25
Median cross-sectional area of disease (cm^2)	69	40

a maximum of 36×10^6 I.U./m^2/day, during the last course), if toxicity allowed. Treatment was carried out in a general oncology ward. Hypotension was managed by the judicious use of intravenous crystalloid solutions, without administration of vasopressor agents. IL-2 toxicity was adequately managed with temporary reduction or stoppage of IL-2 infusion, requiring no intensive care and resulting in no patient mortality.

Clinical Responses to the Combination Therapy

Objective responses exhibited by the renal cell carcinoma and melanoma patients to the presently described combination therapy (Table 2) compares favorably with response rates reported for IL-2/LAK or high dose bolus IL-2 therapy requiring costly intensive supportive care and use of vasopressor agents in most cases (Table 3). In the case of renal cell carcinoma, our results are more encouraging than those reported by most centres except for the NCI Surgery branch[32]. More importantly, the present protocol can be conducted safely in a general oncology ward and thus is more economical than the conventionally practised IL-2 regimens (listed in Table 3), in particular, the IL-2/LAK regimen. In the case of melanomas, the most interesting outcome of our trial was that two patients exhibited objective responses (one complete, one partial) to indomethacin (plus ranitidine) prior to the onset of IL-2 therapy. These patients, at the initiation of the therapy had well-documented progressive disease, thus excluding the possibility that these responses were spontaneous remissions. One of these patients (the complete responder) was not given IL-2 at all, at the patient's own request. In spite of the small sample size, these findings raise the strong possibility that some melanoma patients may respond to indomethacin/ranitidine alone. Since these drugs are often concomitantly used in most IL-2 regimens for symptomatic relief of fever/dyspepsia, they may have accounted for some of the responses ascribed earlier to IL-2 therapy. This scenario is a reminder of that described for primary gliomas, in which corticosteroid-induced CT scan changes may be attributed to anti-cancer interventions, e.g. chemotherapy[42]. Thus indomethacin/ranitidine protocol deserves to be tested in a randomized trial of melanoma patients.

Table 2 Responses to CIT + IL-2 Therapy

	Renal Cell Carcinoma	Melanoma
Objective	5/25 (20%)	3/21 (14%)
Complete	2/25 (8%)	1'/21 (5%)
Partial	3/25 (12%)	2'/21 (9%)
Minor	3/25 (12%)	-
(20-33% reduction of disease)		

'One complete and one partial response occurred with indomethacin/ranitidine alone prior to IL-2 therapy. The complete responder received no IL-2 at the patient's own request.

Present results cannot distinguish between the effects of indomethacin from those of ranitidine (a histamine-type-2 receptor antagonist) or the combination of the two drugs. H-2 receptor antagonists have been reported to reduce histamine-induced T suppressor cell function[43], improve NK function[44], enhance IL-2

Table 3 Reported response rates with IL-2 therapy in renal cell carcinoma and melanoma patients.

Regimen	Objective response rate		Use of intensive care,	Reference
	Renal Ca	Melanoma	vasopressor agents	
Bolus IL-2/LAK	35%	21%	yes	32
	14%	-	yes	33
	-	17%	yes	34
	13%	-	yes	35
Bolus IL-2 plus	9%	-	yes	36
Cont IL-2/LAK	-	14%	yes	37
Cont IL-2/LAK	3%	-	yes	38
	-	2.2%		39
Bolus IL-2	22%	24%	yes	32
	0%	-	yes	40
	8%	-	yes	35
	-	21%	yes	41

production[45] and their effectiveness as single agents has remained highly controversial in cancer immunotherapy[46]. In our *in vitro* studies[47], we have noted that ranitidine augments IL-2 action in the generation of LAK cell activity in the peripheral blood lymphocytes of a minority of healthy subjects or cancer patients, but does not have significant additive or synergistic effect in the presence of indomethacin. The role of ranitidine in combination with indomethacin and IL-2 *in vivo* therefore remains speculative.

Lymphocyte phenotype and function in patients subjected to CIT + IL-2 therapy

We have examined changes in the phenotype[48] and function[49] of peripheral blood lymphocytes during the course of the present combination therapy. Blood samples were drawn prior to the initiation of indomethacin (and ranitidine), after one week (or more) of indomethacin therapy shortly before the onset of IL-2 therapy, and shortly following each 5 day round of IL-2. Phenotyping was done for a large number of markers to identify various subsets of T, B and NK cells as well as IL-2 receptors (55 Kd chain) on these subsets by flow cytometry. Killer function of lymphocytes was measured against NK-sensitive K562 erythroleukemia and NK-resistant, LAK-sensitive Daudi lymphoma targets, in freshly isolated peripheral blood leukocytes (PBL) as well as PBL cultured for three days with IL-2 in the presence or absence of indomethacin. The results can be summarized as follows. Lymphocyte killer function was markedly suppressed in the patient population as compared to normal healthy control subjects, however, this change was not predictable by any change in lymphocyte phenotype. This suppression in NK or LAK cell function was partially reversible by *in vitro* treatment of cells with indomethacin. Indomethacin (plus ranitidine) therapy alone led to a small improvement in killer function in some but not all patients, unrelated to clinical responses, or phenotypic changes. Each round of IL-2 therapy led to marked improvement in killer function of lymphocytes in all patients, which was significantly higher in the responders as compared to non-responders in the case of renal cell carcinoma patients during the first two rounds of IL-2. A similar trend was noticeable in melanomas but no significance could be ascribed to this difference because of the small sample size. The absolute lymphocyte counts (inclusive of all subsets) increased during IL-2 therapy in all patients, more significantly so in the responders as compared to the non-responders in the renal cell carcinoma group. The IL-2 receptor densities also increased more significantly in the responders, in particular, on the CD4+ (T helper) cells. Interestingly, two distinctive features in the pretreatment values of lymphocyte phenotype/function were noted in the responders: (a) renal carcinoma responders had a higher Daudi-killer (LAK-like) activity in unstimulated lymphocytes, and (b) melanoma responders had a higher absolute count of CD8 + (cytotoxic/suppressor T) cells in the blood. Further studies are needed to test whether these features are predictive indicators of clinical responses and thus should be useful in patient selection for this therapy.

SUMMARY

Our animal models have shown that continuous oral administration of indomethacin to abrogate PGE$_2$-mediated immunosuppression in the tumor-bearing host, initiated before IL-2 therapy leads to remarkable improvement of therapeutic efficacy of systemic IL-2 in curing established spontaneous and experimental metastasis in a variety of tumor models, and activating anti-tumor effector cell lineages *in situ*. We have tested this combination therapy (continuous oral indomethacin and ranitidine, initiated before IL-2 therapy; IL-2 therapy given as three courses of continuous venous infusion) in a phase 2 trial of renal cell carcinoma (n = 25) and melanoma (n = 21) patients. Objective response rates were 20% and 14%, respectively. Manageable IL-2 toxicity without the requirement of intensive supportive care or vasopressor agents were important distinctive features. Two melanoma patients achieved objective responses (one complete, one partial) with indomethacin (and ranitidine) alone indicating that these drugs may be of therapeutic value in certain melanomas independent of IL-2. Certain pre-treatment immunological parameters (such as significant LAK-like activity in the PBL of renal cell carcinoma patients and high absolute CD8 + lymphocyte count in the blood of melanoma patients) may be valuable indicators of response to this therapy.

ACKNOWLEDGEMENTS

Studies reported in this article were supported by grants from The National Cancer Institute of Canada with funds provided by the Canadian Cancer Society and performed under the auspices of the Cancer Treatment Evaluation Program, U.S. National Cancer Institute (T87-0151 and T87-0213).

REFERENCES

1. H. Hewitt, E. Blake and A. Walder, A critique for the evidence of active host defense against cancer, based on personal studies of 27 murine tumors of spontaneous origin. Brit. J. Cancer. 33:241-259 (1976).
2. S. Rosenberg, The immunotherapy and gene therapy of cancer. J. Clin. Oncol. 10:180-199 (1992).
3. H.F. Pross and R.S. Kerbel, An assessment of intratumor phagocytic and surface marker-bearing cells in a series of autochthonous and early passaged chemically induced murine sarcomas. J. Nat. Cancer Inst., 57:1157-1167 (1976).
4. V. Santer, J.H. Mastromarino and P.K. Lala, Characterization of lymphocyte subsets in spontaneous mouse mammary tumors and host lymphoid organs. Int. J. Cancer, 25:159-168 (1980).
5. P.K. Lala, V. Santer, H. Libenson and R.S. Parhar, Changes in the natural killer cell population during tumor development.   I. Kinetics and in vivo significance. Cell Immunol., 93:250-264 (1985).
6. R.S. Parhar and P.K. Lala, Changes in the host natural killer cell population during tumor development. II. The mechanism of suppression of NK activity. Cell Immunol. 93:265-279 (1985).
7. J.S. Goodwin and J. Ceuppens, Regulation of the immune response by prosta-glandins. J. Clin. Immunol. 3:295-315 (1983).
8. M.R. Young and S. Knies, Prostaglandin E production by Lewis lung carcinoma: mechanism for tumor establishment in vivo. J. Natl. Cancer Inst., 72:919-922 (1984).
9. A.M. Fulton, H.E. Ownby, J. Frederick and M.J. Brennan, Relationship of tumor prostaglandin levels to early recurrence in women with primary breast cancer: clinical update. Invasion Metastasis, 6:83-94 (1986).

10. P.K. Lala, PGE₂-mediated inactivation of potentially tumoricidal effector cells of the host during tumor development: relevance to metastasis and immunotherapy. In: "Carcinogenesis and Dietary Fat" S. Abraham, ed., Martinus Nijhoff, Publisher, Norwell, MA, pp. 219-232 (1989).

11. R.S. Parhar and P.K. Lala, PGE₂-mediated inactivation of various killer lineage cells by tumor bearing host macrophages. J. Leukocyte Biol., 46:474-484 (1988).

12. J.A.S. Nelson, R.S. Parhar, J.M. Scodras and P.K. Lala, Down-regulation of macrophage 1-A expression in tumor-bearing mice. J. Leukocyte Biol., 48:394-402 (1990).

13. P.K. Lala, T.G. Kennedy and R.S. Parhar, Suppression of lymphocyte alloreactivity by early gestational human decidua. II. Characterization of suppressor mechanisms. Cell Immunol., 116:411-422 (1988).

14. S. Chouaib, K.K. Welte, R. Mertelsman, et al., Prostaglandin E2 acts at two distinct pathways of T lymphocyte activation: inhibition of interluekin-2 production and down-regulation of transferrin receptor expression. J. Immunol., 135:1172-1179 (1985).

15. M. Elkashab, R.S. Parhar and P.K. Lala, Chronic indomethacin therapy reverses PGE₂-mediated suppression of interferon-gamma and IL-2 receptor development on lymphoyctes of tumor-bearing mice and augments receptor development during therapy with IL-2, interferon-gamma or interferon-gamma plus IL-2. XIX International Leukocyte Culture Conference, Banff,AB, p 79 (Abstract) (1988).

16. M.R. Young, M.E. Young and H.T. Wepsik, Effect of prostaglandin E₂ producing nonmetastataic Lewis lung carcinoma cells on the migration of prostaglandin-E₂ responsive metastataic Lewis lung carcinoma cells. Cancer Res., 47:3679-3683 (1987).

17. P.K. Lala, R.S. Parhar and P. Singh, Indomethacin-therapy abrogates prostaglandin mediated suppression of natural killer activity in tumor bearing mice and prevents tumor metastasis. Cell Immunol. 99:108-118 (1986).

18. R.S. Parhar and P.K. Lala, Amelioration of B16F10 melanoma lung metastasis in mice by combination therapy with indomethacin and interleukin-2. J. Exp. Med., 165:14-28 (1987).

19. P.K. Lala and R.S. Parhar, Cure of B16F10 melanoma lung metastasis in mice by chronic indomethacin therapy combined with repeated rounds of IL-2: Characteristics of killer cells generated in situ. Cancer Research, 48:1072-1079 (1988).

20. R.S. Parhar, A. Chambers and P.K. Lala, A comparison of the efficacy of indomethacin, IL-2, IFN-τ or their various combinations in the treatment of experimental murine lung metastases. Proc. 19th Internat. Leucocyte Culture Conf., Banff, AB, Abstract, 79 (1988).

21. P.K. Lala and R.S. Parhar, Chronic indomethacin therapy combined with IL-2 cures primary mammary adenocarcinomas and their spontaneous lung metastases. Proc. Amer. Assoc. Cancer Res. 29:405 (1988).

22. P.K. Lala and R.S. Parhar, Cure of primary adenocarcinomas and their spontaneous lung metastases with chronic indomethacin therapy combined with IL-2. Proc. Can. Fed. Biol. Soc., Abstract, 29:130 (1988).

23. P.K. Lala, M. Elkhashab, R.S. Kerbel and R.S. Parhar, Cure of human melanoma lung metastases in nude mice with chronic indomethacin therapy combined with multiple rounds of IL-2: characteristics of killer cells generated in situ. Internat. Immunol., 2:1149-1161 (1990).

24. R.S. Parhar, R.S. Kerbel and P.K. Lala, Killer cell activation in situ and cure of multi-organ human melanoma metastases in nude mice with chronic indomethacin + IL-2 therapy. Proc. Amer. Assoc. Cancer Res., Abstract, 3:379 (1989).

25. R. Lafreniere and S. Rosenberg, Successful immunotherapy of murine experimental hepatic metastases with lymphokine-activated killer cells and recombinant interleukin-2. Cancer Res., 45:3735-3740 (1985).

26. N.K.S. Khoo, F.P.H. Chan, M.N. Saarloos and P.K. Lala, Immunotherapy of mammary adenocarcinoma metastases in C3H/HeN mice with chronic administrtion of cyclo-oxygenase inhibitors alone or in combination with IL-2. Clin. Exp. Metastasis, 10:239-252 (1992).

27. M.N. Saarloos, N.K.S. Khoo and P.K. Lala, Effects of cancer immunotherapy with indomethacin and IL-2 on murine hemopoietic stem cells. Cancer Res., in press (1992).

28. W.C. Mertens, V.H.C. Bramwell, D. Banerjee, F. Gwardry-Sridhar, N. Al-Mutter, R.S. Parhar and P.K. Lala, Chronic oral indomethacin and ranitidine with intermittent continuous infusion interleukin-2 in advanced renal cell carcinoma. Submitted for publication (1992).

29. V.H.C. Bramwell, W.C. Mertens and P.K. Lala, Continuous oral indomethacin (Indo) and ranitidine (Rant) and continuous venous infusion of interleukin-2 (IL-2) in advanced renal carcinoma. Proc. Amer. Soc. Clin. Oncol., Abstract, 10:171 (1991).

30. W.C. Mertens, V.H.C. Bramwell, F. Gwadry-Sridhar, W. Romano, D. Banerjee and P.K. Lala, Do indomethacin and ranitidine contribute to responses seen in advanced melanoma patients treated with high dose interleukin-2? Lancet, in press (1992).

31. W.C. Mertens, V.H.C. Bramwell and P.K. Lala, Do indomethacin (Indo) and ranitidine (Rant) contribute significantly to responses in advanced melanoma patients treated with high dose interleukin-2? Proc. Amer. Soc. Clin. Oncol. 10:209 (1991).

32. S.A. Rosenberg, Clinical immunotherapy studies in the surgery branch of the U.S. National Cancer Institute. Cancer Treat. Rev. 16(Suppl A):115-121 (1989).

33. R.I. Fisher, C.A. Coltman, J.A. Doroshow, et al., A phase II clinical trial of interleukin-2 and lymphokine activated killer cells (LAK) in metastatic renal cancer. Ann. Intern. Med. 108:518-523 (1988).

34. J.P. Dutcher. S. Creekmore. G.R. Weiss, et al., A phase II study of interleukin-2 and lymphokine activated killer (LAK) cells in patients with metastatic malignant melanoma. J. Clin. Oncol. 7:477-485 (1989).

35. M.S. McCabe, D. Stablein and M.J. Hawkins, The modified group C experience - phase III randomized trials of IL-2 versus IL-2/LAK in advanced renal cell carcinoma and advanced melanoma. Proc. Am. Soc. Clin. Oncol. Abstract, 10:213 (1991).

36. D.R. Parkinson, R.I. Fisher, A.A. Rayner, et al., Therapy of renal cell carcinoma with interleukin-2 and lymphokine-activated killer cells: Phase II experience with a hybrid bolus and continuous infusion interleukin-2 regimen. J. Clin. Oncol., 8:1630-1636 (1990).

37. M. Bar, M. Sznol, M.B. Atkins, et al., Metastatic malignant melanoma treated with combined bolus and continuous infusion interleuken-2 and lymphokine-activated killer cells. J. Clin. Oncol., 8:1138-1147 (1990).

38. R.O. Dillman, R.K. Oldham, K.W. Tauer, et al., Continuous interleukin-2 and lymphokine-activated killer cells for advanced cancer. A National Biotherapy Study Group trial. J. Clin. Oncol. 9:1233-1240 (1991).

39. J.P. Dutcher, E.R. Gaynor, D.H. Boldt, et al., A phase II study of high dose continuous infusion interleukin-2 with lymphokine-activated killer cells in patients with metastatic melanoma. J. Clin. Oncol., 9:641-648 (1991).

40. J.S. Abrams, A.A. Rayner, P.H. Wiernik, et al., High dose recombinant interleukin-2 alone: a regimen with limited activity in the treatment of advanced renal cell carcinoma. J. Natl. Cancer Inst. 82:1202-1206 (1990).

41. D.R. Parkinson, J.S. Abrams, P.H. Wiernik, et al., Interleukin-2 therapy in patients with metastatic malignant melanoma: A phase II study. J. Clin. Oncol. 8:1650-1656 (1990).

42. J.G. Cairncross, D.R. MacDonald, J.H.W. Pexman and J. Ives, Steroid-induced CT changes in patients with recurrent malignant glioma. Neurology, 38:724-726 (1988).

43. D.E. Griswold, S. Alexxi, A.M. Badger, G. Poste and N. Hanna, Inhibition of T suppressor cell expression by histamine type 2 (H_2) receptor antagonists. J. Immunol., 132:3054-3057 (1984).

44. J.I. Allen, H.J. Syropoulos, G. Grant, et al., Cimetidine modulates natural killer cell function of patients with chronic lymphocytic leukemia. J. Lab. Clin. Med., 109:396-401 (1987).

45. F. Aweeka, P. Lizak, M. Garovoy, et al., Interleukin-2 and immunoglobulin increases with H_2-antagonists in humans. Transplant Proc. 21:1718-1721 (1989).

46. T. Smith, Histamine type 2-receptor antagonists in cancer immunotherapy. Compr. Ther., 16:8-13 (1990).

47. P.K. Lala, W. Mertens, R.S. Parhar and N. Al-Mutter, Effects of ranatidine on LAK cell generation with PBL of normal and cancer-bearing subjects. Proc. Am. Assoc. Cancer Res., Abstract, 31:277 (1990).

48. D. Banerjee, W.C. Mertens, V.H.C. Bramwell and P.K. Lala, Sequential changes in lymphocyte subsets in patients on chronic indomethacin + IL-2 therapy for advanced cancer. Proc. Amer. Assoc. Cancer Res., Abstract, 32:247 (1992).

49. P.K. Lala, W.C. Mertens, V.H.C. Bramwell, D. Banerjee and N. Al-Mutter, Correlation of in vitro tumoricidal responses to chronic oral indomethacin therapy and intravenous IL-2 in melanoma and renal carcinoma patients. Proc. Amer. Assoc. Cancer Res., Abstract, 32:248 (1991).

COMBINATION CHEMOTHERAPY AND CYTOKINES IN THE TREATMENT OF ADVANCED PRIMARY LUNG CANCER: RESULTS OF A CONTROLLED CLINICAL TRIAL

G. Sergio Del Giacco[1], Giovanni Mantovani[2], Paola Lai[2], Emiliano Turnu[2], Francesca Locci[1], Anna Carla Scanu[3], Guido Pusceddu[3]

[1]Dept. Internal Medicine and Clinical Immunology
[2]Dept. of Medical Oncology
University of Cagliari Medical School
[3]"R. Binaghi" Hospital,
Cagliari, Italy, 09124

INTRODUCTION

The secondary immunodeficiency present in advanced tumors justifies the use of biological response modifiers, like thymic hormones and/or Interferon (IFN)[1].

A randomized clinical trial was undertaken to evaluate the effects of the addition of Thymostimulin (TS) ± beta IFN to conventional chemotherapy of primary lung cancer. The patients (pts) were randomly assigned to one of three different regimens: the first (A) consisting of Chemotherapy (CH) plus TS, the second (B) of CH + TS + beta IFN (intermittent administration), the third (C) of CH + TS + beta IFN (continuous administration).

Twenty pts with SCLC (2) and with NSCLC (18) entered the study (mean age 57.2 years, range 44-65): 6 in the group A, 8 in the group B and 6 in the group C. The three groups were comparable for histology and TNM staging. An immunological assessment was also carried out both in vivo (skin tests response) and in vitro (response to polyclonal mitogens, to IL 2 and to PHA + IL 2).

The best clinical response has been achieved in the group B (3 PR) compared to C (1 PR, 1MR, 3 NC) and A (1 PR, 1 MR, 3 NC).

The results of this trial have been previously reported by our Group[2,3].

AIM OF THE TRIAL

The suggestions emerging from our previous trial (1988-90), carried out on a small, but well balanced, number of pts, prompted us to prolonge the trial, utilizing only the Arm B (Chemotherapy + TS + intermittent beta IFN), for the years 1990-91.

Patients: The accrual was of 13 pts, all males (mean age: 62 years, range 42-70). The clinical characteristics of pts are shown in Table 1.

Combination Therapies 2, Edited by A.L. Goldstein
and E. Garaci Plenum Press, New York, 1993

Table 1. Clinical characteristics of patients.

Patients Sex	Age	Histologic Type	Stage	Chemoth. n° cicles	Objective response	Protocol Chemo+Ts+IFN-beta
F.L. M	67	SC	ED	3	P	Standard
D.V. M	60	EC	III B	4	PR	Standard
V.A. M	60	EC	IV -	12	P	Standard+MTC-VP16
C.G. M	70	SC	LD	5	PR (CR)	PTC-EPR-VCR
C.L. M	50	AC	IV	9	PR	Standard + 5FU-MTC
A.F. M	70	EC	III B	16	NC	Standard
C.P. M	65	EC	III B	11	PR	Standard + MTC
P.E. M	66	AC	IV	3	NC	Standard + CDDP-VDS
M.A. M	42	SC	LD	3	NC	Standard
C.A. M	65	SC	ED	4	PR	Standard
S.L. M	68	SC	ED	5	P dead (5 months)	CTX - VDS
P.S. M	58	EC	IV	6	P dead (6 months)	Standard + PTC
C.G. M	65	EC	IV	3	P	EPR - VDS

EC: EPIDERMOID CARCINOMA   ED: EXTENDED DISEASE
AC: ADENOCARCINOMA   LD: LIMITED DISEASE
SC: SMALL CELL LUNG CANCER

P : PROGRESSION   CR: COMPLETE RESPONSE
PR: PARTIAL RESPONSE   NC: NO CHANGE

Combination chemotherapy: Cisplatin 70 mg/sqm/i.v. day 1,VP 16 (Etoposide) 120 mg/sqm/days 1,3,5 every 4 weeks for 3 subsequent cycles (induction therapy). If an objective clinical response was obtained, then 2 more cycles were administered. In the event of disease progression, the following alternative non cross-resistant regimen was administered: Epirubicin 55 mg/sqm/i.v., Vindesine 3 mg/sqm/i.v., Cytoxan 500 mg/sqm/i.v. and CCNU 30 mg/sqm/p.o., all the first day every 24 days until progression and in any case for at least 5 cycles.

The pts surviving beyond one year, to whom the total doses foreseen of drugs had been overcome, were given an alternative regimen containing Mytomicin C and Lonidamine.

Immunotherapy

Intermittent Beta IFN (Frone,Serono): The beta IFN, Frone, an human IFN obtained by cultured fibroblasts, was administered at a dosage of 1×10^6 I.U./sqm/i.m. days 7,15,23 for the first month of treatment, 2×10^6 I.U./sqm/i.m. the same days for the second month, 3×10^6 I.U./sqm/i.m. the same days for the third month and then at the same dosage of the third month for the subsequent months.

The following effects have been studied: antiproliferative, antiinfective, immunomodulating, on haemopoiesis, on performance status, on side effects of chemotherapy

RESULTS

Response to therapy: No CR, 5 PR (38.5%), 3 NC (23.05%) (PR + NC 61.5%) and 5 P (38.5%) were achieved, with 1 PR > 12 months and 1 NC > 12 months.

Survival. The pts alive at March 1992 were 11/13 (84.6%).

Treatment's toxicity: The side effects were those generally reported for IFN therapy, the haematologic toxicity were mild.

No pts must delay the chemotherapy due to the side effects of immunotherapy.

Immunological findings: As far as it concerns the in vivo immune response, i.e. skin tests to recall antigens, 3/13 (23%) pts showed a shift of the response from the negative to positive, 9/13 (69%) showed no change (6 remained +, 3 remained -), 1/13 (8%) from positive became negative (Table 2).

Table 2. In vivo immunological evaluation: skin tests (comprehensive results).

No of patients		RESPONSE before treatment		after
3	FROM	−	TO	+
6	FROM	+	TO	+
1	FROM	+	TO	−
3	FROM	−	TO	−

Infections. The infectious episodes were very rare: with reference to this, the results of our previous study are to be stressed[4], showing a striking difference in incidence of infections, mainly pulmonary, between the group of pts treated with chemoimmunotherapy and that of pts treated with chemotherapy only.

CONCLUSIONS

The present trial, still in progress, seems to confirm the results of our previous one. In particular, the addition of an association of thymic hormones plus beta IFN at low dosages intermittently administered to the conventional chemotherapy of primary lung cancer is lacking of untoward side effects, can be beneficial for controlling a further immune depression induced by treatments and for protecting the pts from severe opportunistic pulmonary infections, allowing to them a better "quality of life".

Based on the results so far obtained, a new study was then undertaken to assess the therapeutic activity of the combination chemotherapy with CDDP plus VP16 in association with alpha$_1$ thymosin (TA1) and alpha 2b Interferon (IFN) in NSCLC pts, in terms of: a) response rate; b) duration of response; c) time to progression; d) overall survival of pts. A second purpose was that of assess the treatment's toxicity and the third objective was that of study the immunological profile of the treated pts, mainly the peripheral blood lymphocyte phenotype with monoclonal antibodies (CD3, CD4, CD8, CD25, CD20, DR), the expression of IL 2 receptor and the response to polyclonal mitogen PHA, to IL 2 and to PHA + IL 2. Ten pts with primary NSCLC (mean age 63.5 years, range 42-72) completely fulfilling the selection criteria entered the study and were randomized either to treatment A (only chemotherapy: CDDP 100 mg/m^2 i.v. day 1, VP16 120 mg/m^2 i.v. days 1-3) or to treatment B (the same chemotherapy plus immunotherapy with TA1 1 mg s.c. days 8-11 and 15-18, IFN 3x10^6 I.U./sqm/s.c. day 11 and day 18 of the cycle. 5 pts were assigned to treatment A and 5 pts to treatment B: till now 3 pts have completed 3 cycles, 1 pt 2 cycles and 6 pts have completed only 1 cycle. The study is yet underway.

Acknowledgments

Work supported by 1991 Grant from the Sardinian Region to the "Center for Tumor Immunotherapy".

REFERENCES

1. C. Favalli, A. Mastino, S. Grelli, F. Pica, G. Rasi and E. Garaci, Rationale for therapeutic approaches with thymic hormones, Interleukin 2 and Interferon in combination with chemotherapy, in: "New frontiers in the therapy of malignancies: from biological approaches to clinical trials", G. Mantovani, B. Bonavida, G.S. Del Giacco, G.A. Granger and J.M. Kirkwood, eds., Serono Symposia Review No. 25, Ares - Serono Symposia, Rome (1991), 47-57.
2. G. Mantovani, V. Arangino, F. Locci, A.C. Scanu, A. Podda, G. Salaris, G. Pusceddu and G.S. Del Giacco, Combination chemotherapy and cytokines in the treatment of advanced primary lung cancer: controlled trial three year results, in: "New frontiers in the therapy of malignancies: from biological approaches to clinical trials", G. Mantovani, B. Bonavida, G.S. Del Giacco, G.A. Granger and J.M. Kirkwood, eds., Serono Symposia Review No. 25, Ares - Serono Symposia, Rome (1991), 209-217.
3. G.S. Del Giacco, G. Mantovani, V. Arangino, F. Locci, A.C. Scanu and G. Pusceddu, Combination chemotherapy and cytokines in the treatment of advanced primary lung cancer: Results at three years of a controlled clinical trial, in: "Combination Therapies: Biological Response Modifiers in the treatment of cancer and infectious diseases", A.L. Goldstein and E. Garaci, eds., Plenum Press, New York (1992), 79-85.
4. G.S. Del Giacco, G. Mantovani, G. Piludu, F. Locci, M. Loy, M.C. Piras, L. Cengiarotti, M. Lo Presti, G. Meloni, E. Montaldo and G. Pusceddu, Thymic factors in lung cancer, in: "Thymus Hormones in Oncology", G. Nagel, G. Schioppacassi and P. Schuff-Werner, eds., Serono Symposia Review No. 19, Ares-Serono Symposia, Rome (1988), 149-156.

BIOLOGICAL RESPONSE MODIFIERS AND DIFFERENTIATING

AGENTS IN MYELODISPLASTIC SYNDROMES

Adriano Venditti, Maria Teresa Scimo', Giovanni Del Poeta, Roberto Stasi, Ugo Coppetelli, Mario Masi, Manrico Cecconi, Maurizio Tribalto , Giuseppe Papa, Cartesio Favalli,[1]and Enrico Garaci[1]

Cattedra di Ematologia - Ospedale S.Eugenio - Università di Roma "Tor Vergata"
Piazzale dell' Umanesimo 10 - 00144 Roma- Italy
[1]Cattedra di Microbiologia - Università di Roma "Tor Vergata"
Via Orazio Raimondo - 00174 Roma -Italy

INTRODUCTION

Myelodisplastic syndrome (MDS) includes a spectrum of hematological alterations that have in common the progressive evolution of a monoclonal population of hemopoietic cells, arising from an initial genetic insult, to a preleukemic status and eventually to overt acute leukemia.[1,2,3]

It is likely that most or all of these conditions are caused by mutations,[4,5,6] and chromosome abnormalities[7,8] that affect the growth factor, growth factor receptor, growth factor signal transduction, DNA transcription and/or cell cycle control pathways in hemopoietic precursor.

MDS have been well defined since 1982 when the French-American-British (FAB) group published the study dividing the MDS in five categories of disorders[9] (Table 1) on the basis of morphology and the percentage of the blasts in the bone marrow.

TABLE 1. Classification of Myelodisplastic Syndromes

Refractory Anemia (RA)

Refractory Anemia with Ring Sideroblasts (RARS)

Refractory Anemia with Excess Blasts (RAEB)

RAEB in transformation (RAEB-t)

On clinical point of view the manifestations may vary from mild to incipient acute leukemia; the early stages of MDS are characterized by minimal hematological signs and many cases are discovered by occasional routine examinations.

No specific or generally effective therapy for the MDS exists at this stage, the therapy rlies largely on the administration of blood components to combat cytopenias, and antibiotics to face infection. Obviously those patients requiring a substantial transfusional support are at risk for iron overload and hemocromatosis. As consequence, the treatment of MDS has raised some of the most fundamental questions in the treatment of hematological malignancies and also provided the possibility for throwing light at innovative forms of therapy, especially those forms dealing with the usage of differentiating agents and/or biological response modifiers. Infact a number of physicians agree about the assumption that aggressive chemotherapy is not indicated unless the appearance of an overt acute phase.

Low doses of cytosine arabinoside (LD-ARAc) administered at doses of 5-30 mg/m^2/day encountered the favour of numerous authors.[10,11,12,13] In vitro studies of the human myeloid leukemia cells demostrated ARAc prolongs the time of DNA replication and enhances terminal differentiation.[14] The efficacy of ARAc was therefore, tested in a number of clinical trials[10,11,12,13] of which the results are often in disagreement because of the differences in the schedules and the heterogeneity of the enrolled population.

Even the interferon-alpha (IFN-a) has been explored as potential effective agent in MDS despite the original observation that it provided disappointing results as single agent.[15]

The mode of action of IFN-a is not very well known yet, but it exerts antiproliferative effects on tumor cell lines and on murine tumors in vivo.[16,17,18] Interestingly, non-cycling tumors seem to be more sensitive to the action of IFN-a than those tumors with high percentage of S phase fraction.[19,20] Moreover IFN-a plays a pivotal role in human immunosurveillance since it has immunomodulatory functions; it promotes natural killer activity,[21,22,23] augmentation of antibody dependent cellular toxicity,[24,25,26,27] tumoricidal activity of macrophages,[28,29,30] antibodies production in B-lymphocytes,[31,32,33] expression of cell surface antigens, i.e. HLA-A, B, C and beta-2 microglobulin[34,35,36] finally it decreases oncogene expression.[37,38,39]

Especially fascinating is the connection between MDS, deletion of the long arm of the chromosome 5 (5q- syndrome) and IFN activity; infact the gene controlling the IFN synthesis is located exactly in the 5q and the patients with 5q abnormalities have been found to be deficient in IFN production and in natural killer function.[40]

More recently our attention was drawn to the potential role of thymic hormones for the treatment of preleukemic conditions.

It has been documented that during some hematological malignancies the concentration of thymic factors may be modified;[41] the administration of thymic hormones to tumor-bearing mice prolonged the survival in a significant manner.[42] Evidences exists suggesting that thymic factors stimulate natural killer activity either directly or inducing IFN production.[21,43,44,45] Garaci and co-workers observed that IFN as an adjunct to thymosin alpha1 (T-a1) treatment, restored natural killer activity and prevented cancer progression in tumor-bearing mice pre-treated with cyclophosphamide.[45]

On the basis of the abovementioned biological observations, we recently adopted a schedule of therapy coupling biological response modifiers and differentiating agents in order to treat MDS.

We planned a schema associating the differentiating properties of LD-ARAc with the immunoregularatory activity of IFN-a and T-a1. The aims of the study are: 1) to verify whether this therapy is effective to correct the myelodisplastic features of the disease (morphologically and cytogenetically) 2) to verify whether the therapy may prevent or delay acute transformation 3) to verify how much the therapy may affect the transfusional needs and subsequently the quality of life 4) to verify possible toxicity and side effects.

MATERIAL AND METHODS

Table 2 illustrates the schedule of treatment for MDS patients.

Table 2. Schedule of treatment for MDS patients

ARAc 20 mg/m^2 twice in a day; day 1 to 7

T-alpha1 1 mg subcutaneously; day 8 to 11

IFN-a 3 MU subcutaneously; day 12

The schedule associates in a sequential manner LD-ARAc, T-a1 and IFN-a. Each course of therapy has been delivered every 15 days for twelve courses. Responding patients received a maintenance therapy with T-a1 and IFN-a at the same doses but administered every 28 days. Only those patients aging no more than 75 years and diagnosed as having MDS according to the FAB classification[9] (Table 1) entered the protocol.

So far 11 patients were enrolled, 7 of them being evaluable for an acceptable follow up. The median age was 62 years (range 22 - 68), 4 patients were male and three female. One patients was diagnosed RA, 5 RAEB and the last one RAEB-t (Table 3). None of the patients was previously treated with chemotherapy and/or radiotherapy for his MDS or other malignancies.

Table 3. Clinical characteristics of the patients

PATIENTS	AGE/SEX		DIAGNOSIS	CYTOGENETICS
PW	60	F	RA	46/XX
PML	65	F	RAEB	5q-
DJL	62	M	RAEB	7+/5q-
NM	65	M	RAEB	46/XY
BG	58	M	RAEB-t	46/XY
GG	68	F	RAEB	46/XY
FS	22	M	RAEB	46/XY

Good response was defined as an improvement in at least three of the following parameters: increase in hemoglobin level by 2 gr/dL at least; increase in platelet level by 50×10^9/L at least; increase in granulocyte count by 1×10^9/L at least; decrease in transfusional support by 50%; decrease of blast infiltration in the bone marrow.

Partial response was considered when only two of the previous parameters were fulfilled. Finally we evaluated the number of natural killer in the peripheral blood, during and after the treatment.

RESULTS

Six courses in five patients (72%) were associated with a good response to therapy, good response was still confirmed after twelve courses. One RAEB patient (14%) achieved a partial response after six courses, the response remained stable even after twelve courses; interestingly he was the sole patient showing a complete remission both morphologically, as defined for the acute leukemia, and cytogenetically (disappearance of 5q-). The only RAEB-t patient (14%) failed in achieving any kind of response and he died as consequence of leukemic evolution. Among the good response group one patient developed an acute leukemia and the duration of good response was 6 months, another one died in good response status because of brain cancer (duration of good response 8 months). The remaining good responders are still alive and in good response; duration of good response is respectively 12, 10 and 6 months. Table 4 lists the clinical results.

TABLE 4. Response to therapy

	BEFORE THERAPY				AFTER THERAPY			
	[1]HB g/dL	[2]GR 10^9/L	[3]PLT 10^9/L	[4]BL %	[1]HB g/dL	[2]GR 10^9/L	[3]PLT 10^9/L	[4]BL %
PW	8	3.2	220	4	11	3.3	220	3
PML	6	4.0	450	8	8	3.5	800	4
DJL	9.6	2.0	41	8	13	4.1	120	5
NM	8	3.3	99	8	10	4.5	100	8
BG	6	1.1	81	20	7	0.9	80	25
GG	9.2	1.7	113	9	12	2.0	178	5
FS	8.5	1.3	85	6	13	2.5	101	3

[1]Hemoglobin [2]Granulocytes [3]Platelets [4]Blasts

The absolute number of natural killer in the peripheral blood has been found increased for all the patients but two; for one good responder it remained unchanged, for the unique non responder the absolute number decreased under therapy. Table 5 lists the immunological modifications during the therapy.

The average transfusional support decreased by 10 cc/kg monthly and all of the responder patients reported a better quality of life. Two patients did not need any additional transfusions from the begining of the therapy; one patients decreased by 50% his supportive cares after 6 months of therapy and subsequently he received no more transfusions. Two patients diminished the transfusional needs by 50% and 70% respectively. Finally for two patients the transfusional load was unchanged. All of the responders (3 good responders and 1 partial responder) are still being given maintenance therapy.

The toxicity and side effects were slight and no serious bleeding or infectious episodes were recorded; no prolonged period of intravenous antibiotic therapy was necessary and none patients required ward admission during the treatment.

The most relevant side effect was thrombocytopenia, grade 2 according to the WHO.

Generally the treatment was well tolerated and the patients showed an acceptable compliance even thanks to the simple route of drug administration.

TABLE 5. Immunological features of the patients before and after the therapy

	BEFORE THERAPY			AFTER THERAPY		
	Nk 10^9/L	CD4 10^9/L	T4/T8 Ratio	Nk 10^9/L	CD4 10^9/L	T4/T8 Ratio
PW	0.07	0.75	1.9	0.31	1.08	2.3
PML	0.32	0.L86	2	0.48	1.62	1.9
DJL	0.02	0.34	0.8	0.56	1.10	1
NM	0.21	0.34	0.8	0.43	0.63	1
BG	0.05	0.17	0.9	0.04	0.12	0.9
GG	0.43	0.94	2	0.45	0.92	1.9
FS	0.54	1.37	1.4	0.70	1.60	1.8

DISCUSSION

Therapy of MDS still remains at this time a matter for the physicians and it is largely founded on supportive cares. A number of attempts has been made to treat the disease by differentiation inducer agents[10,11,12,13] or by using IFN as single agent;[15] these efforts were supported by the opinion that MDS do not need to be treated by aggressive chemotherapy unless an acute transformation.

Recently attention has been devoted to functional meaning of thymic hormones during hematological malignancies; some observations proved that thymic factors may vary their concentration during hematological neoplasms.[41]

Following these speculations we planned a schedule of therapy for MDS, associating differentiating properties of LD-ARAc with the immunoregulatory activity of IFN-a and T-a1 (Table 2).

Six out of 7 evaluable patients obtained a response (5 good responders and 1 partial responder) (Table 4). One patient failed in achieving any response and he died for he developed overt leukemia. The partial responder showed even a cytogenetic remission (disappearance of 5q-), two out of 5 good responders died because of brain cancer and leukemic evolution, respectively. Four patients at present are still being followed up; they are still responders and receiving maintenace treatment.

Supportive cares decrease dramatically (by 10 cc/kg monthly average); two patients were transfused no more since they started therapy and another one stopped his transfusion after 6 months of therapy. Moreover, for all the patients but one the number of blasts in the bone marrow was decreased, by contrast the number of natural killer and CD4$^+$ lymphocytes was raised in five patients. Finally all of the responders experienced an improved quality of life.

Although our results are very preliminary the therapy seems to be promising; however a number of important points remain for considerations about the use of combination of LD-ARAc, IFN-a and T-a1. In particular our efforts ought to deal with the following issues: a) correct modalities of schedule administration; IFN-a and T-a1 delivery should mainly addressed, infact they are administrated on the basis of murine-tumor model b) real efficacy of the therapy in the RAEB-t which is an MDS very close to an acute phase c) real efficacy of the LD-ARAc in the RA for which may be sufficient a simple combination of IFN-a and T-a1.

Finally the availability of the recombinant growth factors may lead to alternative approach for MDS treatment, although their safety in terms of blast recruiment has not been clearly demonstrated yet.

REFERENCES

1. K.Foucar, R.M. Langdom, J.O. Armitage, D.B. Olson, T.J. Carroll, Myelodisplastic syndromes, *Cancer* 56:553 (1985).
2. A.Jacobs, Human preleukemia: do we have a model ?. *Br J Cancer* 55:1 (1987).
3. D.G.Oscier, Myelodisplastic syndrome, *Clin Haematol* 1:389 (1987).
4. J.T.Prchal, D.W. Throckmorton, A.J. III Carrol, E.W. Fuson, R.A. Gams, J.F. Prchal, A common progenitor for human myeloid and lymphoid cells, *Nature* 274: 590 (1978).
5. Y.W.Kan, New application for DNA polymorphism, *N Engl J Med* 316:478 (1987).
6. R.A.Padua, G. Carter, D. Hughes, J.Gow, C.Farr, D.Oscier, F.McCormick, A.Jacobs, Ras mutation in myelodisplasia detected by amplification, oligonucleotide hybridization, and transformation, *Leukemia* 2:503 (1988).
7. P.C.Nowell, E.C.Bes, T.Stelmach, J.B.Finan, Chromosome studies in preleukemic states: Prognostic significance of single vs. multiple abnormalities. *Cancer* 58:2571(1986).
8. H.Van den Berghe, K.Vermaelen, C.Mecucci, D.Barbieri, G.Tricot, The 5q- anomaly, *Cancer Genet Cytogenet* 17:189(1982).
9. J.M.Bennett, D.Catovsky, G.Flandrin, D.A.G.Galton, H.R.Gralnick, C.Sultan, Proposals for the classification of the myelodisplastic syndromes, *BR J Haematol* 51:189(1982).
10. J.N.Winter, D.Variakojis, E.R.Gaynor, Low dose cytosine arabinoside therapy in the myelodisplastic yndromes and acute leukemia, *Cancer* 56:443(1985).
11. J.D.Griffin, D.Spriggs, J.S.Wisch, Treatment of preleukemic syndromes with continuos intravenous infusion of low dose cytosine arabinoside, *J Clin Oncol* 3:982(1985).
12. G.Tricot, R.De Bock, A.W.Dekker. Low dose cytosine arabinoside in m.yelodisplastic syndromes, *Br J Haematol* 58:231(1984).
13. L.Degos, S.Castaigne, H.Tilly, Treatment of leukemia with low dose ara-c: a study of 160 cases, *Semin Oncol* 12 (suppl 3): 196 (1988).
14. J.D.Griffin, D.Munroe, P.Major. D.Kufe, Induction of differentiation of human myeloid leukemic cells by inhibitors of DNA synthesis, *Exper Haematol* 10:744(1982).
15. L.Elias, R.Hoffman, S.Boswell, E.Bonnem, A trial of recombinant alpha-2 interferon in the myelodisplastic syndrome, *Blood* 66(suppl) 675 (abstract) (1985).
16. F.R.Balkwill, R.T.D.Oliver, Growth inhibitory effects of interferon on normal and malignant human hemopoietic cells, *Int J Cancer* 20:500(1977).
17. E.C.Borden, T.F.Hogan, J.G.Voelkel. Comparative antiproliferative activity in vitro of natural interferons alpha and beta for diploid and transformed human cells, *Cancer Res* 42:4948(1982).
18. K.C.Chadha, B.I.Srivastava. Comparison of the antiproliferative effects of human fibroblast and leukocyte interferons on various leukemic cell line, *J Clin Haematol Oncol* 11:55(1981).
19. J.S.Horoszewicz, S.S.Leong, W.S.Carter, Noncycling tumor cell are sensitive targets for the antiproliferative activity of human interferon, *Science* 206:1091(1979).
20. A.A.Creasey, J.C.Bartholomew, T.C.Merigan, Role of G0-G1 arrest in the inhibition of tumor cell growth by interferon, *Proc Natl Acad Sci* 77:1471(1980).
21. M.Gidlund, A.Orn, H.Wigzell, A.Senik, I.Gresser, Enhanced NK cell activity injected with interferon and interferon inducers, *Nature* 273:759(1978).
22. R.B.Hebermann, H.T.Holden, Natural killer cells as antitumor effector cells, *JNCI* 62:441(1979).
23. J.Y.Djeu, J.A.Heinbaugh, H.T.Holden, R.B.Hebermann, Augmentation of mouse natural killer cell activity by interferon and interferon inducers, *J Immunol* 122:175(1979).
24. T.Timoten, J.R.Ortaldo, R.B.Hebermann, Characteristics of large granular lymphocytes and relationship to natural killer and killer cells, *J Exp Med* 153:569(1981).
25. M.G.Masucci, R.Sziget, E.Klein, Effect of interferon alpha-1 from E.coli on some cell function, *Science* 209:1431(1980).
26. J.R.Ortaldo, S.Pestka, R.B.Slease, M.Rubinstein, R.B.Hebermann, Augmentation of human k-cell activity with interferon, *Scand J Immunol* 12:365(1980).
27. P.Hokland, K.Berg, Interferon enhances the antibody-dependent cellular cytotoxicity of human polymorphonuclear leukocytes. *J Immunol* 127:1585(1981).

28. S.Sone, T.Utsugi, T.Shirhama, K.Ishii, S.Mutsuura, O.Mitsumasa, Induction by interferon-alpha of tumoricidal activity of adherent mononuclear cells from human blood: monocytes as responder and effector cells, *J Biol Response Mod* 4:134(1985).

29. D.Fertsch, S.N.Vogel Recombinant interferons increase macrophage Fc receptor capacity , *J Immunol* 132:2436(1984).

30. J.R. Sadlik, M.Hoyer, M.A.Leyko, Lymphocyte supernatant-induced human monocyte tumoricidal activity: dependence on the presence of gamma-interferon, *Cancer* 45:1940(1985).

31. B.Harfast, J.R.Huddleston, P.Casali, T.C.Merigan, M.B.A.Oldstone, Interferon acts directly on human B lymphocytes to modulate immunoglobulin synthesis, *J Immunol* 127:2146(1981).

32. M.A.Rodriguez, W.A.Prinz, W.L.Sibbitt, A.D.Bankhurst, R.C.Williams, Alpha-interferon increases immunoglobulin production in cultured human mononuclear leukocytes, *J Immunol* 130:1215(1983).

33. I.Gresser, The effect of interferon on the expression of surface antigens, *in* "Interferons and the Immune System," J.Vilcek, E.DeMaeyer, eds, Amsterdam (1984).

34. G.Sonnefeld, Effects of interferon on antibody formation, *in* "Interferons and the Immune System," J.Vilcek, E.DeMaeyer, eds, Amsterdam (1984).

35. I.Heron, M.Hokland, K.Berg, Enhanced expression of B_2-microglobulin and HLA antigens on human lymphoid cells by interferon, *Proc Natl Acad Sci* 75:6215(1978).

36. V.E.Kelley, W.Fiers, T.B.Strom, Cloned human interferon-gamma, but not interferon-beta or alpha induces expression og HLA-Dr determinants by fetal monocytes and myeloid leukemic cell lines, *J Immunol* 132:240(1984).

37. S.L.Lin, E.A.Garber, E.Wang,Reduced synthesis of pp60 and expression of the transformation-related phenotype in interferon-treated Rous sarcoma virus-transformed rat cells, *Mol Cell Biol* 3:1656(1983).

38. C.H.Dani, N.Mechti, M.Piechaczyk, B.Lcbleu, P.H.Jeanteur, J.M.Blanchard, Increased rate of degradation of c-myc mRNA in interferon-treated Daudi cells, *Proc Natl Acad Sci* 82:4891(1985).

39. D.R.Strayer, D.H.Gillespie, J.Bresseuer, I.Brodsky, Oncogene expression decreased in two patients treated with interferons, *Blood* 64(suppl):293(1984).

40. J.Pedersen-Bjengaard, S.Haahr, P.Philip, Abolished production of interferon by leucocytes of patients with the acquired cytogenetic abnormalities 5q- or -5 in secondary and de novo acute non lymphocytic leukemia, *Br J Haematol* 46:211(1980).

41. E.Garaci, F.Bistoni, C.Favalli, P.Marconi, V.Del Gobbo, C.Rainaldi, B.M.Jaffe, Thymic factors in experimental disease *in* "Immunoregulation," W.A.Mithison eds, N.Fabris, E.Garaci, New York (1983).

42. A.S.Klein, R.Lang, I.Eshel, Y.Sharaby, J.Shoham, Modulation of immune response and tumor development in tumor-bearing mice treated by the factor thymostimulin, *Cancer Res* 47:3351(1985).

43. M.Gidland, A.Orn, A.Wiezell, Enhanced NK cell activity in mice injected with interferon and interferons inducers, 273:759(1978).

44. E.Garaci, A.Mastino, T.Jezzi, C.Favalli, Thymic hormones and cytokines: a synergistic combination with high therapeutic potentialities *in* "Recent advances in autoimmunity and tumor immunology," W.A.Mithison eds, E.Garaci, New York (1988).

45. C.Rinaldi-Garaci, M.R.Torrisi, T.Jezzi, L.Frati, A.L.Goldstein, E.Garaci, Receptors, for thimosin a on mouse thimocyte cells, *Immunology* 91:289(1985).

MYELOID GROWTH FACTORS IN CANCER TREATMENT

Anna Butturini[1] and Robert Peter Gale[2]

[1]Department of Pediatrics,
University of Parma, 43100 Italy
[2] Department of Medicine,
UCLA School of Medicine,
Los Angeles, CA90024-1678 USA

INTRODUCTION

Myeloid growth factors are increasingly used in cancer treatment. Strategies include giving these factors before chemotherapy, to increase sensitivity of cancer cells to cell-cycle specific anticancer drugs, after chemotherapy to accelerate hematopoietic recovery or giving these factors without chemotherapy, to force maturation of cancer cells or to modulate the host immune response to cancer. Here, we consider the conceptual bases of these approaches and whether they are effective in treating human cancers.

Our focus is on myeloid hematopoietic growth factors. Use of lymphokines prevalently acting on immune cells is reviewed elsewhere[1,2].

PRECLINICAL STUDIES

Normal hematopoiesis is hierarchical: totipotent stem cells differentiate to committed progenitors and ultimately to mature end-cells. The system is amplicative: each stem cell gives rise to many progeny. Cell production is closely regulated by cytokines, produced by T-lymphocytes, macrophages, cells of microenvironment (stromal) and natural killer (NK) cells[3]. Those enhancing myelopoiesis are referred to as *myeloid* growth factors.

Several myeloid growth factors were recently molecularly cloned and tested for biological activity in vitro and in animal models. Their site of action is shown in fig.1[3-11]. In many cases, in vivo response to myeloid growth factors differs in magnitude and/or involves cells of different lineages from that predicted by in vitro studies. This results from the complex interactions between cyto-kines and target cells. For example, some growth factors stimulate secretion of other factors regulating bone marrow function. Examples are granulocyte-macrophage colony stimulating factors (GM-CSF), in vitro acting on cells of myeloid lineage, which in vivo increases lymphocytes by causing release of other lymphokines[12] and interleukin-6 (IL-6), which affects pluripotent precursor growth in vitro[7], but in vivo increases prevalently megakariocytopoiesis[13].

Myeloid growth factors also modulate functions of mature myeloid and immune cells. Many of them may have anti-cancer activities. For example, GM-CSF, macrophage-colony stimulating factor (M-CSF) and interleukin-4 (IL-4) increase phagocytosis and antibody dependent cytotoxic activity (ADCC) of neutrophils and macrophages[14-16]; IL-4 and IL-6 affect lymphocytes and other immune cells[17,18]. Also, myeloid growth factors, like GM-CSF, stimulate release of lymphokines with direct anticancer activity, like tumor necrosis factor (TNF) and interferons[15].

Combination Therapies 2, Edited by A.L. Goldstein
and E. Garaci   Plenum Press, New York, 1993

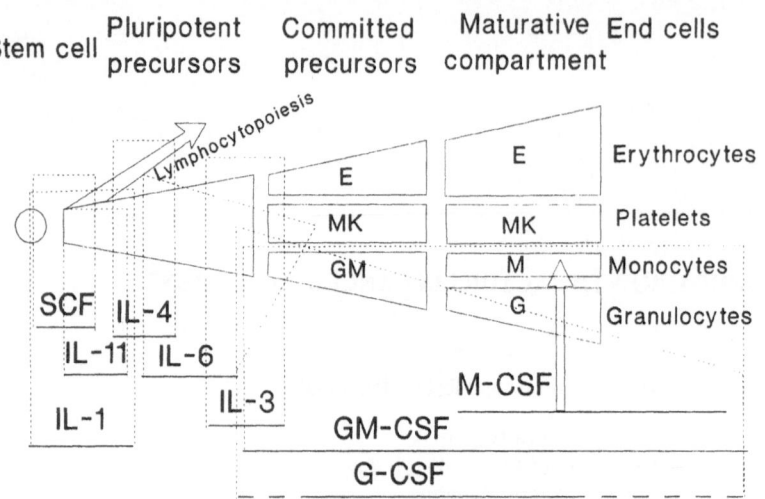

Figure 1. Myeloid growth factor and hematopoiesis.

SCF= stem cell factor; IL-11= interleukin-11; IL-4= interleukin-4; IL-6= interleukin-6; IL-3= interleukin-3; GM-CSF=granulocyte-macrophage colony stimulating factor; G-CSF=granulocyte colony stimulating factor; M-CSF= macrophage stimulating factor.

Results of using myeloid growth factors in animals with experimental cancer are controversial. In some models, GM-CSF, interleukin-3 (IL-3) or IL-4 prevent growth of trans-plantable lymphoid tumors[19,20]. Also, interleukin-1a (IL-1a) and M-CSF potentiate effects of chemotherapy and radiation in animals with syngeneic or allogeneic transplantable cancers[21,22].

Myeloid growth factors can also affect growth of several tumor cell lines including acute myelogenous leukemia (AML)[23-26], and lung, kidney, gastrointestinal and breastcancers[11,27-30]. In most studies, GM-CSF, G-CSF, IL-3, IL-4 or IL-6 increase proliferation of virtually all AML and of a subset of solid tumors. In AML cells, proliferation can be coupled with differentiation[26,31,32]. The effects of myeloid growth factors on cancer cell proliferation have been used to synchronize cancer cells prior to giving cycle-specific drugs. The impact of this might be to increase the effective drug dose. Considerable experimental data suggest that treatment with GM-CSF or IL-3 before cytarabine and anthracyclines increases killing of AML cells[33-35].

CLINICAL TRIALS

Recently, myeloid growth factors were used in persons with cancer. Most studies used GM-CSF or G-CSF. Trials with M-CSF, IL-1b, IL-3, and IL-4 are progressing.

In most studies, myeloid growth factors were given to stimulate hematopoiesis, typically after chemotherapy and/or radiation[36-60], but also as the sole treatment of persons with cancer, mostly in those with neoplastic bone marrow involvement[61-67] or preleukemia (myelodysplastic syndrome-MDS)[37,68-72] (Tables 1,2 & 3).

Studies of myeloid growth factors after chemotherapy show that these factors accelerate neutrophil recovery. Interval to neutrophils >0.5 or 1.0 x 10^9/l decreases typically by 5 to 7 days. This is observed after conventional chemotherapy and after high-dose chemotherapy and radiation followed by auto- or allogeneic transplants. Changes in myeloid growth factor doses are reflected more in the magnitude than speed of recovery.

When given in persons with neoplastic bone marrow involvement or MDS, myeloid growth factors also increase blood neutrophils. Typically, the effects are dose-dependent and transient.

Table 1. Trials of myeloid growth factors in solid tumors.

Factor	Doses[1] (ug/m^2/day)	Tumor[2]	P/T[3]	Previous Therapy[4]	Ref.
GM-CSF	75-<u>750</u>	Br,Mel,NBL.	30/2	AUTO	36
		STS,G.I., GCT,Ov,Br.	167/6	chemo	37-42
G-CSF	40-2500	GCT,Br,Mel.	26/2	AUTO	36
		Ur,Br,Ov, Lung,others	159/7	chemo	36,37, 43-46
M-CSF	**[5]	NBL	3/1	AUTO	36
	0-<u>33000</u>	Various	49/5	-	36,37, 61,62
IL-3	30-<u>1000</u>	SCL,others	46/3	chemo	47-49
IL-1b	0.01-4	G.I.	19/1	chemo	50
		Various	25/2	-	50,63,64
IL-4	10-200	Various	85/3	-	65-67

[1]Doses often requiring treatment interruption for toxicity are underlined

[2]Number of patients/Number of trials

[3]ALLO= High dose chemo- or chemo-radiotherapy followed by allogeneic bone marrow transplant; AUTO= High-dose chemo- or chemo-radiotherapy followed by autologous stem cell transplant; chemo= chemotherapy.

[4]ALL= acute lymphoblastic leukemia; AML= acute myeloid leukemia; CML= chronic myeloid leukemia; CLL= chronic lymphoid leukemia; MDS= myelodysplastic syndrome; Br= breast cancer; Mel= melanoma; NBL= neuroblastoma; GCT= germ cell tumors; Ov= ovarian cancer; MM= multiple myeloma; Ur= transitional cell cancer of urethelium; G.I.= gastro intestinal cancer; SCL= small cell lung cancer; Lung= all lung cancers; STS= soft tissue sarcomas.

[5]Urinary M-CSF, 2 x 10^5-8 x 10^6 units/Kg/day

In these settings, effects of myeloid growth factors on blood cells of non-myeloid lineages is modest. GM-CSF, G-CSF and M-CSF uncommonly affect red blood cells (RBC) or platelets. IL-1b, IL-3 and IL-4 increase RBC and/or platelets in about one half of the patients.

Other studies tested other effects of myeloid growth factors. For example, they were given to sincronize cancer cells before chemotherapy. These trials typically involved persons with AML[73-75].

Adverse effects of treatment with myeloid growth factors are dose-dependent. They graft-failure and graft-versus-host disease (GVHD) are discussed elsewhere[36,52].

As indicated in experimental studies, a possible adverse affect of myeloid growth factors might be to stimulate growth of cancer cells. This is not observed in persons with solid tumors. In persons with MDS and smoldering AML, treatment with GM-CSF, G-CSF or

Table 2. Trials of myeloid growth factors in lymphoid tumors.

Factor	Doses[1] (ug/m²/day)	Tumor[2]	P/T[3]	Previous Therapy[4]	Ref.
GM-CSF	125-<u>500</u>	ALL	18/2	ALLO	51,52
		Lymphoma	14/1	ALLO	52
		ALL	28/2	AUTO	36,53
		Lymphoma	124/5	AUTO	36,53,54
		Lymphoma	23/1	chemo	55
		MM	23/1	chemo	56
G-CSF	40-2500	ALL	21/4	ALLO	36
		ALL	2/1	AUTO	36
		Lymphoma	29/2	AUTO	36
		ALL	12/1	chemo	57
M-CSF	**5	ALL	22/2	ALLO	36,58
		Lymphoma	4/1	ALLO	58
		ALL	5/1	AUTO	36
IL-4	10-200	Lymph/CLL	14/2	-	65,66

for legends, see Table 1.

IL-3 is occasionally associated with transient increase of bone marrow or blood myeloblasts and rarely with disease progression.

EFFECTS ON CURE

There are several means by which using myeloid growth factors might affect cancer cures. For example, their use can allow increased doses of anti-cancer drugs and radiation, shorter intervals between treatment courses or both. Myelod growth factors can also enhance sensivity of cancer cells to cycle specific drugs, induce cell differentiation, increase the function of mature myeloid cells and directly or indirectly modulate the anti-cancer effects of immune cells.

Considerable experimental data indicate that increased doses of drugs and radiation increase cancer cures. Data from clinical trials are less certain[77]. Presently, there is consensus that increasingly intensive treatment affects *response rates* in cancers like breast, ovarian and small cell lung cancers. Recent trials of high-dose therapy are mostly performed in the context of transplants either of autologous bone marrow or blood derived stem cells[78,79]. These data also suggest increased response. However, it is unknown whether these increased responses translate to *cures*.

If high-dose chemotherapy increses cancer cures, what the role of myeloid growth factors. In the context of auto transplants, myeloid growth factors facilitate collection of blood stem cells used for graft[80,81]. As indicated, post transplant treatment with growth factors accelerate neutro-phil recovery. In some studies, this results in shorter hospitalization and decreased bacterial infections; survival was inaffected[36,37,53].

One interesting issue is whether the use of myeloid growth factors might obviate the need of a transplant after high-dose therapy. This could affect the likelihood of cure by avoiding possible infusion of cancer cells with the graft. Considerable data suggest this strategy is possible. For example, some stem cells survive high-dose chemotherapy and/or radiation, as shown by the partial recovery of autologous hematopoiesis in up to 80% recipients of T cell depleted allogeneic bone marrow transplants[82]. Also, some persons receiving high-dose chemotherapy recover bone marrow functions after GM-CSF or G-CSF[46,83]. The anti-cancer efficacy of this approach remains however to be proven in prospective trials.

Table 3. Trials of myeloid growth factors in MDS or myeloid leukemias.

Factor	Doses[1] (ug/m^2/day)	Tumor[2]	P/T[3]	Previous Therapy[4]	Ref.
GM-CSF	125-<u>500</u>	AML	20/2	ALLO	51,52
		CML	6/2	ALLO	51,52
		AML	42/2	chemo	59,60
	5-<u>500</u>	MDS	85/6	-	37,68-70
G-CSF	50-200	AML	33/4	ALLO	36
		AML	30/1	chemo	57
	4-1600	MDS	23/2	-	37,71
M-CSF	**5	AML	23/2	ALLO	36,58
		CML	24/2	ALLO	36,58
IL-3	30-<u>1000</u>	MDS	22/2	-	51,72

for legends see Table 1.

Use of myeloid growth factors might also increase cancer cures by permitting increased dose-intensity by reduce intervals between treatment courses. Whether increased dose-intensity will affect cancer cures is controversial[84-86]; controlled trials are needed.

As indicated, myeloid growth factors may affect the likelihood of cancer cure by other mechanisms. One related to sincronization of cancer cells prior to chemotherapy. Preliminary data in AML are not encouraging[73-75]. Results of trials where myeloid growth factors were given to force maturation of cancer cells, typically in persons with MDS are also unconvincing, with only rare long term remissions reported[87,88]. Myeloid growth factors may also modulate anticancer activity of myeloid and immune cells. Again, in rare case the use of GM-CSF resulted in regression of solid tumors[89]. Results of trials using M-CSF, IL-4 or IL-1b are too preliminary for conclusions.

CONCLUSIONS

Myeloid growth factors are increasingly used in cancer treatment. The most promising use to date is to increase doses and dose-intensity of chemotherapy and radiation. The unanswered question is whether this approach will increase cures. Analysis of this requires randomized trials of large numbers of subjects.

Because of the complex interactions of chemotherapy and growth factors and the fact that multiple anti-tumor mechanisms may be involved, results of these trials must be evaluated with caution. Many variables affect the likeli-hood of cure, such as the individual response of immune and non-immune cells to myeloid growth factors and chemotherapy and the different sensitivity of specific types of cancers to these mechanisms. Since most of these variables are still undetermined, it may be difficult or impossible to detect a clinical impact of myeloid growth factors on cancer cure.

REFERENCES

1. Foon K.A. Biological Response Modifiers. the new immunotherapy. Cancer Res. 49: 1621-39 (1989)

2. Editorial. Interleukin-2: sunrise for immunotherapy. Lancet 2: 308 (1989)

3. Sachs L. The molecular control of blood cell development. Science 238: 1374-9 (1987)

4. Nicola N.A. Hemopoietic cell growth factors and their receptors. Annu. Rev. Biochem. 58: 45-77 (1989)

5. Moore M.A.S. Clinical implications of positive and negative hemopoietic stem cell regulators. Blood 78: 1-19 (1991)

6. Zsebo K.M., Williams D.A., Geissler E.N. et al. Stem cell factor is encoded at the S1 locus of the mouse and is the ligand for the c-kit tyrosine kinase receptor. Cell 63: 213-24 (1990)

7. Ikebuchi K., Wong G.G., Clark S.C., Ihle J.N., Hirai Y., Ogawa M. Interleukin-6 enhancement of interleukin-3-dependent proliferation of multipotential hematopoietic precursors. Proc. Natl. Acad. Sci. USA 84: 9035-9 (1987)

8. Kishi K., Ihle J.N., Urdal D.L., Ogawa M. Murine B- cell stimulatory factor-1 (BSF-1)/interleukin-4 (IL-4) is a multi-CSF which acts directly on primitive hemopoietic precursors. J. Cell. Physiol. 139: 463-8 (1989)

9. Musashi M., Clark S.C., Sudo T., Urdal D.L., Ogawa M. Synergic interactions between interleukin-11 and interleukin-4 in support of proliferation of primitive hematopoietic precursors of mice. Blood 78: 1448-51 (1991)

10. Gasson J.C. Molecular physiology of granulocyte macrophage colony stimulating factor. Blood 77: 1131- 45 (1991)

11. Avalos B.R., Gasson J.C., Hedvat C. et al. Human granulocyte colony stimulating factor: biological activities and receptor characterization on hematopoietic cells and small cell lung cancer cell lines. Blood 75: 851-7 (1990)

12. Faisal M., Cumberland W., Chamlin W., Fahey J.L. Effect of recombinant human granulocyte macrophage colony stimulating factor administration on the lymphocyte subset of patients with refractory aplastic anemia. Blood 76: 1580-5 (1990)

13. Asano S., Okano A., Ozawa K. et al. In vivo effects of recombinant human interleukin-6 in primates: stimulated production of platelets. Blood 75: 1602-5 (1990)

14. Kushner B.H., Cheung N.K.V. GM-CSF enhances 3F8 monoclonal antibody-dependent cellular cytotoxicity against human melanoma and neuroblastoma. Blood 73: 1936-41 (1989)

15. Wing E.J., Magge D.M., Whiteside T.L., Kaplan S.S., Shadduck R.K. Recombinant human granulocyte macrophage colony stimulating factor enhances monocyte cytotoxicity and secretion of TNFa and interferon in cancer patients. Blood 73: 643-6 (1989)

16. Sampson L.L., Heuser J., Brown E.J. Cytokine regulation of complement receptor mediated ingestion by mouse peritoneal macrophages. M-CSF and IL-4 activate phagocytosis by a common mechanism requiring autostimulation by IFN beta. J. Immunol.146: 1005-13 (1991)

17. Paul W.E.Interleukin-4: a prototypic immunoregulatory lymphokine. Blood 77: 1859-70 (1991)

18. Kishimoto T. The biology of interleukin-6. Blood 74: 1-10 (1989)

19. Fabian I., Kletter Y., Slavin S. Therapeutic potential of recombinant granulocyte macrophage colony stimulating factor and interleukin-3 in murine B cell leukemia. Blood 72: 913-8 (1988)

20. Tepper R.I., Pattengale P.K., Leder P. Murine interleukin-4 dysplays potent anti-tumor activity in vivo. Cell 57: 503-12 (1989)

21. Nakamura S., Kashimoto S., Kajikawa F., Nakata K. Combination effect of recombinant human interleukin 1 alpha with antitumor activity on syngeneic tumors in mice. Cancer Res. 51: 215-21 (1991)

22. Lu L., Shen R.N., Lin Z.H., Aukerman S.L., Ralph P., Broxemeyer H.E. Antitumor effects of recombinant human macrophage colony stimulating factor, alone or in combination with local irradiation, in mice inoculated with Lewis lung carcinoma cells. Int. J. Cancer 47: 143-7 (1991)

23. Miyauchi J., Kelleher C.A., Yang Y.C. et al. The effect of three recombinant growth factors, IL-3, GM-CSF and G-CSF on the blast cells of acute myeloblastic leukemia mantained in short term suspension culture. Blood 70: 657-63 (1987)

24. Delwel R., Saleim M., Pelleus C., et al. Growth regulation of human myeloid leukemia: effect of five recombinant hematopoietic factors in a serum-free culture system. Blood 72: 1944-9 (1988)

25. Brach M.A., Lowemberg B., Mantovani L., Schwulera U., Martelmann R., Herrmann F. Interleukin-6 (IL-6) is an intermediate in IL-1 induced proliferation of leukemic human megakaryoblast. Blood 76: 1972-9(1990)

26. Miyauchi J., Clark S.C., Tsunematsu Y. et al. Interleukin-4 as a growth regulator of clonogenic cells in acute myelogenous leukemia in suspension culture. Leukemia 5: 108-15 (1991)

27. Baldwin G.C., Gasson J.C., Kaufman S.E. et al. Non hematopoietic tumor cells express functional GM-CSF receptors. Blood 73:1033-7 (1989)

28. Joraschkewitz M., Depenbrock H., Freund M. et al. Effects of cytokines on in vitro colony formation of primary human tumor specimens. Eur. J. Cancer 26: 1070-4 (1990)

29. Vellenga E., Biesma B., Meyer C., Wagteveld L., Esselink M., de Vries E.G.E The effect of five hematopoietic growth factors on human small cell lung carcinoma cell lines: interleukin 3 enhances the proliferation in one of the eleven cell lines. Cancer Res. 51: 73-6 (1991)

30. Tungekar M.F., Turtley H., Dunnill M.S., Gatter K.C., Ritter M.A. Harris A.L. Interleukin-4 receptor on human lung tumors and normal lung. Cancer Res. 51: 261-4 (1991)

31. Lotem J., Sachs L.In vivo control of differentiation of myeloid leukemia by recombinant granulocyte-macrophage colony stimulating factor and interleukin-3. Blood 71: 375-82 (1988)

32. Shabo Y., Lotem J., Rubinstein M. et al. The myeloid blood cell differentiation-inducing protein MGI-2a is interleukin-6. Blood 72:2070-3 (1988)

33. Miyauchi J., Kelleher C.A., Wang C., Minkin S. Mc Culloch E.A. Growth factors influence the sensivity of leukemic cells to cytosine arabinoside in culture. Blood 73: 1272-8 (1989)

34. Butturini A., Santucci M.A., Gale R.P., Perocco P., Tura S. GM-CSF incubation prior to treatment with cytarabine or doxorubicin enhances drug activity against AML cells in vitro: a model for leukemia chemotherapy. Leukemia Res. 14: 743-9 (1990)

35. Brach M., Klein H., Platzer E., Martelsmann R., Herrmann F. Effect of interleukin-3 on cytosine arabinoside-mediated cytotoxicity of leukemia myeloblasts. Exp. Hematol. 15: 2305-10 (1990)

36. Aurer I., Ribas A., Gale R.P. What is the role of recombinant colony stimulating factors in bone marrow transplantation? Bone Marrow Transpl. 6: 79- 87 (1990)

37. Groopman M.D., Molina J.M., Scadden D.T. Hematopoietic growth factors. N. Engl. J. Med. 321: 1449-59(1989)

38. Steward W.P., Verweij J., Somers R. et al. High dose chemotherapy (CT) with two schedules of recombinant human granulocyte-macrophage colony stimulating factor (rhGM-CSF) in the treatment of advanced adult soft tissue sarcomas (STS). ASCO Proc. 10: 349 (1991)

39. Jost L.M., Pichert G., Stahel R.A. Plecebo controlled phase I-II study of subcutaneous GM-CSF in patients with germ cell tumors undergoing chemotherapy. Ann. Oncol. 1:439-42 (1990)

40. de Vries E.G., Biesma B., Willemse P.H. et al. A double blind placebo controlled study with granulocyte macrophage colony stimulating factor during chemotherapy for ovarian carcinoma. Cancer Res. 51: 116-22 (1991)

41. Bregni M., Siena S., Ravagnani F., Bonadonna G., Gianni A.M. High-dosecyclophosphamide in patients with operable breast cancer: recombinant human GM- CSF amiliorates drug-induced leukopenia and thrombocytopenia. Haematologica 75 (suppl.1): 95-8 (1990)

42. Steward W.P., Scarffe J.H., Dirix L.Y. et al. Granulocyte-macrophage colony stimulating factor (GM-CSF) after high dose melphalan in patients with advanced colon cancer. Br. J. Cancer 61: 749-54 (1990)

43. Bronchud M.H., Howell A., Crowther D., Hopwood P., Souza L., Dexter T.M. The use of granulocyte colony-stimulating factor to increase the intensity of treatment with doxorubicin in patients with advanced breast and ovarian cancer. Br. J. Cancer 60: 121-25 (1989)

44. Crawford J., Ozer H., Stoller R. et al. Reduction by granulocyte colony stimulating factor of fever and neutropenia induced by chemotherapy in patients with small cell lung cancer. N. Engl. J. Med. 325: 164-70 (1991)

45. Eguchi K., Sasaki S., Tamura T. et al. Dose escalation study of recombinant human granulocyte-colony stimulating factor (KRN8601) in patients with advanced malignancy. Cancer Res. 49: 5221-4 (1989)

46. Neidhart J., Mangalik A., Kohler W. et al. Granulocyte colony stimulating factor stimulates recovery of granulocytes in patients receiving dose-intensive chemotherapy without bone marrow trans plantation. J. Clin. Oncol. 7: 1685-92 (1989)

47. Ganser A., Lindemann A., Seipelt G. et al. Effects of recombinant human interleukin-3 in patients with normal hematopoiesis and in patients with bone marrow failure. Blood 76: 666-76 (1990)

48. Kurzrock R., Talpaz M., Estrov Z., Rosenblum M.G., Gutterman J.U. Phase I study of recombinant human interleukin-3 in patients with bone marrow failure. J. Clin. Oncol. 9: 1241-50 (1991)

49. Postmus P.E., Gietema J.A., Damsma O., Willemse P. H. B., de Vries E.G.E., Vellenga E. Phase I trial of RH-interleukin-3 s.c. in patients with relapse of small cell lung cancer treated with chemotherapy. Asco Proc. 10: 248 (1991)

50. Crown J., Jakubowski A., Kemeny N. et al. A phase I trial of recombinant human Interleukin-1b alone and in combination with myelosupressive doses of 5-fluorouracil in patients with gastrointestinal cancer. Blood 78: 1420-7 (1991)

51. Powles R., Smith C., Milan S. et al. Human recombinant GM-CSF in allogeneic bone marrow transplantation for leukemia: double blind, placebo controlled trial. Lancet 336: 1417-20 (1990)

52. Nemunaitis J., Buckner C.D., Appelbaum F.R. et al. Phase I/II trial of recombinant human granulocyte-macrophage colony stimulating factor following allogeneic bone marrow transplantation. Blood 77: 2065-71 (1991)

53. Nemunaitis J., Rabinowe S.N., Singer J.W. et al. Recombinant granulocyte-macrophage colony stimulating factor after autologous bone marrow transplantation for lymphoid cancer. N. Engl. J. Med. 324: 1773-8 (1991)

54. Lazarus H. M., Andersen J., Chen M. G. et al. Recombinant granulocyte macrophage colony stimulating factor after autologous bone marrow transplantation for relapsed non-Hodgkin's lymphoma: blood and bone marrow progenitor growth studies. A phaseII Eastern Cooperative Oncology Group Study. Blood 78: 830-7 (1991)

55. Ho A.D., Del Valle F., Haas R. et al. Sequential studies of the role of mitoxantrone, high-dose cytarabine and recombinant human granulocyte-macrophage colony stimulating factor in the treatment of refractory non Hodgkin's lymphoma. Sem. Oncol. 17 (supp.10): 14-8 (1990)

56. Barlogie B., Jagannath S., Dixon D.O. et al. High- dose melphalan and granulocyte macrophage colony stimulating factor for refractory multiple myeloma. Blood 76: 677-80 (1990)

57. Ohno R., Tomonaga M., Kobayashi T. et al. Effect of granulocyte colony stimulating factor after intensive induction chemotherapy in relapsed or refractory acute leukemia. N. Engl. J. Med. 323: 871-7 (1990)

58. Masaoka T., Shibata H., Ohno R. et al. Double blind test of human urinary macrophage colony stimulating factor for allogeneic and syngeneic bone marrow transplantation: effectiveness of treatment and 2 year follow up for relapsed leukemia. Br. J. Haematol. 76: 501-5 (1990)

59. Buechner T., Hiddemann W., Koenigsmann M. et al. Recombinant human granulocyte macrophage colony stimulating factor after chemotherapy in patients with acute myeloid leukemia at higher age or after relapse. Blood 78: 1190-7 (1991)

60. Estey E.H., Dixon D., Kantarjan H.M. et al.Treatment of poor prognosis, newly diagnosed acute myeloid leukemia with AraC and recombinant human granulocyte macrophage colony stimulating factor. Blood 75: 1766-9 (1990)

61. Budd J.T., Thomassen M.J., Murthy S.V. et al. Phase I trial of recombinant monocyte macrophage colony stimulating factor in patients with refractory malignancy. AACR Proc. 32: 172 (1991)

62. Zamkoff K., Hudson J., Groves E. et al. A phase I trial of recombinant macrophage stimulating factor, human (rM-CSF),by rapid intravenous infusion in patients with refractory malignancy. ASCO Proc.10: 93 (1991)

63. Tewari A., Buhles W.C., Starnes H.F. Preliminary report: effects of interleukin-1 on platelet count. Lancet 336: 712-4 (1990)

64. Steis R., Smith J., Janik J. Phase I study of recombinant interleukin-1b (Sintax). Asco Proc. 10: 211 (1991)

65. Davis I., Maher D., Cebon J. et al. Pharmacokinetic and clinical studies of interleukin-4 (IL-4) in patients with malignancy. ASCO Proc. 10: 287 (1991)

66. Freimann J., Estrov Z., Itoh H. et al. Phase I study of recombinant human interleukin-4. ASCO Proc. 10: 216 (1991)

67. Lotze M.T. Presented at the UCLA Symposium on Cellular Immunity and the Immunotherapy of Cancer. Park City (Utah). Jen.Feb. 1990

68. Thompson J.A., Lee D.J., Kidd P., Rubin E., Kaufmann J., Bonnem E.M., Fefer A. Subcutaneous granulocyte macrophage colony stimulating factor in patients with myelodysplastic syndrome: toxicity, pharmacokinetics, and hematological effects.J. Clin. Oncol. 7: 629-37 (1989)

69. Antin J.H., Weinberg D.S., Rosenthal D.S. Variable effect of recombinant human granulocyte macrophage colony stimulating factor on bone marrow fibrosis in patients with myelodysplasia. Exp. Hematol. 18: 266-70 (1990)

70. Estey E.H., Kurzrock R., Talpaz M., et al. Effect of low doses of human granulocyte macrophage colony stimulating factor in patients with myelodysplastic syndrome. Br. J. Hematol. 77: 291-5 (1991)

71. Negrin R.S., Haeuber D.H., Nagler A. et al. Maintanance treatment of patients with myelodysplastic syndromes using recombinant human granulocyte colony stimulating factor. Blood 76: 36-43 (1990)

72. Ganser A., Seipelt G., Lindemann A. et al. Effects of recombinant human interleukin-3 in patients with myelodysplastic syndromes. Blood 76: 455-62 (1990)

73. Bettelheim P., Valent P., Andreeff M. et al. Recombinant human granulocyte macrophage colony stimulating factor in combination with standard induction chemotherapy in de novo acute myeloid leukemia. Blood 77: 700-11 (1991)

74. Cannistra S.A., DiCarlo J., Groshek P., et al. Simultaneous administration of granulocyte macrophage colony stimulating factor and cytosine arabinoside for treatment of relapsed acute myeloid leukemia. Leukemia 5: 230-8 (1991)

75. Buchner T., Hiddemann W., Wormann B et al. Multiple corse chemotherapy and GM-CSF from day minus one until neutrophil recovery versus chemotherapy alone in newly diagnosed AML. Ann. Hematol. 64 (suppl.1): A78 (1992)

76. Donatini B., Krupp P., Jones T. Ecogramostatim and pre-existing autoimmune thyroid disease. Lancet 338: 1526-7 (1991)

77. Canellos G.P. The case for high-dose chemotherapy: it is chemotherapy's last gamble? Eur. J. Cancer Clin. Oncol. 4: 351-5 (1987)

78. Dicke K.A., Armitage J.O., Dicke-Evinger B. "Autologous Bone Marrow Transplant V". University of Nebraska Press. Omaha (1990)

79. Armitage J.O., Antman K.M. High-dose Cancer Therapy: Pharmacology, Hemopoietins And Stem Cells. William and Wilkins. New York (1991)

80. Korbling M., Holle R., Haas R. et al. Autologous blood stem cell transplantation in patients with advanced Hodgkin's disease and prior radiation to the pelvic site. J. Clin. Oncol. 8: 978-85 (1990)

81. Gianni A.M., Siena S., Bregni M. et al. Granulocyte-macrophage colony stimulating factor to harvest circulating hematopoietic stem cells for autotransplantation. Lancet 2: 580-4 (1988)

82. Lawler M., Humphries P., McCann S.R. Evaluation of mixed chimerism by in vitro amplification of dinucleotide repeat sequences using the polymerase chain reaction. Blood 77: 2504-14 (1991)

83. Laporte J.P., Fonillard L., Donay L. et al. GM-CSF instead of autologous bone marrow transplantation after the BEAM regimen. Lancet 338: 601-2 (1991)

84. Klasa R.J., Murray N., Coldman A.J. Dose-intensity meta-analysis of chemotherapy regimens in small cell carcinoma of the lung. J. Clin. Oncol. 9: 499-508 (1991)

85. Meyer R.M., Hryniuk W.M., Goodyear M.D. The role of dose-intensity in determining outcome in intermediate grade non-Hodgkin lymphoma. J. Clin. Oncol. 9: 339-47 (1991)

86. Dodwell D.J, Gurney H., Thatcher N. Dose intensity in cancer chemotherapy. Br. J. Cancer 61: 789-94 (1990)

87. Vadhan-Raj S., Broxmeyer H.E., Spitzer G. et al. Stimulation of non-clonal hematopoiesis and suppression of the neoplastic clone after treatment with recombinant human granulocyte-macrophage colony stimulating factor in a patient with therapy-related myelodysplastic syndrome. Blood 74: 1491-8 (1989)

88. Toki H., Matsutomo S., Okabe K., Shimokawa T. Remission in hypoplastic acute myeloid leukemia induced by granulocyte colony stimulating factor. Lancet 1: 1389-90 (1989)

89. Steward W.P., Scarffe J.H., Austin K. et al. Recombinant human granulocyte-macrophage colony stimulating factor (rhGM-CSF) given as daily short infusion in a phase I dose-toxicity study. Br. J. Cancer 59: 142-5 (1989)

EFFICACY OF THE COMBINED TREATMENT WITH FLUCONAZOLE AND THYMOSIN α 1 AGAINST *Candida albicans* INFECTION IN MORPHINE-TREATED MICE

Paolo Di Francesco, Roberta Gaziano, Francesca Pica,
Ida Casalinuovo, Anna Teresa Palamara, Luisella Belogi,
Cartesio Favalli and Enrico Garaci

Department of Experimental Medicine and Biochemical
Sciences, University of Rome, Tor Vergata, Rome, Italy

INTRODUCTION

Pulmonary infections, viral hepatitis, bacterial endocarditis, bacteremia, abscesses at the site of injection, cellulitis and thrombophlebitis are reported to be common in intravenous drug abusers[1] (Table 1). Parallely, there is evidence that has demonstrated that morphine, cocaine and marijuana can affect a variety of immunological functions in humans and in experimental models[2,3,4], suggesting that the drug-induced inhibition of natural resistance mechanisms may represent an important risk factor in increasing susceptibility of abusers to opportunistic infections (Table 1).

Candida albicans is a dimorphic fungus whose importance as an opportunistic agent of human disease is increasingly considered. The microorganism is usually harboured as harmless commensal in the gastrointestinal tract, but candidosis occurs in severely debilitated hosts undergoing immunosuppressive treatments or conditions. These include broad-spectrum potent antibacterials, complicated surgeries, burns injuries, illicit intravenous drug

Combination Therapies 2, Edited by A.L. Goldstein
and E. Garaci Plenum Press, New York, 1993

use, pregnancy, frequent and prolonged use of indwelling devices, organ transplants, chemoterapy-induced neutropenia and acquired immunodeficiency syndrome (AIDS)[5].

In recent years, outbreaks of candidiasis with an unusual presentation have been reported in heroin addicts[6]. Skin lesions (deep-seated scalp nodules and folliculitis in hairy zones) and eye lesions (mainly chorioretinitis) developed sequentially within 10 days of injection of brown heroin. The rapid development of nodules secondary to folliculitis suggests a depressive action on cellular immunity of heroin[6]. Opioid administration was associated with immune abnormalities such as defective mitogenesis, antibody responses and altered lymphocyte distribution[2,7] (Table 1). A general depression of phagocyte activity, number of thymocytes and white blood cells and delayed hypersensitivity reactions have been reported[7]. Morphine also suppresses cytotoxic cell activities, mediated by Natural Killer (NK) cells, and Interferon (IFN) production[7]. In particular, it seems that brown heroin may have a specific depressive action on cellular immunity directed against C.*albicans*, confirming that the negative impact of morphine on innate resistence mechanisms is at least one of the reasons for its effects on the development of fungal infection[6].

New specific therapies or regimens to help the host immune system in the control of fungal infection have been recently used in experimental models and in certain high-risk patients[3]. However, the therapeutic potential of Biological Response Modifiers (BRMs) should be further explored in the face of the poor results often afforded by conventional antifungal therapy in severe systemic infections of the immunocompromised host.

In this paper we present results on a new specific combination therapy between an antifungal agent (*i.e.*, fluconazole) and an immunomodulator of thymic origin [*i.e.*, thymosin alpha one (Tα1)].

Tα1, a synthetic peptide originally isolated in its native form from thymosin fraction 5 (TF-5) modulates *in vitro* T-cell and NK-mediated cytotoxic activities[8,9]. *In vivo* studies indicated that thymic hormones can correct experimental or clinical immunodeficiencies[7]. Combination therapies with several BRMs (Tα1, IFN α/β, IL-2) have recently been proposed in the treatment of cancer to normalize and potentiate cellular immune responses depressed by the disease itself or cancer therapy[10] (see also Garaci and Favalli in this book). The use of BRMs may also be useful in the treatment and control of immune disorders induced by drug abuse. As a result of this observation we have recently shown that Tα1 accelerates the recovery of normal cytotoxicity when administered during *in vivo* cocaine treatment and after the suspension of drug administration[11] (see also Ravagnan *et al.* in this book).

Fluconazole is a recently licensed bis-triazole that inhibits fungal cytochrome P-450, blocks the demethylation of lanosterol and inhibits the synthesis of ergosterol[12].

This compound has been approved by the US Food and Drug Administration to treat oropharyngeal and esophageal candidiasias, peovide maintenance-phase therapy of cryptococcal meningitis, and the failures of primary candidal infection[12].

Table 1. *Effects of illicit drugs on the immune system and infectious diseases.*

Drug of abuse	Immunosuppressive effects	Infections
Cocaine	IL-2, IL-4 and IFN-γ induction. NK and CTL activities, antibody formation, macrophages activities and O_2 production.	Influenza virus, HBV, HIV, HSV1, HSV2
Morphine, heroin	Peritoneal phagocyte counts, phagocytosis and killing and O_2 production. NK cell activity, IFN-γ and IFN-α production. Total number of circulating lymphocytes, rosette formation and antibody production, T cell blastogenesis.	Influenza virus, HBV, HSV1, HSV2, HIV. *Klebsiella pneumoniae*, *Pneumocistis carini*, *Staphylococcus aureus*, *Cryptococcus neoformans*, *Candida albicans*
Marjiuana	NK and CTL activities, IFN induction, PFC responses, blastogenesis.	HSV1, HSV2, HIV *Listeria monocytogenes*.

RESULTS AND DISCUSSION

Table 2 show the effect of fluconazole (FLU) against a C. *albicans* infection in normal and morphine-treated mice. Six- to eight-week-old CD1 mice were infected i.v. with 1.0×10^6 C. *albicans* cells (strain ATCC 2091) on day 0. Morphine was administrated s.c. (75 mg/kg/day) before (on day -3,-2,-1), during and after (on day +1,+2,+3,+4,+5) intravenous challenge with C. *albicans*. Our data indicate that the administration of fluconazole 6, 24 and 48 hours after fungal infection was more effective in normal mice in comparison with morphine-treated mice. In contrast, significant protection against letal infection resulted when Tα1 (200 μg/kg/day) was administered in fluconazole-treated mice before (on day -3,-2,-1) and after (on day +1,+2,+3,+4,+5) C. *albicans* challenge (Fig. 1). In the present study we confirm that morphine can adversely affect the outcome of infectious diseases. It is well known that morphine and its related narcotic agents drastically reduce phagocytes count, killing properties and superoxide anion production in PMNLs and macrophages, suggesting that the negative impact of morphine on phagocytic function is at least one of the reasons for its effect on the development of infection.

Table 2. *Comparison of different Fluconazole treatments against a systemic C. albicans infection in normal and morphine-treated mice.*

Groups[1]	No. animals	M.S.T. (days)	P< [2]	D/T[3]
Vehicle	15	11.53	-	15/15
...+ FLU[4] 0.5 mg/kg	15	16.2	0.003	10/15
..+ FLU 2.5 mg/kg	15	17.53	0.001	7/15
Morphine[5]	15	5.53	-	15/15
.. + FLU 0.5 mg/kg	15	8.8	0.166	13/15
..+FLU 2.5 mg/kg	15	13.66	0.001	12/15

Morphine *vs.* Vehicle: P<0.001

[1] Four to six week-old CD1 mice received i.v. 1.0×10^6 viable C. *albicans* cells (strain ATCC 2091) on day 0.
[2] By Mann-Whitney *U* test.
[3] Dead mice at 30 days over total animals injected.
[4] Fluconazole (FLU, Sigma Tau, Italy) s.c. at the concentrations indicated on days 0,+1,+2.
[5] Morphine (SALARS, Italy; 75 mg/kg/day, s.c) on days -3,-2,-1,0,+1,+2,+3,+4,+5.

Here we present a new combination therapy between an antinfungal drug and $T\alpha1$, in view of the immunomodulatory effects of thymic hormones. Our data show that fluconazole when used at low and non-toxic doses is insufficient to produce protection against *Candida* infection in morphine-depressed mice. However, the same doses of fluconazole significantly increase the survival time of morphine-treated mice when administered in combination with $T\alpha1$. In particular, a significant resistance to lethal challenge was obtained by treatment with $T\alpha1$ during morphine administration, suggesting that action can be taken against the immunosuppressive effects of morphine by the appropriate employment of BRMs. The finding that $T\alpha1$ increases the resistance against C. *albicans* seems to suggest that mature T cells may be involved in resisting infection. It is possible that increased levels of T cells induced by $T\alpha1$ treatment can potentiate the activation of fungicidal effectors *via* release of soluble mediators (IL2, IL4, GM-CSF, IFN γ)(see Romani *et al.* in this book). Since macrophages and PMNLs play a significant role in resistance to C. *albicans*, a possible direct activation of phagogytes cannot be ruled out. These hypotheses are currently under investigation in our laboratory.

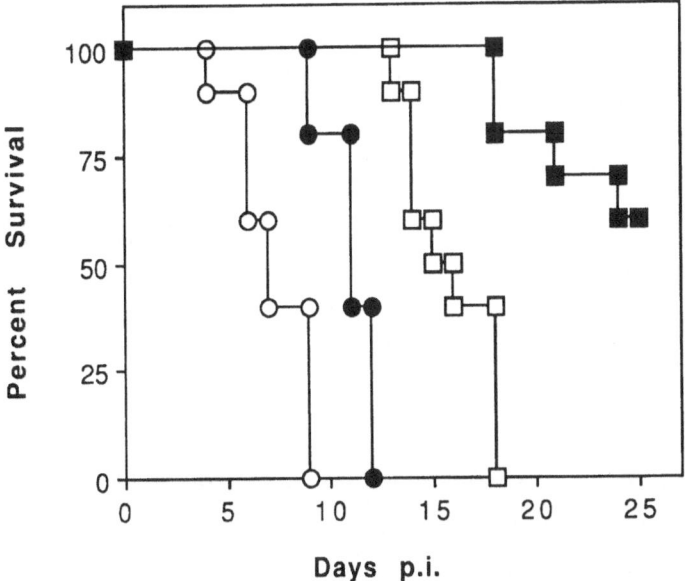

Figure 1. Effect of the combined treatment with fluconazole and Tα1 on the survival of *Candida*- infected and morphine-treated mice. Four- to six-week-old CD1 mice were divided into four experimental groups (20 mice/group) and treated as follows: control diluent (●); morphine (75 mg/kg/day, s.c) on days -3/+5 (○); Fluconazole (0.5 mg/kg/day, s.c.) on days 0,+1,+2 (□); Fluconazole plus Tα1 (200 μg/kg/day, i.p) on days -3/+5 (■). On day 0, all mice were inoculated i.v. with 1.0×10^6 viable C. *albicans* cells. Survival curves represent the values of one representative out of two independent experiments. P<0.01 *vs* control diluent for the mortality ratio on the 30th day (Fisher exact test).

In conclusion, we can suggest that the use of BRMs in combination with direct chemoterapy may be useful in achieving an anti-infection effect without the toxic side-effects associated with high and repeated doses of an antifungal drug.

In fact, the possibility of controlling infection and improving the quality of life without the need for massive, debilitating treatments could serve as a significant encouragement to embark on disintoxicating and rehabilitation manegement, the succes of which depends solely on the willingness and general physical condition of the addict.

ACKNOWLEDGMENTS

We would like to thank Enrico Salvatore Pistoia for his excellent technical assistance. This work was supported by CNR, CT04 and M.U.R.S.T., grant 60%.

Corresponding author: Paolo Di Francesco, Department of Experimental Medicine and Biochemical Sciences, University of Rome, Tor Vergata, Via O. Raimondo, I-00173, Rome, Italy.

REFERENCES

1. H. W. Haverkos and W. R. Lange. Serious infections other than human immunodeficiency virus among intravenous drug abusers. *J. Infect. Dis.* 161: 894-902 (1990).

2. G. G. Nahas and C. Latour. Physiopathology of illicit drugs: cannabis, cocaine, opiates. Advances in the biosciences, Pergamon Press, Oxford (1990).

3. P. Di Francesco, F. Pica, C. Croce C. Favalli, E. Tubaro, and E. Garaci.. Effect of acute or daily cocaine administration on cellular immune response and virus infection in mice. *Nat. Imm.Cell Growth Reg.* 9: 397-405 (1990).

4. P. Di Francesco, Marini, S., Pica, F., Favalli, C., Tubaro, E. and Garaci, E. *In vivo* cocaine administration influences lymphokine production and humoral immune response. *Immunol. Res.*, 11, 74-79, (1992)

5. J. Cohen. Infections of the immunocompromised host. Current Opinion in Infectious Diseases. Vol.5, No 3 (1992).

6. P. Elbaze, J. P. Lacour, J. Cottalorda, Y. Le Fichoux and J. P. Ortonne. The skin as the possible reservoir for *Candida albicans* in the oculo-cutaneous candidiasis of heroin addicts. *Acta Derm. Venereol.* 72: 180-181 (1992).

7. Fischer, G. Opioid peptides modulate immune functions. *Immunopharmacol. Immunotoxicol* , 10 (3): 265-277 (1988).

8. K.K. Oates and M. C. Coss. The role of thymosin as biological response modifiers. *Med. Sci. Res.* 17: 793-796 (1989).

9. A.L. Goldstein, Low, T.L., Adoo, M., Mc Clure, J., Thurman, G.B., Rossio, G., Lay, C.Y., Chang, D., Wang, S.S., Harwey, C., Ramel, A.H. and Meienhofer, J. Thymosin alpha one: isolation and sequence analysis of immunological active polypeptide. *Proc. Natl. Acad. Sci.*, 74: 725-731 (1977)

10. C. Favalli, A. Mastino, S. Grelli, F. Pica, G. Rasi, and E. Garaci. Rationale for therapeutic approches with thymosin α1, interleukin 2 and interferon in combination with chemotherapy. Combination Therapies. Eds. A. G. Goldstein and E. Garaci, Plenum Press, New York. 275-281 (1992).

11. P. Di Francesco, F. Pica, S. Marini C. Favalli, E. Garaci.. Thymosin alpha one restores murine T-cell mediated responses inhibited by in vivo cocaine administration. *Int. J. Immunopharmac.* 14: 1-9 (1992).

12. T. G. Evans, J. Mayer, S. Cohen, D. Classen, and K. Carroll. Fluconazole failure in the treatment of invasive mycoses. *J. Infect. Dis.* 164: 1232-1235 (1991).

ANTI-CYTOKINE THERAPY OF MURINE CANDIDIASIS

Luigina Romani, Elio Cenci, Antonella Mencacci, Roberta Spaccapelo,
Enrico Schiaffella, Laura Tonnetti, Paolo Puccetti, and Francesco Bistoni

Department of Experimental Medicine and Biochemical Sciences, University
of Perugia, Via del Giochetto, 06100 Perugia, Italy

INTRODUCTION

One major feature of antimicrobial resistance in human and experimental settings is the dichotomy of the response against intracellular and extracellular pathogens. The major mechanism in resistance to intracellular pathogens is cytotoxicity occurring through the activity of cytotoxic or phagocytic cells, or mediated by antibody. In contrast, resistance to extracellular pathogens mostly relies on antibodies with neutralizing or opsonizing activity. These two types of response are primarily characterized by the induction of delayed type hypersensitivity (DTH) and help for antibody synthesis, respectively, thus providing a possible explanation for the separate and often reciprocal regulation of humoral and cell-mediated responses to microbial pathogens. Indeed, in most microbial infection models, cellular and humoral responses seem to be reciprocally regulated both in time and intensity (1). As a matter of fact, either type of response is governed by one of the two major T cell subsets known as Th1 and Th2 (2, 3). Strong DTH and low antibody responses are associated with the activation of Th1 cells, whereas high antibody levels, including IgE, and poor or absent footpad responses, mainly result from Th2 cell activation. Such an orchestrated picture derives largely from studies of murine cutaneous *Leishmania major* infection, where susceptibility or resistance are genetically determined. As a result, resistant mice are characterized by strong DTH responses and production of cytokines of the Th1 secretion profile, whereas susceptible mice have high antibody levels and produce a preponderance of Th2 cytokines (4). Although less clearly defined, a similar situation may apply to other infectious disease models, including those with bacteria, protozoa and viruses (5). In contrast, no data are available on Th responses to fungi.

This issue, however, seems to be important because human responses to *Candida albicans* include DTH and humoral responses, as demonstrated by the occurrence of a positive skin test reaction in most healthy adults and by the presence of *Candida*-specific IgE in sera and vaginal fluids of women with recurrent candidal vaginitis (5). To study the possible occurrence of Th1 and Th2 responses to *Candida* in mice, we have used two mutagenized yeast variants that, although both agerminative and avirulent, differ in their ability to elicit protective immunity (7). When mice were infected with either of these variants of *C. albicans*, both variants established chronic infection, but only one, Vir⁻3, resulted in the induction of protective immunity. This was associated with the detection of strong DTH reactivity, high levels of the Th1 cytokines, IL-2 and IFN-γ and low levels of

Combination Therapies 2, Edited by A.L. Goldstein
and E. Garaci Plenum Press, New York, 1993

Table 1. Immunity to *C. albicans* as a consequence of Th subset activation.

- Infection with Vir⁻3 (protective immunity)

        high IFN-γ   low IL-4
        strong DTH   low IL-6

- Infection with Vir⁻13 (non-protective immunity)

        low IFN-γ   high IL-4
        poor DTH   high IL-6, and antibody

---

the Th2 cytokines, IL-4 and IL-6. The reverse was true for the non-protective variant Vir⁻13 (Table 1).

Pattern of Susceptibility and Resistance to *C. albicans* Infection as a Consequence of Differential Th Subset Activation.

To find out whether genetically determined susceptibility and resistance correlate directly with Th subset activation, we used mice of different haplotypes as the recipients of an intravenous challenge with *C. albicans* cells. A strain distribution of resistance versus susceptibility is known to exist in mice of different haplotypes, with BALB/cByJ mice being the most resistant and DBA/2J mice the most susceptible upon systemic infection (8). We injected mice of different strains intravenously with 10^5 live cells of the variant of *C. albicans*, PCA-2. This yeast variant results in chronic infection in immunocompetent hosts associated with persistent colonization of different organs (9), and the selective activation of the Th1 subset (10), capable of conferring long-lived, acquired anticandidal resistance. The different strains of mice were examined for: a) resistance to PCA-2 challenge; b) resistance to reinfection with the wild-type CA-6 cells, and c) development of DTH and antibody production. The results are summarized in Table 2. It is apparent that: 1) The different strains behaved differently in terms of resistance to primary challenge and ability of survivors to mount a secondary protective response. In particular, mice of C57B1/6 and BALB/c strains were found to survive primary infection with PCA-2 cells and subsequent challenge with virulent CA-6 cells. These mice exhibited strong DTH reactivity to *Candida* cells and a prominent antibody response mediated by Ag-specific IgG2a antibodies. These data strongly suggest the selective activation of the Th1 subset in response to *C. albicans* infection in C57B1/6 and BALB/c mice; 2) Mice of C3H/He and CBA/J strains, while able to survive PCA-2 infection, were nevertheless incapable of resisting later challenge with CA-6 cells. In this case, Th1- and Th2-like functions were variably detected, such that DTH reactions developed in C3H/He but not in CBA/J mice, while *Candida*-specific antibodies of both IgG2a and IgG1 isotypes were detected in both strains of mice. The concomitant expression of Th1 and Th2 functions in these strains is compatible with the hypothesis that both subsets are activated during *C. albicans* infection, or the Th0 phenotype is expressed; 3) Finally, elevated serum IgG, IgA and IgE responses and no DTH reactions were detected in infected DBA/2 mice that were incapable of resisting primary challenge with PCA-2 cells. Thus, the Th2 status is associated with susceptibility to systemic *C. albicans* infection. All together these data can be taken to indicate that the Th2 status which predominates in mice after *C. albicans* infection correlates with genetically determined, non-H-2-linked, susceptibility or resistance.

Table 2. Pattern of susceptibility and resistance to systemic *C. albicans* infection in different strains of mice: correlation with Th responses.

Strain	Haplotype	Infection with:		Th responses	
		PCA-2	CA-6	DTH	Antibody
C57B1/6	b	R	R	++	IgG2a
BALB/cCr	d	R	R	++	IgG2a
C3H/He	k	R	S	+	IgG1+IgG2a
CBA/J	a	S	-	-	IgG1+IgG2a
DBA/2Cr	d	S	-	-	IgE

R, resistant; S, susceptible; ++ and +, high to moderate DTH reactivity; -, no DTH.
For antibody, the relevant isotype of antigen-specific antibody is indicated.

Cytokine and Anti-Cytokine Modulation of Th Status during *C. albicans* Infection

It was previously demonstrated (7, 12) that protection against *C. albicans* infection correlates with sustained production of the Th1 cytokine, IL-2 and IFN-γ by CD4$^+$ cells, whereas the non-protective state was associated with release of high amounts of the Th2 cytokines, IL-4 and IL-6. Interestingly, both types of cytokines could be detected as early as three days after infection, both in terms of specific biological activities in the supernatants from in vitro cultured T cells and in terms of specific mRNA transcripts (7, 12). This finding is particularly relevant considering that the quality and, perhaps the quantity, of cytokines present soon after infection might trigger polarized CD4$^+$ Th responses (13). This behavior is thought to reflect cross-regulation between Th1 and Th2 subsets and in fact Th1 cells produce IFN-γ that inhibits the proliferation of Th2 lymphocytes allowing the former population to dominate (15), and vice versa. Th2 cells produce IL-10 that inhibits Th1 cytokine synthesis, thereby releasing Th2 cell expansion from control by IFN-γ (16).

To assess the role of early Th1 and Th2 cytokine production during *C. albicans* infection, neutralizing monoclonal antibodies (Mabs) to specific cytokines were injected into mice in occurrence with infection. CD2F1 mice [known to be Th1 responders to the infection with low-virulence PCA-2 and Th2 responders to infection with virulent CA-6 cells (7, 12)] were given 1 mg intraperitoneally of purified Mab specific for IFN-γ or IL-4. The former Mabs were injected as a single injection 6 h before infection during the first week with the intent of preventing the development of polarized and stabilized Th1 responses. On the contrary, anti-IL-4 Mab was administered into mice infected with virulent CA-6 cells to prevent the differentiation and proliferation of Th2 CD4$^+$ cells upon which IL-4 acts both as differentiation and a growth factor (17). Mice were monitored for mortality parameters, quantitative yeast cell recovery from kidneys and pattern of cytokine production by CD4$^+$ splenocytes in vitro upon restimulation with specific antigen. These results can be summarized as follows: 1) treatment with anti-IFN-γ Mab does not modify mouse susceptibility to PCA-2 infection in that all mice survived challenge (Table 3). However, the animals were unable to resist subsequent challenge with virulent CA-6 cells, thus suggesting that neutralization of endogenous IFN-γ prevents the development of acquired anti-*Candida* immunity. Quantitative yeast cell recovery from the kidneys revealed a higher number of yeast cells in mice treated with Mab to IFN-γ than in control mice (data not shown).

When the pattern of cytokine production was examined in mice treated with Mab to IFN-γ, it was found that CD4+ T cells produced in vitro less IFN-γ and IL-2 than cells from control mice; in contrast, the production of IL-4 in IFN-γ-depleted mice was markedly increased. These data indicate that neutralization of endogenous IFN-γ in a murine model of systemic candidiasis does not affect the outcome of a primary infection with attenuated cells but interferes with the generation of acquired protective immunity, and is associated with a predominant Th2 status. We have previously shown that anti-IFN-γ treatment also blocked the effector functions mediated by IFN-γ in immunized mice (11). Altogether these results point to a crucial role of IFN-γ both in the generation and maintenance of acquired anti-*Candida* immunity. 2) Anti-IL-4 Mab treatment initiated at the time of infection resulted in cure of a high percentage of mice injected with virulent CA-6 cells (Table 3), with establishment of long-lasting protective immunity. The phenomenon was associated with clearance of the fungus from the kidneys of cured animals. CD4+ T cells from anti-IL-4-treated animals produced in vitro high levels of IFN-γ and IL-2, as opposed to the high levels of IL-4 and IL-6 by CD4+ cells from control, non-healer mice. These results indicate that anti-Il-4 treatment of mice infected with *C. albicans* could convert the animals from the susceptible to the resistant phenotype by inhibiting the expression of the Th2 subset and up-regulating the functions associated with Th1 cells.

Table 3. Effect of anti-cytokine Mab treatment on course of primary and secondary infection with *C. albicans*.

| | Infection with: | | | | |
| | PCA-2[2] | | CA-6 | | |
Treatment[1]	MST	D/T	MST	D/T	Th status
Control Mab	>60	0/8	-	-	Th1
Control Mab	-	-	9	8/8	Th2
Mab anti-IFN-γ	>60[3]	0/8	-	-	Th2
Mab anti-IL-4	-	-	>60[4]	0/8	Th1

[1] CD2F1 mice were injected with 1 mg of purified anti-IFN-γ Mab (IgG1 antibody from hybridoma R46A2) or anti-IL-4 Mab (IgG1 antibody from hybridoma 11B11) during the first week of infection. Control Mab, isotype-matched antibody used at the same dose.
[2] 10^6 and 10^5 PCA-2 and CA-6 cells, respectively, were injected i.v.
[3] These mice were unable to survive subsequent challenge with the lethal CA-6 cells.
[4] These mice survived subsequent lethal challenge with CA-6 cells.

CONCLUSIONS

The division of CD4+ T cells into distinct subsets based upon cytokine production is a major advance in our understanding of immune responses, particularly those associated with infectious disease. Studies in animal models have revealed that T lymphocytes and the cytokines they produce play a crucial role in determining the outcome of parasitic infections in terms of both protective immunity and immunopathology (18). In the murine *C. albicans* infection model, we found that: a) genetically determined susceptibility and vaccine-induced resistance (19) directly correlate with the Th status of the host, Th1 responses being associated with resistance and Th2 responses with susceptibility; b) appropriate anti-cytokine treatment at the time of infection can alter the outcome of the infection by interfering with cytokine-mediated cross-regulation of Th subsets. These data suggest that Th1-Th2 cross-regulation contributes to resistance and susceptibility to *C. albicans* infection in mice, and strongly indicate that an understanding of the mechanisms of immune defense may be useful in explaining patterns of disease, in possibly protecting individuals at risk (20) and also in attempting new strategies of immune intervention in fungal infections.

ACKNOWLEDGMENT

The authors are grateful to Eileen Zannetti for careful preparation of the manuscript. This work was supported by Progetto Finalizzato FATMA, contract no. 92.00023.PF41, Consiglio Nazionale delle Ricerche, Italy.

REFERENCES

1. P.H. Lagrange, G.B. Mackness, and T.E. Miller, Influence of dose and route of antigen injection of the immunological induction of T cells, *J. Exp. Med.* 139:528 (1974).
2. T.R. Mosmann, and R.L. Coffman, Heterogeneity of cytokine secretion patterns and functions of helper T cells, *Adv. Immunol.* 46:111 (1989).
3. P. Scott, E. Pearce, A.W. Cheever, R.L. Coffman, and A. Sher, Role of cytokines and CD4+ T-cell subsets in the regulation of parasite immunity and disease, *Immunol. Rev.* 112:161 (1989).
4. R.L. Coffman, R. Chatelain, L.M.C.C. Leal, and K. Varkila, *Leishmania major* infection in mice. A model system for the study of CD4+ T-cell differentiation. *Res. Immunol.* 142:36 (1991).
5. P. Scott, and S.H.E. Kaufmann, The role of T-cell subsets and cytokines in the regulation of infection, *Immunol. Today* 12:346 (1991).
6.. S.S.Witkin, J. Jeremias, and W.J. Ledger, Vaginal eosinophils and IgE antibodies to *Candida albicans* in women with recurrent vaginitis, *J. Med. Vet. Mycol.* 27:57 (1989).
7. L. Romani, S. Mocci, C. Bietta, L. Lanfaloni, P. Puccetti, and F. Bistoni, Th1 and Th2 cytokine secretion patterns in murine candidiasis: association of Th1 responses with acquired resistance, *Infect. Immun.* 59:4647 (1991).
8. R.F. Hector, J.E. Domer, and E.W. Carrow, Immune responses to *Candida albicans* in genetically distinct mice, *Infect. Immun.* 38:1020 (1982).
9. A. Vecchiarelli, R. Mazzolla, S. Farinelli, A. Cassone, and F. Bistoni, Immunomodulation by *Candida albicans*: crucial role of organ colonization and chronic infection with an attenuated agerminative strain of *Candida albicans* for establishment of anti-infectious protection, *J. Gen. Microbiol.* 134:2583 (1988).
10. E. Cenci, L. Romani, A. Vecchiarelli, P. Puccetti, and F. Bistoni, Role of L3T4+ lymphocytes in protective immunity to systemic *Candida albicans* infection in mice, *Infect. Immun.* 57:3581 (1989).
11. L. Romani, E. Cenci, A. Mencacci, R. Spaccapelo, U. Grohmann, P. Puccetti, and F. Bistoni, Gamma interferon modulates CD4+ subset expression in murine candidiasis, *Infect. Immun.* 60:4950 (1992).
12. L. Romani, A. Mencacci, U. Grohmann, S. Mocci, P. Mosci, P. Puccetti, and F. Bistoni, Neutralizing antibody to interleukin 4 induces systemic protection and Th1-associated immunity in murine candidiasis, *J. Exp. Med.* 170:19 (1992).

13. P. Scott, IFN-γ modulates the early development of Th1 and Th2 responses in a murine model of cutaneous leishmaniasis, *J. Immunol.* 147:3149 (1991).
14. A. Sher, R.T. Gazzinelli, J.P. Oswald, M. Clerici, M. Kullberg, E.J. Pearce, J.A. Berzofsky, T.R. Mosmann, S.L. James, H.C. Morse, and G.M. Shearer, Role of T-cell derived cytokines in the downregulation of immune responses in parasitic and retroviral infection, *Immunother.* 127:1 (1992).
15. T.F. Gajewski, S.R. Schell, G. Nan, and F.W. Fitch, Regulation of T-cell activation: differences among T-cell subsets, *J. Immunol.* 140:1555 (1988).
16. D.F. Fiorentino, M.W. Bond, and T.R. Mosmann, Two types of mouse T helper cell IV: Th2 clones secrete a factor that inhibits cytokine production by Th1 clones, *J. Exp. Med.* 170:2081 (1989).
17. S.L. Swain, L.M. Bradley, M. Croft, S. Tongonogy, C. Atkines, A.D. Weinberg, D.D. Duncan, S.M. Hendrick, R.W. Dutton, and G. Huston, Helper T-cell subsets: phenotype, function and the role of lymphokines in regulating their development, *Immunol. Rev.* 123:115 (1991).
18. A. Sher, and R.L. Coffman, Regulation of immunity to parasites by T cells and T cell-derived cytokines, *Annu. Rev. Immunol,* 10:385 (1992).
19. L. Romani, A. Mencacci, E. Cenci, R. Spaccapelo, P. Mosci, P. Puccetti, and F. Bistoni, CD4[+] subset expression in murine candidiasis, *J. Immunol.* 150:925 (1993).
20. G.M. Shearer, and M. Clerici, T helper cell immune dysfunction in asymptomatic, HIV-1-seropositive individuals: the role of Th1-Th2 cross-regulation, *Chem. Immunol.* 54:21 (1992).

THE BASIC RESEARCH AND CLINICAL APPLICATION

OF THYMOPEPTIDIN

Chang Xue Zheng, Cheng Su Xu*, Shilian Liu*

Dept. of Bio-Sci. and Biotech. Tsinghua University
*Dept. of Molecular Biology and Biochem. Institute
of Basic Medical Sciences, Chinese Academy of Medical
Sciences, Beijing,china.

Ample evidence has shown that the thymus gland is the major and central organ of immune system. The thymus produces many hormone-like factors and provides an environment for the differentiation and maturation of the thymocytes.In the past three decades, a number of thymic factors with hormone-like activity have been isolated and prepared from thymus gland and serum, such as thymosin fraction 5, thymosin $\alpha 1$, thymopoietin, thymulin, and thymic humoral factor(1). some of them are being under clinical trail to treat the patients with different diseases related to immune deficiency.In the present paper We would like to report research works on thymic peptides conducted by us and our Chinese colleagues.

We first started our work on thymic factor by methods of Allan Goldstein .We modified the isolation and the in vitro bioassay of thymosin fraction 5 and applied the preparation to treat patients with immuno disorder diseases since 1973.The results of clinical trails were encouraging.For the molecular weights of most thymic factors that had been described were lower than 10 KD, We isolated and prepared the small thymic peptides from supernatant of homogenized fetal calf thymus by method of Liu (2,3). Then We purified the preparation by gel filtration with Sephadex G-15, DEAE-Sephadex A-25, Sephadex G-10, and two dimensional paper chromatography.

Fetal Calf Thymus
↓
Homogenization
in PH2 buffer
↓
Heating to 85°C
Centrifugation
↓
Supernatant
↓
Ultrafiltration
↓
Gel filtration sephadex G-15
↓
Gel filtration DEAE-Sephadex A-25
↓
Gel filtration Sephadex G-10
↓
CTP-8aa

Finally We got a pure peptide (CTP-8aa) consisting of Glu,Asp,ang Gly at a molecular ratio 3:3:2 with molecular weight less than 1 KD. The E-rosette augmenting activity of the peptide is 150 to 500 times higher than that of original mixed peptides.

We have developed a procedure to prepare the thymic peptides with a purpose as a drug for clinical trail. The preparation, named thymopeptidin (TP), is a mixture of small thymic peptides, The molecular weight of component peptides of the preparation is less than 5KD. The immunological experiments showed that TP is very active in stimulating E-rosette formation of thymocytes and human umbilical cord blood lymphocytes. TP is able to enhance the proliferation of lymphocytes in the presence of ConA and PHA. For example,Chen et al (4) showed that in the presence of ConA, TP was demonstrated to promote the proliferation of PNA-negative thymocytes and cortisone resistant thymocytes (CRT).It indicates that the functionally more mature thymocyte subpopulations are more susceptible to the TP.

Chen et al (5) also described that low concentration of TP (1-10 g/ml) was able to enhance the cytotoxic T cell lytic activity of ConA-induced CRT and spleen cells (Table 2).

Table 1. Effect of TP on proliferation of cortisone-resistant thymocytes

TP Conc.	Corporation of ^{3}H-TdR (cpm/well)		
(μg/ml)	− Con A	+ Con A	P
100	90±17	13748±991	<0.001
10	129±12*	57472±5704	<0.01
1	204±39*	56110±3645	<0.001
0.1	157±25*	45700±3078	<0.02
0	135±21	35928±1993	

* P > 0.05

Table 2. Effect of TP on the generation of CTL from Con A-induced cortisone-resistant thymocytes

Dose of TP (μg/ml)	Con A (3μg/ml)	specific lysis %		
		Exp.1	Exp.2	Exp.3
100	+	9.0±0.13*	13.7±0.3*	13.3±1.1*
10	+	31.2±0.7*	39.4±1.2*	40.9±1.8
1	+	27.4±1.8*	43.3±0.6*	51.5±0.2*
0	+	18.3±0.9	21.8±0.1	38.7±3.0

Values of each group are the mean±SD of 6 replicates.
* P < 0.05

Table 3. Effect of tp on IL2 production of cortisone resistant thymocytes(CRT)

Group	Activity of IL2 (^{3}H-TdR incorporation,cpm/w)			
	Exp.1	Exp.2	Exp.3	Exp.4
TP100-CRT	20980±4099*	37446±294*	2661±121*	3438±293*
TP 10-CRT	65575±6558*	36063±1389*	2051±303*	1074±186*
TP 1-CRT	69223±7076*	31996±2489*	2236±79*	801±92
TP 0-CRT	7745±1489	6159±1044	1402±81	661±83

CRT were incubated with TP (0-100µg/ml) for 3.5 hrs at 37°C.
Wash with PBS, added ConA (3.0µg/ml) and incubated for 24 hrs
The IL2 activity of supernatant was detected.
* $P<0.05$

Zhang(6) reported that TP itself was not enough to stimulate CRT to produce IL2, but together with ConA TP did stimulate the IL2 production of CRT (Table 3).

It was shown that TP could enhance the production of TCF by PHA induced human peripheral blood T lymphocytes.

Feng et al(7)observed that treatment of tumor-bearing mice with TP plus cyclophosphamide was more effective in inhibition of tumor growth than that with only cyclophosphamide . The macrophage cytotoxicity of these two groups is 16.5% and 5.8% respectively.The possible explanation was that TP indirectly effects on anti-tumor activity of macrophages (Table 4).

Table 4. EFFECTS OF TP ON MOUSE EXPERIMENTAL TUMOR

Group*	Treatment	No of mouse	Survival time(day)	Weight Tumor(g)
1	No	31	21.7± 15.7	1.6 ± 1.1
2	CP	31	32 ± 20	0.48 ± 0.32
3	TP	31	21.6± 11.1	1.78 ± 1.13
4	TP+CP	31	40.4± 16.8	0.33 ± 0.25

* All the mice were inoculated with $2x10^6$ of S180 by S.C.

In the studies of protection of mice from radiation damage by TP,Chi et al(8) showed that under radiation dose of 800 and 900 rad. the rate of survival of control group was 15.4% and 0 respectively,while the survival rates of TP treated group were 50% and 37.5% respectively .(Table 5).

Xu et al(9) observed the effect of TP on E-RFC % of peripheral blood lymphocytes

Table 5. Protection of mice from radiation damage

GROUP	NO OF ANIMAL	DOSE OF RADIATION (RAD)	NO OF SURVIVOR	RATE OF SURVIVAL (%)
TP Treat.	14	800	7	50
CONTROL	13	800	2	15.4
TP Treat	8	900	3	37.5
CONTROL	68	900	0	0

from normal monkeys and monkeys with acute diarrhea. The result showed that E-RFC of lymphocytes from monkeys with acute diarrhea was significantly lower than that of the control and the treatment with TP by I.V. normalized the E-RFC of sick monkeys to the level of the control (Table 6).

Table 6. Comparison of E-RFC% of peripheral blood between normal monkeys and monkeys with acute diarrhea before or After Treatment

Monkeys	Treatment	No	X(%)±SD	Range %
Normal(1)		45	43±13.9	18-69
Sick	AB* + TP			
Before(2)		20	14±14.0	5-43
After (3)		20	57± 8.1	36-71
Sick	AB			
Before(4)		10	29±11.0	13-42
After (5)		10	32±15.0	8-56

* Antibiotics
   2:1 = P <0.001   3:2 = P <0.001
   5:4 = P <0.02   5:3 = P <0.001

Gao and Wang reported that TP was effective in anti infection of candida albicans and bacillus leprae in experiments with mice.

Because it is easy to scale up the production of TP, in past decade patients with secondary immunodeficency disease, autoimmune disease, infectious disease and cancer have been treated with TP .

Viral Hepatitis B type is a very popular infectious disease in China. TP was employed to treat patients with hepatitis B ,the results were inspiring .For example,Du et al(10) treated 75 HBsAg positive carriers with TP, 35 patients (47%) became HBsAg negative. In contrast, only 3 of 53 HBsAg positive patients(6%) treated with non-specific transfer factor became HBsAg negative. The mortality of fulminant viral hepatitis so far has been reported is still very high (around 70%).Recent investigation of the pathogenesis indicated that most patients of this disease are complicated with severe acquired deficiency of cellular immunity. Su et al(11) treated 25 fulminant viral hepatitis patients with intravenous administration of TP plus routine treatment(infusion glucose and electrolytes, injection of glucagon and insulin,prednisolon) 20 of them (80%) were survival. But at same time 9 (50%) of 18 patients treated routinely (as control) died.It showed that adding TP to the combination therapy of fulminant viral hepatitis is probable of benefit to the patient's resistance to secondary infection and thereby may prevent the development of fatal complication of infection.   TP has been recommended as a routine medicine for the treatment of viral hepatitis B patient by the Committee of Evaluation of Medicine for hepatitis in China .

Histocytosis X in children is a very serious   cancer-like disease.The mortality of this disease treated with chemotherapy (cyclophosphamide) is still very high. Yan et al(12) in Beijing Children Hospital treated 40 histocytosis (Letterer Siwe disease) patients with cyclophosphamide, the mortality was 45%. But when they treated 24 patients with cyclophosphamide plus TP, the mortality decreased to 20.8%.

Zuo et al(13) applied TP to treat patients with systemic lupus erythromatosus(SLE). They found that for 40 patients treated with TP plus regular medicine, and for 74 patients treated with hormone only, the mortality rates were 6.9% and 36.5% respectively. 62.1% of patients from first group and 39.2% of patients from second group released from syndrome respectively more than two years.

Chen et al(14) reported that 106 children with asthmatic bronchitis and bronchial asthma were treated with TP and were observed for more than 12 months. 75% of patients were found to improved and cured (Table 7).

Table 7.TP treatment of patients with bronchial asthma and asthmatic bronchitis

Group	No of Patient	Cured	Significantly improved	Improved	No effect
A.B.*	20	2	5	8	5
B.A.#	86	6	19	40	21

* ASTHMATIC BRONCHITIS
# BRONCHIAL ASTHMA

They also did EaRFC% assay for peripheral lymphocyte from healthy children and children with asthma. The result showed the EaRFC% of lymphocyte from sick kids significantly lower than that of lymphocyte from the healthy kids. But The lymphocytes from sick kids were more sensitive to the activation in vitro by TP. It means that TP functions as an active immuno-regurator.Likewise,Yu reported that 20 kids with asthma were treated with TP, 95% Of patients had significant improvement.(Table 8)

Zhang et al (15) reported the result of observation on effect of TP treatment in 11 patients with myasthenia gravis. The clinical effect of TP in these patients was 54.5%. Landi et al (16) showed that IgM and IgD positive lymphocyte subpopulation in patients with myasthenia gravis is higher than in healthy people.They thought it i due to the increase of B cell subpopulation.Zhang showed that a absolute B cell counts(EAC-RFC)were reduced to 60.8% after treatment increase in REFC%,decrease in immuno-complex and C3 in serum were noticed in 9 patients.

Chen (17) employed TP in treatment of patients with herpes zoster . There were two groups: TP treated and placebo(saline solution). The average age of patients and days of illness onset in these two groups are comparable. Days of lesion disappearance, days of illness course and incidence of reminiscent neuralgia of the TP treated group was significantly improved than that of the placebo group (Table 9).

Table 8. ERFC assay of peripheral lymphocyte from healthy children and children with asthma

Group	No of Child	EaRFC %	EaRFC %	Activation %
Healthy	31	27.1±3.4	7.5±3.4	28.4±8.4
Asthma	30	19.1±5.0	10.7±2.9	63.1±26.8

Table 9. Result of TP treatment of patients with herpes zoster

	Group		
	TP Treatment	Placebo	P value
No of cases	35	13	
Average age (year)	36.1	37.3	
Days of illness onset*	4.5	3.7	>0.05
Days of lesion disappearance*	7.6	13.4	<0.01
Days of illness course*	12.1	17.0	<0.05
Incidence of reminiscent neuralgia (%)	8.5	21.0	<0.01

* Average days

Sjögren's syndrome is an immune deficiency disease. Cellular immunity malfunction is one of the major pathogenic cause. Wen et al(18) treated 12 patients with typical Sjögren's syndrome, all of them were women. The average illness course was 4.7 year. After treatment with TP , the syndrome in 3 patients completely disappeared, in 5 patients was significantly improved. The sialochemical analysis showed that flow of saliva of patients was significantly lower than that of control(11 normal women were chosen as control) .while IgA and Na+ were higher than those of the control. After treatment with TP, The flow of saliva of patients increased and Na+ concentration decreased statistically significantly (Table 10).

Zhang et al(19) treated 80 cancer patients (including breast cancer,lung cancer,digestive organ cancer,malignant lymphoma and so on) with TP. Most patients were treated with surgery(34 cases),radiation(11 cases), chemotherapy(3 cases), combination therapy (32 cases) before TP treatment. T lymphocyte subsets in the peripheral blood of the patients were determined by indirect immunoenzyme staining method with OKT monoclonal antibodies before and after TP treatment. The result showed that the proportion of OKT3 (total T cell) cells,OKT4 (helper/inducer) cells, and T4/T8 ratio were lower than the levels of healthy control adults (P<0.005) before TP treatment. After TP treatment ,The proportion of OKT3,OKT4 and T4/T8 ratio all significantly increased (P,0.005).

and the proportion of OKT8 cells remained at pre-treatment level (P > 0.05). The authors pointed that the TP increased the proportion of T4 cell and significantly ameliorated immune functions in these patients with cancer (Table 11).

Table 10 .Result of sialochemical analysis of patients with Sjögren's syndrome at pre-treatment and post-treatment with TP

Group♣	Flow of saliva (ml/min)	IgA (u/ml)	Na$^+$ (mEq/L)	K$^+$ (mEq/L)
Control	0.146±0.066	3.17±1.0	6.0±2.35	16.55±2.18
TP treat.				
Pre-	0.034±0.029*	17.72±12.92*	38.9±18.26*	23.0±10.12
post-	0.069±0.050#	11.49±8.40	21.04±14.03#	17.2±5.19

♣ There were 11 cases patients in both of groups.
* pre-treat./control : P <0.01 - 0.001
# post-treat./pre-treat. : P <0.05-0.01

Table 11 .Evaluation of T Lymphocyte Subset in the peripheral Blood of Patients with Cancer at Pre-treatment and Post-treatment of Thymopeptidin

Parameter*	Healthy♣ group	Pre-treatment	Post-treatment	P value#
OKT3	63.20±5.5	49.7±11.7	54.8±8.3	<0.005
OKT4	40.9±4.5	27.2±7.5	33.6±6.5	<0.005
OKT8	26.0±2.7	25.5±7.5	24.1±4.3	>0.05
T4/T8	1.6±0.3	1.1±0.3	1.4±0.3	<0.005

* The data are expressed as Mean SE.OKT3,OKT4,OKT8 are expressed as %.
♣ 50 cases of healthy adult as control
The values were tested for significantly different for post- and pre-treatment of TP.

The dose of clinical use of TP depended on the severeness of immune disorder. Generally speaking, 0.1mg /Kg body weight, daily or once per two days.20 mg of TP daily, I.V. were used for treatment of patients with fulminant viral hepatitis. No any side effects and toxic effects were observed in the clinical uses of TP till now.

The clinical application of TP in China continued for about 10 years. In 1984, TP was proved by Chinese Medicine Administration, and has been produced since 1984. Now about 10 Chinese pharmaceutical factories are producing TP .The yield is about 5 million ampules per year.

The physiological function of thymus is very complex, and the maturation and function of thymocytes are believed to be regulated by multi-factors.The characters and mechanism of action of thymic hormone-like factors are still unclear. From our experience the preparation containing mixture of thymic peptides is an effective and safe clinical medicine for primary and acquired immune diseases.

REFERENCES

1. Allan L. Goldstein et al; Thymic Factors, in "Biological Response Modifiers and Cancer Therapy", Marcel Dekker,Inc. (1988).
2. Liu Shilian et al; Studies on Thymic Peptide Factors. 1: Isolation, Purification and in vitro E-rosette Augmentation Activity of calf Thymic Peptide Factors.Acta Academiae Medicinae Sinicae,4,No.4,202,(1982).
3. Cui Lian Xian et al;Isolation ,Purification, Biochemical property and E-rosettee Activity in vitro of Porcine Thymic Factors.ibid. 6,No4, 170,(1984).
4. Chen Wei Feng et al; Effect of Thymic Peptides on The Mitogen induced Proliferation of Murine Thymocyte Subpopulation.Acta Biologiae Experimentalis Sinica, 18, No3, 341, (1985).
5. Chang Hui Hua et al; Effect of Thymic Peptides on Production of IL2 of ConA-induced Spleen Cells and CRT Cells. Shanghai J. of Immunology. 5, No4, 211, (1985).
6. Chen Wei Feng et al;The Enhancement Effect of Calf Thymic Peptides on The Mitogen Induced Murine Cytotoxic T Cell Response.Chinese J. of Microbiology and Immunology. 5, No6. 337, (1985).
7. Feng Qi et al;Effect of Thymic Peptide(TP) on the Antitumor Activity of Murine Macrophage,Acta Biologiae Experimentalis Sinica,16,No4,377,(1983).
8. Chi Ze Rong et al; Effect of Thymic Peptide on Protection of Mice from Radiation.Kexue Tongbao. 18, 1428, (1987).
9. Xu Cheng Su et al; Effect of Thymic Peptides on T Lymphocyte Function of Rhesus Monkeys with Acute Diarrhea. Chinese J.of Microbiology and Immunology. 4, No5, 324, (1984).
10. Du Fei Li; Clinical Application of TP in Treatment of Patients with Hepatitis B. Selected Papers on TP . Chinese Academy of Medical Science . No2, (1983).
11. Su Sheng et al; Clinical Application of TP in Treatment of Fulminant Viral Hepatitis. Chinese J.of Internal Medicine,26,No4,223.(1987).
12. Yang shiyuan et al; Clinical Application of TP in Treatment of Children with Histocytosis. Selected Papers on TP. Chinese Academy of Medical Sciences, No2,(1983).
13. ZhoDa Bon et al; Treatment of SLE patients with TP. Selected paper of Tp,Chinese Academy of Medical Sciences, No2, (1983).
14. Chen Yu Zhi; Observation of Effect of TP for Treatment of Children with Bronchial Asthma and Asthmatic Bronchitis.
Chinese J . of Respiratory Disease. 9,No4,211,(1986).
15. Zhang Zhenxin; Preliminary Observation on Effect of TP in Myasthenia Gravis. Acta Academiae Medicinae Sinicae.6,No5,366,(1984).
16. Landi G et al;J.Neurosurg. Psych.45:158,(1982).
17. Chen Xue Rong; Observations of the Effect of TP on Herpes Zoster. Immunology Communication. No2,37,(1984).
18. Wen Zhuxian ; Preliminary Observation of Effect of TP in treatment of Sjogren's Syndrome, Chinese J. of Oral Disease.21:219,(1986).
19. Chang Shan wen et al;Effect of thymic peptide on T lymphocyte subsets of patients with cancer. Selected Paper of Japan-China Medical Scholarship Fellows,P112, Ministry of Public Health of China and Japan-China Medicine Association, (1991).

TREATMENT OF HEPATITIS C VIRUS-ASSOCIATED CHRONIC LIVER DISEASE WITH ß-INTERFERON AND INOSINE PRANOBEX: COMBINATION SCHEDULE VS MONOTHERAPIES

Domenico Sansonno, Claudio Azzolini, and Franco Dammacco

Department of Biomedical Sciences and Human Oncology
Section of Internal Medicine and Clinical Oncology
University of Bari Medical School
Policlinico, Piazza G. Cesare 11, 70124 Bari, Italy

INTRODUCTION

The recently identified hepatitis C virus (HCV)[1] is responsible for almost 90% of cases of chronic post-transfusion non-A, non-B hepatitis and for more than 70% of sporadic cases[2]. Acute NANB hepatitis becomes chronic in 50% of cases[3] and 20-30% of them progress to cirrhosis[4].

Currently, no therapy for chronic hepatitis C has been shown to be effective. However, encouraging results have been reported using interferons, a family of proteins produced by virus-infected cells and endowed with antiviral properties and various immunomodulatory activities[5]. Earlier studies on the treatment of chronic hepatitis with ß-interferon (ß-IFN) did not yield satisfactory responses, possibly because only crude and unstable preparations were available[6]. Subsequently, highly purified ß-IFN preparations became available, capable of inducing systemic interferon levels sufficient to exert reproducible antiviral effects. By using these stable preparations of ß-IFN, clinical responses were achieved that greatly exceeded the spontaneous remission rate. However, clinical remissions were only transient and immediate relapse after discontinuation of therapy was shown in the majority of patients[7,8].

Inosine pranobex (IP) is an antiviral molecule with inhibitory effects either on DNA or RNA viruses, which also possesses some immunomodulating properties resulting in an enhanced direct antiviral activity by interference with interleukin-2 production and receptor expression[9]. Recently, IP has been used in the treatment of HCV-associated chronic liver disease and clinical improvement has been found to parallel the inhibitory effect of the drug on the circulating levels of the HCV RNA as detected by polymerase chain reaction[10]. In order to verify the potential therapeutic effect of a combination therapy which included ß-IFN and IP, we started a clinical trial

Combination Therapies 2, Edited by A.L. Goldstein
and E. Garaci   Plenum Press, New York, 1993

in HCV-associated chronic liver disease in which combined administration of these two agents was compared with the effects of ß-IFN and IP monotherapies.

MATERIALS and METHODS

Forthy-eight patients were enrolled at our Institution between June and December, 1991. All suffered from histologically documented chronic NANB hepatitis, with serum alanine aminotransferase (ALT) 2-4 times higher than the upper limit of the normal range for at least 12 months. A history of parenteral exposure was obtained for 15 patients (31.2%). Patient characteristics are given in table 1.

Table 1. Baseline characteristics of patients with chronic Non-A, Non-B hepatitis randomly allocated to Inosine Pranobex or ß-Interferon or combination of ß-Interferon plus Inosine Pranobex

Clinical Features	No Treatment Group	Inosine Pranobex Group	ß-Interferon Group	Inosine Pranobex plus ß-Interferon Group
Women/men	4/3	5/4	10/8	8/6
Mean age[a] ± SD	50.7±8	54.6±7	52.3±9	49.7±11
CPH	1	1	3	3
CAH	3	3	7	6
CAH/Cirrhosis	3	5	8	5
History of blood transfusion or acupuncture	1	3	6	3
Mean ALT level at start ± SD (Nx)[b]	4.4±2.7	4.2±2.7	3.8±1.8	4.7±2.2
Anti-HBc, Anti-HBs or both	3	4	8	8

CPH: Chronic persistent hepatitis; CAH: Chronic active hepatitis; Anti-HBc: Antibody to hepatitis B core antigen; Anti-HBs: Antibody to hepatitis B surface antigen
[a] Range: 29-70; [b] Results are expressed as times the upper limit of the normal range

All cases were negative for serum hepatitis B surface antigen (HBsAg) and hepatitis B virus DNA[11] as well as for anti-nuclear and anti-smooth muscle antibodies. All were anti-human immunodeficiency virus (HIV) negative. Furthermore, Wilson's disease and alfa-1-antitrypsin deficiency were ruled out. No patient gave a history of drug or alcohol abuse. No patient had ascites or encephalopathy. All serum samples were tested for antibody to HCV (anti-HCV) using enzyme-linked immunosorbent assay (ELISA) and confirmed by the second generation immunoblotting assay (4-RIBA) provided by Ortho Diagnostic Systems (Raritan, NJ, USA). After giving informed consent to their participation into the trial, which was approved by local ethics commission, all patients were randomly allocated to one of three groups to receive oral IP (Viruxan[R], Sigma Tau, Pomezia, Rome) 3 gr a day in three doses 3 times weekly, or ß-IFN (Frone[R], Serono, Rome) 3 MU by subcutaneous injection three times weekly for 16 weeks, or the combination of IP and ß-IFN at the same doses as above in alternate days so that IP was administered in the days free from ß-IFN.

Blood samples were obtained before entering the study, and then every two weeks during the treatment and the follow-up periods. Routine tests included erythrocyte, leucocyte and thrombocyte counts, measurements of serum urea, creatinine, and alkaline phosphatase levels, prothrombin time. Liver biopsy specimens were obtained just before entry into the study.

Patients were classified according to the evolution of their serum ALT levels. "Failure response" was defined as an absent or a poor decrease of ALT concentration, whereas "partial response" was defined as a decrease of 70% or more of the pretherapeutic values without normalization. In addition, "transient response" was defined as the normalization of ALT levels on treatment followed by an increase to more than the upper limit of normal before discontinuation of therapy. Finally, "complete response" was defined as sustained normalization of ALT during the entire period of therapy.

All patients were observed for at least 12 weeks after the stoppage of the therapy by regular monitoring of liver enzymes and anti-HCV antibodies. Statistical analysis was performed using the Student's t-test and frequency rates were compared by Fisher's exact test.

RESULTS

Patients included in the study groups were comparable as regards sex, age, race, history of blood or parenteral exposure, anti-HCV or HBV serology, mean ALT values, pictures of histological liver disease. All 48 patients completed the study.

Frequency of clinical responses evaluated by the changes in serum ALT levels during the treatment period are described in fig.1.

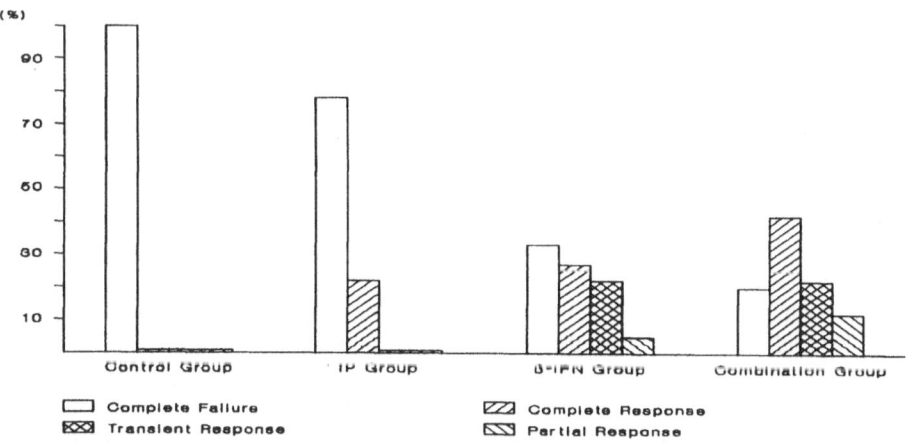

Figure 1. Percentages of clinical responses in treated groups and control group.

Six (42.3%) patients achieved complete response in the combination group (IP+ß-IFN) compared with no patient in the placebo group (p<0.0001), 2 (22.2%) patients in the IP group (p<0.001) and 6 (33.3%) patients in the ß-IFN group (p=NS). A statistically significant difference was found when the ß-IFN group was compared with the IP group (p=0.05). Transient response (transient ALT normalization) was demonstrable in 3 (21.4%) patients of the combination group, in 4 (22.2%) patients of the ß-IFN group and in no patient of the IP group. Furthermore, other 2 (14.3%) patients in the combination group and 1 (5%) patient in the ß-IFN group demonstrated a partial response (significant decrement of ALT without normalization). Complete failure to respond was found in 3 (21.4%) patients in the combination group, in 7 (38.9%) (p<0.05) patients in the ß-IFN group, in 7 (77.9) (p<0.01) patients in the IP group and in 7 (100%) patients in the control group (p<0.0001).

As reported in fig.2, complete response occurred relatively quickly after starting IFN treatment.

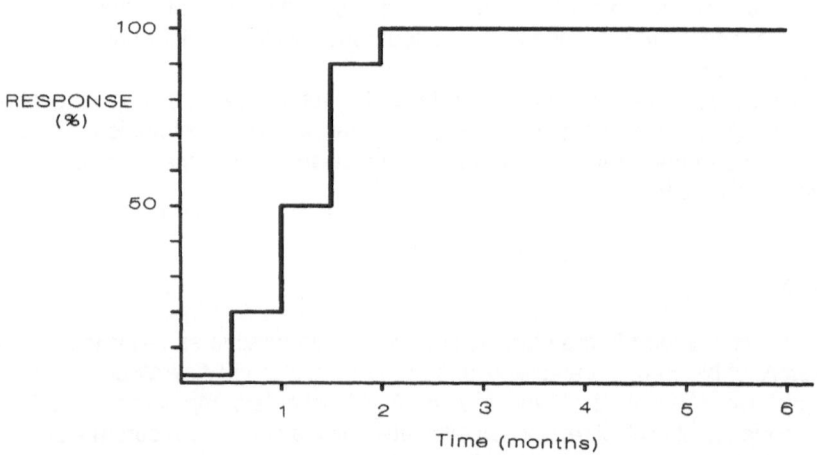

Figure 2. Percentage of response in relation to the duration of the therapy.

Almost 90% of patients of the combination group and the ß-IFN monotherapy group showed clinical amelioration within 6 weeks of treatment. A different behavior was observed in 2 patients of the IP group whose clinical response was obtained after at least 3 months of therapy.

Analysis of patients at the end of terapy led us to identify some predictive parameters of therapeutic responsiveness. When patients with complete response were compared with the remaining patients in each group, ALT levels at the beginnig of the treatment were significantly lower (55±21 vs 117±36; mean±SD; p<0.01).

In addition, a significant difference was observed between responder and non-responder or partially responder patients in terms of pretreatment duration of the disease (3.1±1.7 vs 9.7±4.5 years; mean±SD, p<0.01).

A histological picture of cirrhosis was found in 2/14 (14.3%) patients with complete response, whereas it was present in 19/34 (55.9%) (p<0.01) of non-responder and partially responder patients.

After discontinuation of therapy, patients were followed up and relapse was found to occur in 12/14 (85.7%) patients. In all patients an immediate exacerbation of ALT was demonstrable after therapeutic stoppage and in every case relapse occurred within 12 weeks (fig.3). The 2 non-relapsing patients belonged to the combination therapy group.

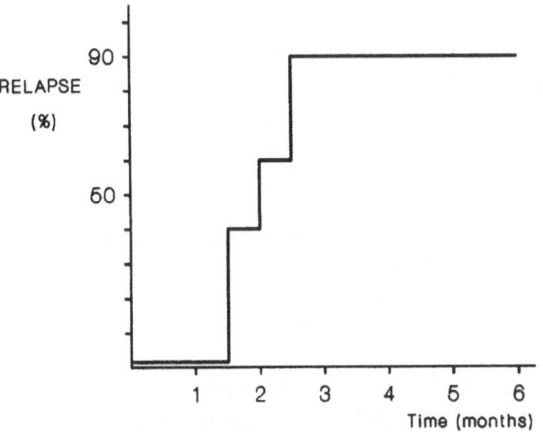

Figure 3. Percentage of relapse after discontinuation of therapy.

No side effects (with the exception of nausea and gastralgia in 1 patient) were demonstrated in the IP group. Moderate adverse reactions including fever, myalgia, headache, arthralgia, depression, leukopenia and thrombocytopenia occurred in both IP+β-IFN and β-IFN groups. However, in no case adverse reactions required discontinuation of therapy. The frequencies of side effects in patients treated with either β-IFN or IP+β-IFN were compared. No differences were found except for nausea that occurred in 6 (42.3%) patients treated with the combination schedule (p<0.05). Leukocytopenia and thrombocytopenia occurred only in patients with accompanying cirrhosis.

DISCUSSION

This study demonstrates that fibroblast interferon (β-IFN) at a dose of 3 MU thrice weekly is well tolerated and is able to induce transaminase normalization in more than a third of patients with HCV-related chronic active hepatitis. These results do not significantly differ from those obtained with the use of recombinant α2b interferon by Davies et al.[12] who described a complete response in 22 of 58 (38%) patients with chronic hepatitis C. However, although IFN therapy has been shown to be effective in reducing biochemical and histological activity of chronic liver disease, it is unable to achieve complete eradication of the virus and discontinuation of therapy is followed by relapse in the great majority of patients. This warrants a search for optimal IFN regimen(s) and/or combination therapies by which antiviral and immunomodulatory effects of IFN might be enhanced.

In this study, we tested the use of a combination schedule in which an antiviral molecule such as IP is associated to ß-IFN. Our results indicate that combination of ß-IFN and IP induces a complete response with higher frequency. The positive clinical effects of this combination were further emphasized by much lower clinical responses obtained with ß-IFN or IP monotherapies. As expected, high basal ALT value, long duration of chronic liver disease, and superimposed cirrhosis[13] were confirmed to be unfavourable conditions which do not draw advantage from ß-IFN monotherapy.

Therapeutic responses occur very quickly and in our experience almost 90% of patients achieved complete responses within 6 weeks of therapy, thus suggesting that it is useless to protract IFN therapy behind this time. However, the rate of relapse has been very high after therapy stoppage in this study.

These results indicate, furthermore, that patients with HCV infection are prone to respond to ß-IFN therapy and that clinical response is immediate suggesting that HCV is an agent highly sensitive to ß-IFN. However, this rapid improvement is followed by an equally rapid relapse after therapy discontinuation, indicating that ß-IFN is unable to induce a complete recovery. On the other hand, the synergistic effect of IP is suggested by the higher frequency of complete response and stabilization of therapeutic response, as well as by the lower frequency of response failure in the combination group.

The occurrence of a relatively large proportion of non-responsive or partially responsive patients clearly indicates that other types of therapies are urgently needed. Likely, they represent a peculiar biological condition in which some resistant factors such as intercellular adhesion molecules could play an important role in the virus-cell interactions by preventing and/or neutralizing the action of cytokines on the target cells[14].

REFERENCES

1 Q.L. Choo, G. Kuo, A.J. Weiner, L.R. Overby, D.W. Bradley, M. Houghton, Isolation of a cDNA clone derived from a blood-borne non-A, non-B viral hepatitis genome, *Science* 244: 359 (1989).

2. D.Sansonno, F. Dammacco, Antibodies to hepatitis C virus in non-A, non-B post-transfusion and cryptogenic chronic liver disease, *Lancet* ii: 798 (1989).

3. H.J. Alter, Transfusion-associated non-A, non-B hepatitis: the first decade, in: *"Viral hepatitis and liver disease"*, A.J. Zuckerman, ed, A.R. Liss, New York (1988).

4. R.L. Koretz, O. Stone, M. Mousa, G.L. Gitnik, Non-A, non-B post-transfusion hepatitis. A decade later, *Gastroenterology* 88: 1251 (1985).

5. W.H. Caselmann, J. Eisenburg, P.H. Hofschneider, R. Koshy, ß and γ-interferon in chronic active hepatitis B. A pilot trial of short term combination therapies, *Gastroenterology* 96: 449 (1989).

6. A. Biliau, The clinical application of fibroblast interferon. An overview, *Med Oncol & Tumor Pharmacother* 1: 87 (1984).

7. K. Ohnishi, F. Nomura, S. Lida, Treatment of post-transfusion non-A, non-B acute and chronic hepatitis with human fibroblast ß-interferon: A preliminary report, *Am J Gastroenterol* 84: 596 (1989).

8. K. Chayama, S. Saiton, Y. Arase, K. Ikeda, T. Matsumoto, Y. Sakai, M. Kobayashi, M. Unakami, T. Morinaga, H. Kumada, Effect of interferon administration on serum hapatitis C virus RNA in patients with chronic hepatitis C, *Hepatology* 13: 1040 (1991).

9. D.M. Campoli-Richards, E.M. Sorkin, R.C. Heel, Inosine pranobex: a preliminary review of its pharmacodynamics and pharmacokinetics properties, and therapeutic efficacy, *Drugs* 32: 383 (1986).

10. W. Prohasca, K. Kleesiek, Treatment of chronic hepatitis C with inosine pranobex, *Lancet* 338: 390 (1991).

11. D. Sansonno, P. Detomaso, M.A. Papanice, G. Fiore, G. Bufano, O.G. Manghisi, Correlation between hepatitis B virus deoxyribonucleic acid and receptors for polymerized human albumine in HBV chronic infection, *Digestion* 37: 206 (1987).

12. G.L. Davis, L.A. Balart, E.R. Schiff, K. Lindsay, H.C. Bodenheimer, R.P. Perrillo, W. Carey, I.M. Jacobson, J. Payne, J.L. Dienstag, D.H. Vanthiel, C. Tamburro, J.Lefkowitch, J. Albrecht, C. Meschievitz, T.J. Ortego, A.Gibas, Treatment of chronic hepatitis C with recombinant interferon alfa. A multicenter randomized, controlled trial. *N Engl J Med* 321: 1501 (1989).

13. X. Causse, H. Godinot, M. Chevallier, P. Chossegros, F. Zoulin, D. Ouzan, J-P. Heyraud, T. Fontanges, J. Albrecht, C. Meschievitz, C. Trepo, Comparison of 1 or 3 MU of Interferon alfa-2b and placebo in patients with chronic non-A, non-B hepatitis. *Gastroenterology* 101: 497 (1991).

14. D. Sansonno, V. Cornacchiulo, P. Gatti, F. Dammacco, Circulating levels and liver tissue distribution of intercellular adhesion molecule-1 during ß-interferon therapy of hepatitis C virus-associated chronic active disease, *Int J Clin Lab Res* 22: 100 (1992).

SUSTAINED RESPONSE TO THYMOSIN THERAPY IN PATIENTS

WITH CHRONIC ACTIVE HEPATITIS B

Milton G. Mutchnick,[1] J.I. Jaurequi[2]
and David A. Shafritz[2]

[1]Department of Medicine, Wayne State University
School of Medicine, Detroit, MI 48201; [2]Liver
Research Center, Albert Einstein College of
Medicine, NY 10461

INTRODUCTION

Chronic hepatitis B (CHB) is a widespread disease associated with significant morbidity and mortality. At least 300 million people worldwide are chronically infected with the hepatitis B virus (HBV) with carrier rates as high as 20% in some populations (1).

The increased incidence of cirrhosis, liver failure and hepatocellular carcinoma in HBV infected individuals provides justification for aggressive therapeutic intervention to favorably influence the natural course of the disease. Alpha interferon is now licensed in the United States as the sole therapeutic agent in the treatment of HBeAg(+), CHB. Interferon induced disease remission occurs in approximately one third of patients. After a follow up period of 3-7 yrs, a sustained response is reported in 87% of individuals showing an initial remission with interferon therapy (2). Thus, 25%-30% of patients with HBeAg(+), CHB show a long-term response to alpha interferon. Moreover, the majority of the patients with sustained response lose the HBsAg (2).

We have previously reported on the results of a Phase II study assessing the efficacy of thymosin fraction 5 (TF5) and thymosin α_1 (Tα_1) in the treatment of CHB (3, 4). Nine of 12 patients (75%) receiving thymosin had a response to treatment, while 2 of 8 (25%) patients given placebo experienced spontaneous remission of disease. We now report on the long term follow up of the 12 patients treated with thymosin.

Combination Therapies 2, Edited by A.L. Goldstein
and E. Garaci   Plenum Press, New York, 1993

PATIENTS AND METHODS

Study Population

A double-blind and placebo controlled Phase II study was conducted between 1986 and 1990 to assess the efficacy of thymosin in the treatment of CHB (3, 4). A total of twenty patients between the ages of 18 and 70 yrs were randomized into one of three treatment arms after meeting entry criteria. These included the presence of the hepatitis B surface antigen (HBsAg) and elevated serum alanine aminotransferase (ALT) levels for at least 6 months; hepatitis B virus DNA (HBV DNA) seropositivity; histologic confirmation of chronic active hepatitis (5) and compensated liver disease. Previously known hepatic encephalopathy, bleeding esophageal or gastric varices, intravenous drug abuse, homosexuality and pregnancy were causes for exclusion. Previous history of malignancy, the presence of hepatitis D antibody or antibody to HIV were additional causes for exclusion.

Study Protocol

The initial 12 patients (Group I) were randomly assigned to receive TF5 (90mg/M^2 body surface area), $T\alpha_1$ (900μg/M^2) or placebo (1.4% sodium bicarbonate) by subcutaneous injection, twice weekly for 6 months. The remaining 8 patients (Group II) were randomized to receive higher doses of TF5 (120mg/M^2), $T\alpha_1$ (1200μg/M^2), or placebo.

If patients reported local discomfort at the injection site, the independent study monitor would determine if treatment would continue or, in the event the patient was receiving TF5, change the treatment to $T\alpha_1$. The clinicians remained blinded to reports of injection site discomfort and to changes in treatment. No patients discontinued therapy and in no instance was the change over from TF5 to $T\alpha_1$ instituted more than 2 weeks after treatment was initiated.

A positive response to treatment was defined as loss of detectable serum HBV DNA by blot hybridization using a ^{32}P-labeled, cloned HBV DNA probe (6) and normalization or near normalization of ALT levels at 1 year. The number of patients entered into each arm for the two doses of TF5 and $T\alpha_1$ are shown in Table 1. Nine (75%) of the 12 patients treated with thymosin demonstrated response to treatment.

All 12 patients treated with thymosin have been evaluated at varying intervals following completion of the 6 month treatment period. The 9 patients responding to thymosin were last seen at intervals ranging from 1 to 5 yrs (mean 3.5 yrs) after completion of injections. Serum biochemical tests, assays for HBV markers (HBsAg, anti-HBs, HBeAg, anti-HBe) and HBV DNA by blot hybridization were performed. In addition, serum samples were subjected to the polymerase chain reaction (PCR), using a method (JIJ, DAS unpublished) which detects HBV DNA at the 10^{-15}-10^{-16} gm level.

Results

Of the 9 patients (1 woman, 8 men; mean age 47 yrs at initiation of treatment) who responded to thymosin treatment, 7 were White, 1 was Black and 1 was Hispanic. Two responders received TF5, (90mg/M^2), 4 responders received $T\alpha_1$ (2 each at 900μg and 1200μg/M^2), and the remaining 3 received 1 or 2 weeks of TF5 initially, followed by 24 or 25 weeks of Tα_1 (2 patients received the lower dose and a single patient, the higher dose). At the conclusion of the initial one year study, all 9 responders were negative for serum HBV DNA by blot hybridization, however, 3 patients remained HBV DNA positive by PCR. During the follow up period there was disease reactivation in 2 (22%) of the responders characterized by significant elevations in ALT and reappearance of HBeAg and serum HBV DNA.

Table 1. Treatment groups

Thymosin fraction 5	Number
90mg/M^2	2
120mg/M^2	1
Thymosin alpha 1	
900μg/M^2	3
1200μg/M^2	2
Thymosin fraction 5 (1 or 2 weeks)	
Thymosin alpha 1 (24 or 25 weeks)	4
Placebo	8

Seven (78%) of the 9 patients responding to thymosin treatment had a sustained remission remaining negative for HBeAg and serum HBV DNA at the 10^{-15}-10^{-16} gm level (PCR). ALT levels in all 7 patients remained normal with 5 patients seroconverting to HBsAg(-) and anti-HBs(+) status (Table 2).

Serum HBV DNA was positive by PCR but not dot blot in 2 of the 7 responders at the conclusion of the 12 month study. Both became negative by 3 and 12 months respectively, following the 1 year study (Table 3).

Table 2. Characteristics of thymosin responders at last assessment

Patient	Follow up (mos)	ALT[a]	HBsAg	Anti-HBs	HBeAg	Anti-HBe
1	60	14	-	+	-	-
2	54	30	-	+	-	(+)
3	56	7	-	+	-	ND
4	40	13	-	+	-	-
5	31	17	-	+	-	-
6	60	24	+	-	-	+
7	13	25	+	-	-	-

[a]Normal value: ALT <50 IU/L; (+), trace positive; ND, not done

Table 3. HBV DNA status at last assessment

	12 Months		Follow up
Patient	Dot Blot	PCR	PCR
1	0	-	-
2	0	-	-
3	0	1+	-
4	0	-	-
5	0	-	-
6	0	-	-
7	0	1+	-

Three of 12 patients treated with thymosin (1 woman, 2 men) did not respond and were considered treatment failures at 1 year. One non-responder died 25 months following completion of the injections ($T\alpha_1$, $900\mu g/M^2$) while awaiting orthotopic liver transplantation. A second patient continued to show mild ALT elevations and was asymptomatic 34 months following completion of treatment (TF5, $120mg/M^2$). The third patient who received TF5 ($120mg/M^2$) initially followed by $T\alpha_1$ ($1200\mu g/M^2$), subsequently cleared the HBeAg and HBV DNA (PCR) and normalized his ALT levels. This "delayed" response to treatment occurred at between 15 and 37 months following completion of treatment. A flow chart summarizing the outcome for the 12 patients treated with thymosin is shown in Figure 1.

In the placebo group of 8 patients, 2 patients experienced a spontaneous remission of disease with normalization of the ALT and loss of serum HBV DNA by both dot blot and PCR during the study period. One patient who seroconverted to a HBsAg(-), anti-HBs(+) status, later developed hepatocellular carcinoma and died 48 months after treatment. Of the remaining 6 patients, 1 was lost to follow up, 1 patient died following orthotopic liver transplantation, 1 patient had active disease 38 months following treatment and 1 patient died of a drug overdose during the 1 year study. Two patients were entered into an open crossover protocol and were treated with $T\alpha_1$ (1 each at $900\mu g/M^2$ and $1200\mu g/M^2$) for 6 months. Both patients responded to treatment, clearing the HBeAg and HBV DNA (PCR). ALT levels in both patients returned to normal.

DISCUSSION

Initial response to thymosin treatment occur in 75% of patients with CHB and long term remission occurred in almost 80% of these patients. Moreover, 7 (58%) of 12 patients given thymosin appeared disease free at a mean follow up of 3.7 yrs. Five of the 7 patients with sustained remission seroconverted to HBsAg(-) and anti-HBs(+): Two lost HBsAg during the 12 month study period and the remaining 3 patients at from 2.5 - 3.5 yrs following treatment. One responder to thymosin first lost detectable HBsAg after 5 months of therapy but remained HBeAg(+) for an additional 7 months. The HBV DNA in this patient was negative by dot blot after 4 months of treatment and was continuously negative for HBV DNA by PCR after 6 months of treatment.

The HBsAg loss occurred over an extended period following thymosin therapy and resembled the rate of HBsAg clearance observed in patients responding to alpha-interferon (2).

Two initial responders to thymosin therapy experienced reactivation of disease between 2 and 3 years after completion of treatment with reappearance of HBV DNA (PCR) in one. HBV DNA by PCR had remained continuously positive throughout the study and follow up period in the second patient, although the dot blot assay was negative at the conclusion of the 12 month study. No predictive factor was identified for disease reactivation.

The observation in this Phase II study, demonstrating a 75% initial response to thymosin treatment and a high proportion of sustained remissions (80%), must be viewed as preliminary. It is clear, however, that thymosin is a safe drug which to date has not been associated with any known adverse effects. A Phase III, multicenter study is now in its concluding stage and should yield additional information on the efficacy of $T\alpha_1$ in the treatment of CHB.

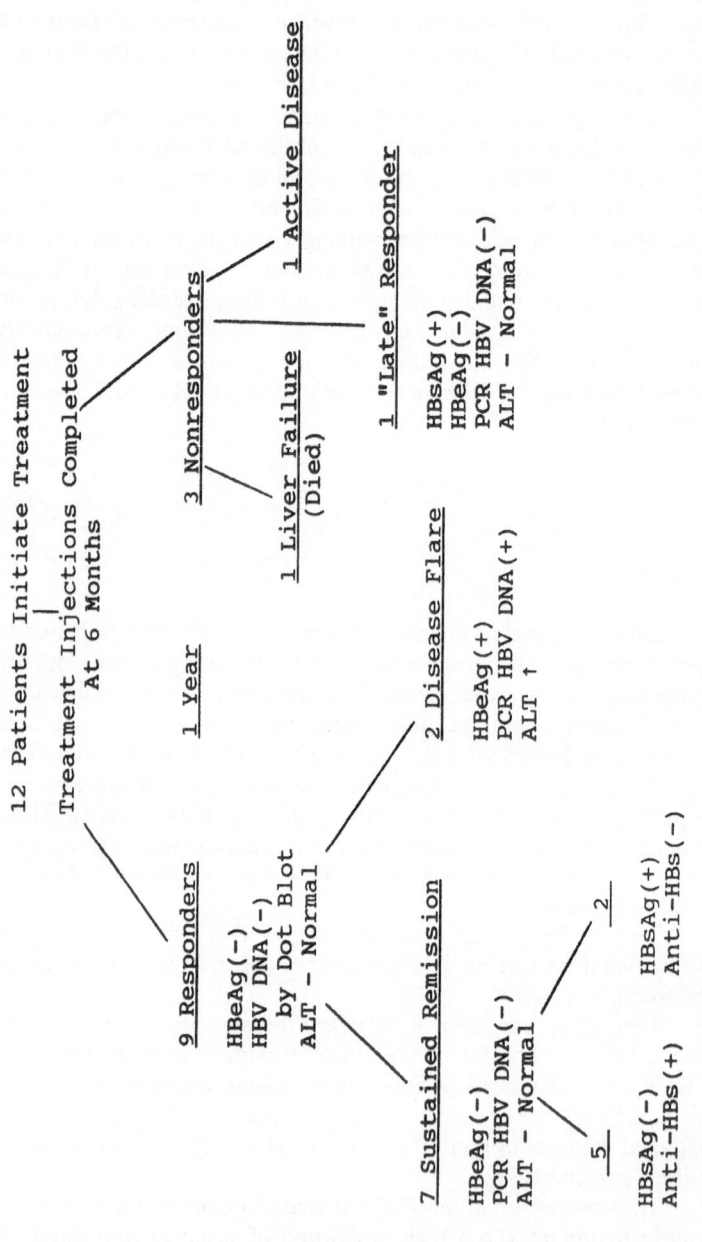

Figure 1. Response to Thymosin Treatment

REFERENCES

1. Davis GL: Chronic hepatitis. In: Kaplowitz N, ed. Liver and Biliary Diseases. Baltimore: Williams & Wilkins, 292-294, 1992
2. Korenman J, Baker B, Waggoner J, et al: Long-term remission of chronic hepatitis B after alpha-interferon therapy. Ann Int Med 114:629-634, 1991
3. Mutchnick MG, Appelman HD, Chung HT, et al: Thymosin treatment of chronic hepatitis B: A placebo-controlled pilot trial. Hepatology 14:409-415, 1991
4. Mutchnick MG, Cummings GD, Hoofnagle JH, Shafritz DA: Thymosin: An innovative approach to the treatment of chronic hepatitis B. In: Goldstein AL, Garaci E, eds. Combination Therapies. Biological Response Modifiers in the Treatment of Cancer and Infectious Diseases. New York: Plenum Publishing Corp., 149-156, 1992
5. Knodell RG, Ishak KG, Black WC, et al: Formulation and application of a numerical scoring system for assessing histological activity in asymptomatic chronic active hepatitis. Hepatology 1:431-435, 1981
6. Lieberman HM, LaBrecque DR, Kew MC, et al: Detection of hepatitis B virus DNA directly in human serum by a simplified molecular hybridization test: comparison to HBeAg/anti-HBe status in HBsAg carriers. Hepatology 3:285-291, 1983

COMBINATION ANTI-HIV THERAPY: QUESTIONS AND ANSWERS

Thomas C. Merigan

Center for AIDS Research
Stanford University School of Medicine, Stanford, California 94305

INTRODUCTION

It seems clear, given the ability of the HIV virus to produce variation in its structure, it's presently deeply imbedded nature in our population, and its chronic asymptomatic carriage, this virus is not going to be durably impacted upon by any single modality or type of individual agent. Instead, we must combine a number of approaches to control it within a given patient and in society as a whole. Combination therapy includes intelligent sequencing of drugs in the individual as well as concomitant administration. The principles covering this approach can be taken from control strategies with other chronic diseases (tuberculosis or cancers) as well as the special possibilities that evolve from the nature of this viral infection and our host responses to it. Insights in pathogenesis coming from the study of untreated and treated patients must govern rational selection of therapy. At present, only $CD4^+$ T cell level governs drug selection, whereas we must move to studies of an individual's virus and more details of the immune system responses in order to select the most appropriate immediate and longterm therapy.

This presentation will demonstrate wide differences in an individual's ability to mount these responses or for their virus to change to drug resistant reverse transcriptase genotypes associated with rapid disease progression in the face of therapy. Of course, before clinicians will accept such factors as important, one must be able to show that they influence the outcome of therapy and must be readily available to individual clinicians who are treating patients.

DISCUSSION

The last two years, we have completed a study on immunization of HIV seropositive individuals early in infection, that is when $CD4^+$ T cell levels are greater

Combination Therapies 2, Edited by A.L. Goldstein
and E. Garaci   Plenum Press, New York, 1993

than 400 CD4$^+$ T cell/mm^3 with recombinant HIV-1 gp160 vaccine or a control (hepatitis B vaccine). This study involved 52 patients, half of whom were seen at New York University and half at Stanford University. The results in these patients will be reported elsewhere (Valentine, et al. In preparation, 1992, Kundu et al, Submitted 1992). Those studies demonstrated an enhanced lymphocyte proliferation to an envelope antigen of HIV-1 in those receiving a range of gp160 dosages without concomitant rise in the response of patients receiving hepatitis B vaccine. In the Stanford group of patients, increases in two other important lymphocyte responses were documented which differed in the patients who received gp160 vaccine versus those receiving hepatitis B vaccine, that is the T helper cell responses namely, interferon gamma and interleukin-2 production on gp160 stimulation in vitro and HIV-1 envelope specific HLA class I and class II restricted cytotoxic T cell activities. Finally, in the group as a whole, in close relationship to the enhanced HIV specific proliferation and cytotoxicity, delayed type hypersensitivity to immunizing gp160 as measured by skin test reactivity was also enhanced in those who received gp160 vaccine versus those who received hepatitis B vaccine (Katzenstein, et al, in preparation, 1992). There was an apparent requirement for repeated immunization with proliferation response falling when immunization less frequently. It was interesting that a few of the patients before treatment had both skin test reactivity and proliferative responses to gp160 and that some of the patients after immunization did not show enhancement of both of these responses. Therefore, there are clearly individual differences in individual responses to both initial infection and to immunotherapy. This means that successful widespread use of immunotherapy or even proper staging of patients will require better insights into these responses and how they correlated with prognosis. Such insights will come from studies currently underway, which are controlled to look at the effect of enhancement of HIV envelope specific helper and cytotoxic and memory T cell responses to see if they are associated with long term protection against opportunistic infections, neoplasms and a reduction in virus load in the controlled trial (Redfield, Personal Communication, 1992).

My group has been interested in a new strategy for treatment of patients who are late in HIV infection, that is when CD4$^+$ T cells are less than 200 and above 50. We have been perfecting a schedule for intravenous injection of polyethylene-glycolated (PEG) interleukin-2, together with nucleoside therapy. In previous efforts, our group looked at recombinant interleukin-2 given with nucleoside therapy in early infection and noted striking CD4$^+$ and CD8$^+$ T cell elevations caused by the therapy (Swartz, 1991). When we studied the function of the CD4$^+$ and CD8$^+$ cells there appeared to be enhancement of both class I and II restricted HIV envelope specific cytotoxic responses. There is no evidence of increase in serum P24 or serum HIV RNA levels, or proviral DNA levels in CD4$^+$ cells as measured by PCR (Clark, G., 1992). On this basis, we decided to treat patients later in infection and when or other long acting interleukin-2 became available for clinical studies, we studied it acutely in patients at a range of disease stages to develop an optimum dosage and schedule. We found that one or three million units of PEG-IL-2 given every other week was capable of producing 25 to 50 CD4$^+$ T cell elevations /mm^3 in the circulation which could be sustained for many weeks (Wood, R., Submitted, 1992). Again, we observed enhancement of natural killer and HIV envelope specific HLA class I and II restricted cytotoxic T cell activities without enhanced HIV proviral levels. Because the three million dosage produced a greater response but yet was associated with reversible hypotension in up to 30% of our patients in the first few hours after injection, we thought it was useful to try and combine another agent with the one million unit dosage level to see if we could get further elevation from this lower dosage. We recently became aware of the thymosin alpha 1 work of Professor Garaci and associates in Rome and we are planning to evaluate whether it will further enhance our lymphocyte levels after PEG-IL-2.

There are questions as to whether enhanced lymphocyte levels by this methodology is just redistribution of lymphocytes from central sites to the peripheral circulation and hence, whether or not this approach will be associated with increased resistance to disease. We think that only if a safe regimen is evolved which can be tested against a control group in a randomized double-blind trial, can we determine whether these T cells will be capable of controlling opportunistic infections and cancers similarly to those produced by acute inhibition of HIV replication by nucleosides.

The third major direction my laboratory is pursuing is whether the dideoxy compounds with different cross resistance mechanisms initiated early in infection will prevent significant falls in CD4+ T cell levels. Recent work in our laboratory has demonstrated that presence of HIV with amino acid changes in position 215 in the HIV reverse transcriptase, which are selected for by AZT administration are associated with declining CD4$^+$ T cell levels (Kozal, M., Submitted, 1992). The lowered CD4$^+$ T cell level was associated with these changes in reverse transcriptase position 215, both in virion RNA in the circulation and proviral DNA within CD4$^+$ cells. The most interesting finding is that the RNA change precedes the same change in DNA by several months. It is as though virus replicating in deep sites gained entrance to circulation and ultimately this led to becoming the viral form most common in the CD4$^+$ T cell proviral DNA population which turned over less rapidly. As the appearance of the mutation was seen in the RNA at a high levels of CD4$^+$ T cell, it could be used to predict the CD4$^+$ T cell fall and hence could drive rational drug manipulation. However, we need data as to whether changes of drug at this point will prevent the subsequent CD4$^+$ T cell fall and that can only be seen with empiric trials. Fortunately, there are several ACTG and pharmacutical company sponsored trials which might give the answer to this question in the next few years. Another important question is whether combination antiviral therapy will prevent the appearance of the mutation. Again, several studies are underway with the addition of ddI and ddC to use them both early and late in infection in people to see if it will prevent the occurrence of this AZT selected mutation.

SUMMARY

Our laboratory is interested in development of new antiretrovirals mono and combination therapy as monitored by new methods for measurement of viral load, immunity and disease status. We are attempting to determine if there is a role for combination therapy within dideoxy compounds or with one given in combination with either specific (gp160) or non-specific (PEG IL-2) immunomodulators. We believe that such therapy needs to be individualized in each patient at least according to stage of disease and perhaps according to various host or viral factors.

We found that immunization of HIV seropositive individuals very early in infection (CD4+ T cells >400/mm^3) with HIV-1 envelope protein gp160 enhanced

HIV-1 envelope specific HLA class I and class II restricted cytotoxic T lymphocyte (CTL) activities as well as gp160 stimulated lymphocyte proliferation, and interferon gamma and interleukin-2 production in vitro as well as delayed type hypersensitivity to immunizing gp160 measured by skin test reactivity. Gp160 stimulation increased both function and number of HIV-1 envelope specific CTLs. The question remaining is whether immunoenhancement of specific helper and cytotoxic T cells will be associated with long term protection against opportunistic infections, neoplasms and/or reduction of virus load.

In regard to PEG IL-2 given late in HIV infection (when CD4+ T cells are less than 200), we observe up to 50% enhancement of $CD4^+$ T cell levels for many weeks if injections are continued. Again the same questions remains, will these T cells will be capable of controlling opportunistic infections and cancers?

Finally, the third major direction we are pursuing is whether dideoxy compounds with different cross resistance mechanisms initiated early in infection ($CD4^+$ T cell 200-500/mm²) will prevent significant falls in $CD4^+$ T cell levels. The presence of the amino acid changes at position 215 in reverse transcriptase provoked by AZT is associated with waning $CD4^+$ T cell levels and in fact, the presence of the mutation appears to precede the fall in $CD4^+$ T cells. The question remaining is whether combination antiviral therapy, that is either ddI or ddC in combination with AZT will prevent the appearance of the mutation. Several ACTG studies, including ACTG 175, are directed toward answering the latter question.

REFERENCES

Schwartz, D.H., Skowron, G. and Merigan, T.C., 1991, Safety and Effects of Interleukin-2 Plus Zidovudine in Asymptomatic Individuals Infected With Human Immunodeficiency Virus. Journal of Acquired Immune Deficiency Syndrome. 4:11-23.

A.G.B. Clark, Holodniy, M., Schwartz, D.H., Katzenstein, D.A. and Merigan, T.C., 1992, Decrease in HIV Provirus in Peripheral Blood Mononuclear Cells During Zidovudine and Human rIL-2 Administration. Journal of Acquired Immune Deficiency Syndrome, 5:52-59.

MECHANISMS OF DISEASE PROGRESSION AND CD4 DEPLETION IN HIV-1 INFECTION

F. Aiuti[1], E. Scala[1,] I. Mezzaroma[1], G.P. D'Offizi[1], R. Ferrara[1], G. Ricci[1], and F. Pandolfi[2]

[1]Department of Allergy and Clinical Immunology, University of Rome "La Sapienza", Viale Dell'Universita', 37, 00185 Rome, Italy
[2] Chair of Metodologia Clinica, Catholic University of Rome, Rome, Italy

INTRODUCTION

The pathogenesis of HIV (Human Immunodeficiency Virus) disease is still obscure and a central question is related to the mechanisms responsible for CD4 depletion. Two major groups of causes should be considered: those which are virus mediated and others which may be due to immune mechanisms.

HIV-type 1 is in part responsible for CD4 cell death due to ENV proteins that induce cell fusion of infected and uninfected cells. Fusion of these cells leads to the formation of multinucleated syncytia that ultimately die.[1] The cells expressing low levels of CD4 receptors appear less susceptible to this form of cell death. Other proposed, but less documented, mechanisms of cytopathicity induced by HIV-1 include high levels of viral replication with associated membrane injury, accumulation of unintegrated DNA, altered second-messenger production and changes in membrane permeability.[2,3] The amount of CD4 depletion induced by HIV virus varies during the stages of HIV infection and is correlated to the number of infected cells, to the virus particles and to the different strains of HIV-1. High cytopathic viruses are correlated with rapid CD4 cell decline.[4] Coinfection with other viruses such as HTLV-I, HTLV-II, HHV-6, CMV or mycoplasma may also accelerate the course of HIV infection and these conditions have also been considered as possible cofactors in the decline of CD4 cells.[2,5]

In addition to the viral cofactors, the time of progression from infection to full-blown AIDS is also influenced by host co-factors. Among these, we have recently investigated the role of age and found that younger infected subjects have a slower progression to AIDS than aged people.[6] On the contrary, the different categories at risk such as drug abusers, bi-sexuals, homosexuals are not relevant for HIV disease progression.[6]

Intriguing data have been obtained for hemophiliacs who show a low tendency to progression in contrast to HIV subjects infected by blood transfusion that have a higher tendency to develop AIDS in a short time.

The risk of Kaposi's sarcoma is present mainly in homosexuals or bi-sexuals and rarely in heterosexuals with a past history of sexual practices associated with fecal contact.[7,8] Genetic factors are also known to play a role and HLA-B7 is considered to be a negative prognostic factor, while HLA-A3 is associated with a less progressive course.[9]

THE ROLE OF THE IMMUNE SYSTEM

The immune system also plays an important role in the pathogenesis of HIV infection and in the mechanisms of CD4 lymphocyte depletion.

One mechanism that has been proposed to account for the loss of T helper function to recall antigens is that CD4+ cells expressing the memory phenotype are selectively lost in the first stages of HIV infection, whereas *naive* T cells usually remain functionally intact[10]. We also found that a small percentage of CD4 cells, negative both for *naive* and memory cell markers, are preserved until the last stages of HIV infection (R. Paganelli - unpublished observations). Other factors are implicated in the loss of T helper function. One important mechanism is represented by MHC restricted cytotoxic T cells (CTL) that kill HIV infected cells, but may also lyse the uninfected cells carrying the ENV gp120 on their membrane. These cytotoxic cells are also considered as important positive factors since they may control HIV replication. CTL are very efficient in the first stages of HIV disease and decline in patients with full-blown AIDS, before the increase of viral replication.[10]

Another important factor that could interfere with the T-cell receptor may be an autoantibody that has been detected in 35% of AIDS patients and in 5% of asymptomatic HIV positive individuals.[11] This antibody is directed against HIV gp41, a protein which shares homology with the non-polymorphic portion of the HLA class II molecules. Other autoantibodies are present in the sera of AIDS patients and may react with HIV infected CD4+ cells or inhibit mitogen induced T-cell proliferation.[12]

Both the TAT protein and the gp120 HIV products could be responsible for inhibition of T helper responses. In our experiments we found that gp120 at concentrations of 0.5-2 μg is responsible for inhibition of antigen driven proliferation of lymphocytes from HIV positive or negative subjects and T cell clones (O. Pontesilli, unpublished observations).

NK cells may also be inhibited by gp120 through interference with microtubule reorganization.[13] However, we believe that gp120 concentrations used in our and other experiments are rarely reached *in vivo*. Probably this occurs only in some tissues, such as lymphnodes, where HIV replication is very high. Soluble factors such as cytokines were also involved in AIDS pathogenesis and may play an important role in stimulating a latent or low level chronic HIV infection to full productivity. Induction of HIV expression by Granulocyte Monocyte Colony Stimulating Factor(GM-CSF) and other cytokines have been shown in acute HIV infection. There is evidence that Tumor Necrosis Factor (TNF)-alpha and monocyte-derived cytokines may play an important role in the pathogenesis of HIV infection. Folks et al.[14] showed that recombinant TNF-alpha and TNF-beta can augment HIV expression in cell lines. AIDS patients have been shown to express high levels of TNF- alpha in their sera. Since TNF-alpha is also known to function in the normal regulation of immune responses, it may play a role in the gradual progression of HIV disease.

TWO ADDITIONAL MODELS OF IMMUNE DEPLETION: SUPERANTIGENS AND APOPTOSIS

Two other models have been proposed to explain the destruction of CD4 cells. The first is related to the super antigen hypothesis. HIV-related super antigens may induce proliferation of T cells bearing specific T cell receptors followed by death and clonal depletion.[5]

The second hypothesis is related to virally induced programmed cell death or apoptosis which lead to cell death without proliferation.[15] According to Newell et al.,[16] T lymphocyte activation causes programmed cell death when the CD4 antigen is co-stimulated. Anti alpha-beta TCR receptor stimuli increase proliferative responses while anti immunoglobulin block proliferative responses and induces apoptosis. In addition Mittler et al.[17] described that gp120 and anti gp120 generate a block of T cell activation induced by an anti T cell receptor alpha-beta monoclonal antibody. We performed experiments with CD4 cells that were cultured in the presence of anti T cell receptor, staphylococcal enterotoxin B (SEB) and murine anti-Ig. According to previous data, we found that addition of anti CD4 and anti immunoglobulin reduces activation obtained by anti T cell receptor. In contrast, we could not confirm the inhibitory effect of CD4 cross- linking by anti CD4 on activation induced by SEB (M. Fiorilli et al, unpublished observations). Other experiments using gp120 also failed to show inhibitory effects of CD4 cross-linking on the activation of these cells by anti TCR. We conclude that the binding of CD4 and of gp120 (or the multivalent cross-linking of CD4 by gp120 and anti gp120 polyclonal antibodies) does not seem to modify the proliferative response to anti TCR antibody or super antigen.

Another important factor accounting for CD4 depletion and for total lymphopenia during HIV infection may be represented by the high spontaneous mortality rate (MR) of T cells in HIV infected individuals as suggested by Montagnier.[5] The MR of HIV infected individuals is significantly increased in vitro in comparison to normal subjects. In our experiments,[18] we confirmed that the mean percentage of cell death in HIV patients range is between 30-50% in different experimental conditions in contrast to 8-10% in normal subjects. The mortality rate increases in the last stage of AIDS, and also in subjects with a number of CD4 cells in vivo below 400/mm³. We also evaluated if several known cytokines may reduce the spontaneous MR in vitro. Only IL-2 and fibroblast cell derived factors (FDF)[19] were capable of reducing the percentage of dead cells in vitro.

To study the role played by apoptosis in T-cell death of HIV derived peripheral cells, we evaluated the low MW fragmentation of DNA characteristic of apoptosis.[18] Apoptosis was observed in about 50% of cases and it is more frequent in cells derived from patients with advanced disease. Of course apoptosis is not the only mechanism of T cell death. Other models have been reported. These include the selective depletion of T cells expressing a defined set of Vβ sequences,[20] but these data have not been confirmed by other groups (Wigzell H. and Essex M. separate personal communications). Thus, the mechanisms leading to T-cell depletion are not yet completely understood.

CONCLUSIONS

In conclusion: 1) HIV plays an important role in the pathogenesis of HIV disease and CD4 depletion especially at sites where it is actively replicating. 2) Autoimmune mechanisms, programmed cell death and super antigens may also play a significant (but still poorly understood) role. 3) CTL play a role in controlling HIV-1 replication, but after several years, the beneficial activity of the immune system declines and there are not enough new cytotoxic T cell clones to control the escape of viral mutants. In this regard we believe that the administration of vaccines in seropositive subjects (therapeutical vaccine),[21] may be useful for increasing and inducing specific cell-mediated immunity, thus contributing to delay the progression of CD4 depletion. All the available experiments both in monkeys and in humans, demonstrate that recombinant gp120 or gp160 vaccines are safe. The answer to the question whether these vaccines are useful in protection of HIV transmission and for the control of the progression of HIV disease lies in the future.

ACKNOWLEDGMENTS

This study was supported in part by a grant from the Istituto Superiore di Sanita' (Ministero della Sanita') n. 7204-01 and in part by the World Laboratory Project 1991-92.

REFERENCES

1. J. Sodroski, W.G. Goh, C. Rosen, K. Campbell, W.A. Haseltine. Role of the HTLV-III/LAV envelope in syncytium formation and cytopathicity. Nature. 322:470 (1986).
2. W.C.Greene. The molecular biology of human immunodeficiency virus type 1 infection. N.Engl. J. Med. 324:308 (1991).
3. J.A. Levy, L.S. Kaminsky, W.J. Marrow, K. Steinerk, P. Lucw, D.Dina, J. Maxie, L. Oshiro. Infection by the retrovirus associated with the acquired immunodeficiency syndrome. Clinical, biological and molecular features. Ann. Int. Med. 103:694 (1985).
4. A.S. Fauci. The human immunodeficiency virus: infectivity and mechanisms of pathogenesis. Science 239:617 (1988).
5. L. Montagnier, M.L. Gourgeon, R. Olivier, S. Garcia, C. Dauguet, M. Adams, J.M. Bechet, D. Guetard, A. Laurent, A. Hovanessian, M. Kirstetter, R. Roue, G. Pialoux, B. Dupont. Factors and Mechanisms of AIDS pathogenesis. In Science challenging AIDS. G.B. Rossi, E. Beth-Giraldo, L. Chieco-Bianchi, F. Dianzani, C. Giraldo, P. Verani Eds. S. Karger, Basel (1991).
6. G. Rezza, A. Lazzarin, G. Angarano, F. Aiuti. Risk of AIDS in HIV seroconverters: a comparison between intravenous drug users and homosexual males. Eur. J. Epidemiol. 6: 101 (1991).

7. V. Beral, D. Bull, S. Darby, I. Weller, C. Carne, M. Beecham, H. Jaffe. Risk of Kaposi's sarcoma and sexual practices associated with faecal contact in homosexual or bisexual men with AIDS. Lancet 1,339, (1992).
8. J.W. Curran, H.W. Jaffe, A.M. Hardy, R.M. Selik, T.J. Dondero. Epidemiology of HIV infection and AIDS in the United States. Science 239: 610 (1988).
9. Z.F. Rosenberg, A.S. Fauci. The immunopathogenesis of HIV infection. Advances in Immunology. 47: 377 (1989).
10. G.M. Shearer, M. Clerici. Early T-helper cell defects in HIV infection. AIDS. 5:245 (1991).
11. H. Golding, F.A. Robey, F.T. Gates, W. Londer, P.R. Bernning, T. Hoffman, B. Golding. Identification of homologous regions in human immunodeficiency virus I, gp41 and human MHC class II, beta 1 domain. I. Monoclonal antibodies against the gp41-derived peptide and patients'sera react with native HLA class I antigens suggesting a role for autoimmunity in the pathogenesis of acquired immune deficiency syndrome. J. exp. Med. 167:914 (1988).
12. B. Dorsett, W. Cronin, V. Churma, H.L. Ioachin. Anti-lymphocyte antibodies in patients with the acquired immunedeficiency syndrome. Am. J. Med. 78: 621-6 (1985).
13. M.C. Sirianni, S. Soddu, W. Marorini, G. Arancia, F. Aiuti. Mechanism of defective natural killer cell activity in patients with AIDS is associated with defective distribution of tubulin. J. Immunol. 140, 2565 (1988).
14. T.M. Folks, K.A. Clause, J. Justement, A. Robson, E. Duh, J.M. Kehrl, A.S. Fauci. Tumor necrosis factor alpha-induced expression of human immunodeficiency virus in a chronically infected T cell clone. Proc. Natl. Acad. Sci. USA 86: 2365 (1989).
15. J.C. Ameisen, A. Capron. Cell dysfunction and depletion in AIDS: the programmed cell death hypothesis. Immunol. Today 12: 102 (1991).
16. M.K. Newell, L.J. Haughn, C.R. Meran, M.H. Julius. Death of mature T cells by separate ligation of CD4 and the T-cell receptor for antigen. Nature 347: 286 (1990).
17. R.S. Mittler, M.K. Hoffman. Synergism between HIV gp120 and gp120-specific antibody in blocking human T cell activation. Science 245: 1380 (1989).
18. F. Pandolfi, A. Oliva, G. Sacco, V. Polidori, D. Liberatore, I. Mezzaroma, A. Giovannetti, J.T. Kurnick, F. Aiuti. Fibroblast-derived factors preserve viability in vitro of mononuclear cells isolated from subjects with HIV-1 infection. AIDS 7:323 (1993).
19. A. Scott, F. Pandolfi, J.T. Kurnick. Fibroblasts mediate T cell survival: A proposed mechanism for retention of primed T cells. J. Exp. med. 172, 1873 (1990).
20. L. Imberti, A. Sottini, A. Bettinardi, M. Puoti, D. Primi. Selective depletion in HIV infection of T cells that bear specific T cell receptor V beta sequences. Science 254: 860 (1991).
21. Redfield R, Birx D.L., Ketter N. A phase one evaluation of the safety and immunogenecity of vaccination with recombinant gp160 in patients with early human immunodeficiency virus infection. N. Engl. J. Med. 324:1783 (1991).

COMBINED THERAPY WITH ZIDOVUDINE, THYMOSIN α1 AND α-INTERFERON

IN THE TREATMENT OF HIV-INFECTED PATIENTS

Enrico Garaci[1], Giovanni Rocchi[2], Luigi Perroni[3], Cartesio D'Agostini[1], Fabrizio Soscia[3], Antonio Mastino[1], Sandro Grelli[1], Carlo Federico Perno[1], and Cartesio Favalli[1]

[1]Department of Experimental Medicine and Biochemical Sciences, University of   Rome "Tor Vergata", Via O. Raimondo 00173 Rome, Italy

[2]Department of Public Health, University of Rome, "Tor Vergata"

[3]S. Maria Goretti Hospital, 04100 Latina, Italy

INTRODUCTION

Infection caused by human immunodeficiency virus (HIV) is characterized by the progressive emergence of a complex form of immune dysfunction in patients. However, the exact mechanisms by which HIV damages the immune system are still not fully understood. It is known that depletion of CD4+ cells and decline in CD8+ specific and natural killer aspecific cytotoxic functions are strictly connected with HIV-infection (1-3). Regarding to CD4+ cell depletion, it was considered, until recently, exclusively due to a direct cytopathic effect of the virus. However there is now growing evidence that other mechanisms could be involved. Among them, autoimmune disorders could play a role (4). Moreover apoptosis of lymphocytes seems to be involved in CD4+ cell depletion (5). Finally, not only the quantitative fall in CD4+ cells but also their functional impairment, characterizes the immunodeficiency caused by HIV-infection. This impairment is partly explained by the reduction of cytokine production, particularly IL-2 (6), and appears to be, at least in part, independent of the decline in the CD4+ cell count. In fact the decrease in cellular immune functions (measured as IL-2 production) precedes a significant reduction in CD4+ cell number by at least 12 months (7,8).

Combination Therapies 2, Edited by A.L. Goldstein
and E. Garaci   Plenum Press, New York, 1993

TABLE 1. Effect of combination treatment in vitro with thymosin α1 and interferon on cytotoxicity in PBMC from HIV seronegative or seropositive volunteers.[a]

	% NORMALIZED CYTOTOXICITY (MEAN ± S.D.)[b]			
	IN VITRO TREATMENT			
	Control	Tα1	IFN	Tα1+IFN
GROUP				
HIV- volunteers	100.0±15.6	89.3±15.3	124.9±20.7[c]	169.3±4.7[d]
HIV+ volunteers	100.0±26.0	99.1±32.0	147.7±27.1[e]	174.6±48.0[f]

a) Separated peripheral blood mononuclear cells from 10 HIV seronegative or seropositive volunteers were cultured (2 x 10.6/ml in 1ml/well) in complete culture medium alone (control) or in complete medium with addition of thymosin α1 (Tα1, 100 ng/ml), interferon-α (IFN, 500 units/ml) or both (Tα1+IFN).
b) Cytotoxicity against K-562 cells was tested after 24 hrs of culture with a 4 hr ^{51}Cr release assay. Results are expressed as mean values per group calculated from individual values of cytotoxicity obtained for each patient from quadruplicate wells at effector/target ratio of 50:1 ± S.D as follows:

$$\frac{\text{\% cytotoxicity treated culture}}{\text{\% cytotoxicity control culture}} \times 100$$

Statistics by paired Student's t-test: c, P=0.0025 against control; d, P=0.0018 against control and P=0.0169 against IFN; e, P=0.0001 against control; f, P=0.0001 against control and P=0.0156 against IFN.

The availability of drugs able to efficiently inhibit HIV replication in vitro as well as in vivo has resulted in the increase of the median survival of HIV infected patients (9-11). But antiretroviral therapy, even in combination with other drugs able to counteract opportunistic infections, does not appear to provide long-term efficacy. Zidovudine (AZT), for example, delays disease progression, but seems to have minimal effect on the decline of immunologic functions. In addition a number of studies show that antiviral therapy is made vain by the appearance of drug-resistant HIV-strains (12,13). As a consequence, the use of agents able to restore immune responses should be considered in association with antiretroviral drugs. In fact, restored immune activity is important both in avoiding opportunistic infections and tumors, and in destroying HIV infected cells. On the other hand the use of antiretroviral therapy is important to avoid the possibility of the HIV virus, released by lysed cells, infecting other non infected cells.

Our previous studies demonstrated the high immunopotentiating efficacy of combination therapy with thymosin α 1 (Tα1) plus interferon in experimental animal models of immunodepression (14-16). We have thus decided to examine the potential beneficial effects of this combination immunotherapy in association with AZT on HIV-infection.

IN VITRO PRELIMINARY STUDIES

Before testing the effects of combination therapy with Tα1 and IFN in association with AZT in HIV-infected patients, we have performed a series of experiments in order to answer the following questions: i) does combination treatment with Tα1 and IFN in vitro exert a restoring activity on cytotoxicity of lymphocytes collected from HIV patients similar to that observed in animal models? ii) does combination treatment with Tα1 and IFN modify HIV replication in untreated or AZT-treated lymphocytes in vitro?

Results, reported in table 1, showed that pretreatment with Tα1 was able to significantly potentiate the cytotoxic activity of IFN-α stimulated peripheral blood mononuclear cells (PBMC) collected from HIV-positive patients. PBMC from healthy controls also responded to Tα1 pretreatment. Treatment with Tα1 alone exerted no effect on NK activity in both groups. In contrast, treatment with IFN alone was able to stimulate the cytotoxic activity of cells collected from healthy donors, as expected, as well as from HIV-patients. Also under the experimental conditions utilized in our studies we observed an impairment of NK activity associated to HIV infection, which had been previously described by other authors when tested on fresh PBMC. Interestingly, in vitro pretreatment with Tα1 of PBMC collected from HIV-patients was able to increase the IFN-induced cytotoxic activity to levels which were higher than those observed in PBMC from healthy donors when stimulated by IFN-α alone, showing a complete restoration of the NK cell responses to this cytokine.

Table 2 shows the results of combination treatment with Tα1, IFN-α and AZT on HIV replication, when tested as viral antigen production in the supernatants, by human primary cultures of PBMC infected in vitro with HIV. Data indicate that AZT exerted its well known antiviral effect when used as single agent, while no or very low antiviral effects were exerted by Tα1 or IFN-α at sub-optimal doses, when used as single agents or in combination. The addition of Tα1 or IFN-α or both to AZT treatment only modified slightly the antiviral action of this drug. The results of these experiments showed that a combination treatment with Tα1 in vitro did not potentiate the direct antiviral activity of IFN-α at a sub-optimal dose, whether associated or not with AZT. On the other hand, no evident negative interference with the direct antiviral activity of AZT was observed following Tα1 and IFN-α treatment when used alone or in combination, thus opening the way to their potential use in association in vivo in HIV-patients.

EFFECTS OF COMBINATION TREATMENT WITH THYMOSIN α1, IFN-α AND AZT ON HIV-INFECTED PATIENTS

We have thus started a pilot clinical study on the effects of combination treatment with Tα1, IFN-α and AZT in HIV-infected patients. In this report we present some of the results after one year. The cohort of the enrolled patients

TABLE 2. Effects of zidovudine alone or in combination with Ta1 and/or IFN-α[a] on HIV replication in vitro.

TREATMENT[b]	% VIRAL YIELD[c]	
	No AZT	Plus AZT
Control	100 ±13.5	17.6± 4.3
IFN-α	82.6± 8.6	7.0± 0.2
Ta1	96.9± 1.1	21.9± 0.6
Ta1+IFN-α	91.4±14.1	9.4± 1.8

a) Viral yield was evaluated after 12 day culture in IL-2 (10 U/ml) of PHA stimulated PBMC from healthy donor in vitro infected with HIV.
b) Drugs were added to the cultures every three days at the following concentrations: AZT 0.2 μM, Ta1 100 μg/ml, IFN-α 20 U/ml.
c) Results are expressed as mean values from triplicate cultures ± s.d., calculated as follows:

$$\frac{\text{p24 sample}}{\text{p24 control}} \times 100$$

The p24 concentrations were evaluated by a commercial kit.

was composed by forty subjects (23 M and 17 F, age 22-43) HIV seropositive. Of the forty patients, twenty-seven were drug abusers, 9 were homosexuals, and 4 were heterosexuals. Of the 4 heterosexual, 2 had sexual partners who were drug abusers. The study inclusion criteria for the patients was: 1) positive test for HIV, made by ELISA and confirmed by Western blot (Dupont de Nemours, Bruxelles, Belgium); age 18 or older; 2) CD4+ lymphocytes ranging from to 200 - 500/mmc; 3) CDC classes II or III; Karnosky >70; 4) no previous antiretroviral or immunomodulator treatment; and 5) normal hematologic, hepatic, renal, and coagulation function. Written informed consent was obtained from each patient. The subjects were randomly assigned to four groups which were homogeneous in terms of age, risk factors, and sex. After one year 28 patients had completed the cycle of treatment and were ready for evaluation. None of the individuals which did not complete the one-year cycle of treatment, equally distributed into the four groups (3 patients each), withdrew because of treatment-side effects, but rather due to either admission to therapeutic communities or their lack of compliance.

The first group received AZT 500 mg/day in two administrations; the second group AZT plus natural human lymphoblastoid interferon alpha (IFN-α, The Wellcome Foundation ltd.) 2 MU i.m. twice weekly; the third group AZT plus Ta1 (Sclavo Pharmaceuticals, Siena, Italy) 1 mg s.c. twice weekly ; the fourth group AZT plus Ta1 plus IFN-α. At entry and at intervals of 4 weeks the patients were evaluated by interviews, symptom questionnaire, physical examination, and by laboratory testing which included hematologic, immunologic and virologic studies. Laboratory evaluation included complete blood count with differential, platelet count, glucose, electrolytes, blood urea nitrogen, liver function test, cholesterol, triglycerides, coagulation profile, beta-2 microglobulin assayed by turbidimetric immunoassay. Virologic studies included determination of serum antibody by ELISA, polymerase chain reaction (PCR) assay (only at the end point of one year). Immunological studies included the phenotypic characterization of peripheral blood lymphocyte subpopulations by monoclonal antibodies and flow cytometry, and NK assay.

Regarding toxicity, no adverse effects or major toxicity were observed in any patient of any group, and none of the volunteers had to interrupt the treatment or reduce the dosage of drugs they were receiving. Also other biochemical parameters tested were not modified in any of the patients (data not shown). None of the patients progressed to AIDS during the treatment. Results shown in figure 1 indicate the absolute CD4+ cell counts at time 0 and after 3, 6 and 12 of the treatment in the patients which completed the one-year treatment cycle, expressed as change from baseline at time 0. CD4+ lymphocytes in the AZT group averaged from 382+61 (mean±S.D.) before treatment to 331+63 after 12 months. In the group receiving AZT and IFN-α, the CD4+ cell count changed from 396+98 to 392+140, and in the group receiving AZT and Tα1 cell count changed from 411+84 to 446+115. However, in all these groups of patients, CD4+ values at time 0 and after 12 months were not significantly different when tested by the paired Student's t-test. In contrast, in the group treated with AZT plus Tα1 and IFN-α, the CD4+ cell number averaged from 309+77 before treatment to 496+230 after 12 months, with a statistically significant difference (P value = 0.029 at paired Student's t-test). Moreover, the HIV-DNA analysis by PCR, performed only in patients belonging to the groups which received AZT alone or AZT plus combination treatment with Tα1 and IFN-α at the one-year end-point, demonstrated that the calculated number of viral copies per CD4+ cells was statistically significantly lower in the patients receiving the combined treatment (data not shown).

A smaller cohort of patients have been followed also after the one year end-point, considering that combination treatments did not cause any undesirable effect. Until now (24 months after the beginning of treatment), results confirm the trend previously observed, without any sign of adjunctive toxicity in patients which received immunotherapy in association with AZT and with a difference among patients receiving AZT plus Tα1 and IFN-α and those receiving all the other treatments which was even more evident than that observed after 12 months of therapy.

CONCLUSIONS

Our previous studies in the murine experimental model have shown that treatment with Tα1 followed by low doses of IFN-α was highly effective in restoring cytotoxic activities in animal models of immunosuppression induced by tumors, and/or cytostatic drugs (14-19). Here we show that a similar synergistic effect between Tα1 and IFN-α on cytotoxic activity can be observed in vitro in PBMC collected from HIV-infected patients. Moreover the results of a pilot clinical study demonstrate that neither Tα1 or IFN-α show significant side effects or toxicities when administered either as single agents with AZT or in combination. In addition the immunological monitoring of patients indicates that the combination of AZT+Tα-1+IFN-α seems to be more effective than AZT or AZT with either single agent alone in the control of CD4+ cell fall which is caused by HIV infection. At the one-year end-point, indeed, patients treated with a combination of AZT+Ta-1+IFN-α showed 61% increase in the absolute number of CD4+ cells, whereas in the group treated with AZT+Ta-1 alone it was 8% . There was no evident change in the group treated with AZT+IFN-α alone while a decrease of 13% in the CD4+ cells was observed in the group with AZT alone. Over the first six months of treatment with AZT and IFN-α there was demonstrated an increase in CD4+ cells but this effect declined in the following 6 months. It is not possible at moment to evaluate the effect of combination therapies versus AZT alone on disease progression since none of the patients in any of the groups has yet progressed to AIDS. However, the increase in the CD4+ cell number and the restoration of some immune functions, (parameters usually utilized for the prognosis of the progression of the

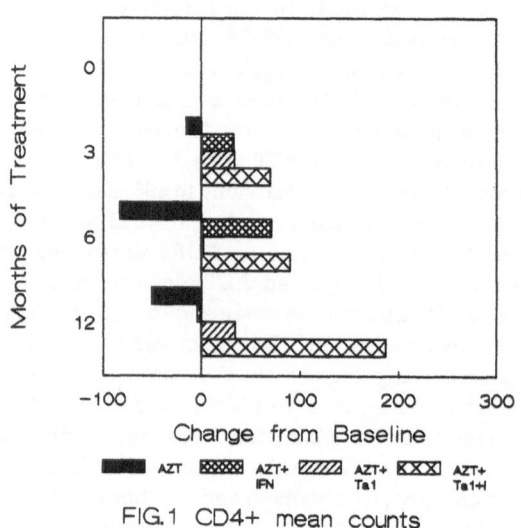

FIG.1 CD4+ mean counts

disease), in the group treated with AZT+Ta-1+IFN-α, is encouraging and suggests a possible beneficial impact on the disease. Regarding the mechanism of action of combination immunotherapy, the fact that we did not observe in vitro antiviral activity induced by either Ta1 IFN-α or by the combination of Ta1+ IFN-α, suggests an indirect effect mediated by an improvement in immune function. Thus it is reasonable to presume that combination therapy would potentiate the cytotoxic responses against HIV infected cells, as a result of the combined effect of the two cytokines. Moreover, Ta1 should exert a beneficial effect in inducing thymic maturation of the CD4+ population from more immature T-cell populations and in increasing production of IL-2 and αIFN from CD4+ mature cells.

In conclusion, our results although preliminary, suggest that the combination of AZT+Tα1+IFN-α was well tolerated for at least 24 months and was associated with a substantial and sustained increase in the number of CD4+ T cells. These data indicate the need for a controlled, double blind clinical trial in a larger cohort of patients, to assess the potential advantage and efficacy of the combination AZT+Tα1+IFN-α in comparison with groups of patients treated with AZT alone or with single agents. Such a multi-center trial has recently been initiated by the Ministry of Health of Italy.

ACKNOWLEDGEMENT

This work was supported by National Research Council (C.N.R.), Project "Prevention and Control of Disease" and by Healthy Ministry "AIDS Research Project".

REFERENCES

1. Fauci AC. The human immunodeficiency virus: infectivity and mechanism of pathogenesis. Science 1988; 239:617-623.

2. Bonovida B, Katz J, Gottlieb M. Mechanism of defective NK cell activity in patients with acquired immunodeficiency syndrome (AIDS) and AIDS-related complex. J Immunol 1986; 137:1157-1163.

3. Sherer GM, and Clerici M. How human immunodeficiency virus ravages the immune system. Curr Opin Immunol 1992; 4:463-465.

4. Via CS, Shearer GM. Autoimmunity and the acquired immune deficiency syndrome. Curr Opin Immunol 1989; 1:753-756.

5. Ameisen JC, Capron A. Cell dysfunction and depletion in AIDS: the programmed cell death hypothesis. Immunol Today 1991; 12:102-105.

6. Murray HW, Lane CH, et al. Impaired production of lymphokines and immune (gamma) interferon in the acquired immunodeficiency syndrome. N Eng J Med 1988; 310:883-889.

7. Lucey DR, Melcher GP, Hendrix CW, Zajac RA, Goetz DW, Butzin CA, Clerici M, Warner RD, Abbadessa S, Hall K, et al. Human immunodeficiency virus infection in the US Air Force: seroconversion assay to predict change in CD4+ T cell counts. J Infect Dis 1991; 164:631-637.

8. Shearer GM, Clerici M. Early T-helper cell defects in HIV-1 infection. AIDS 1991; 5:245-253

9. Fischi MA, Richman DD, Grieco MH, et al. The efficacy of azidothymidine (AZT) in the treatment of patients with AIDS and AIDS related complex: a double-blind, placebo controlled trial. N Engl J Med 1987; 317:185-191.

10. Graham NM, Zeger SL, Park LP, Vermund SH, Detels R, Rinaldo CR, Phair JP. The effects on survival of early treatment of human immunodeficiency virus infection. N Engl J Med 1992; 326:1037-1042.

11. Yarchoan R, Mitsuya H, Broder S. The immunology of HIV infection: implication for therapy. AIDS Res Hum Retroviruses 1992; 8:1023-1031.

12. Larder BA, Kelliam P, Kemp SD. Zidovudine resistance predicted by direct detection of mutation in DNA from HIV-infected lymphocytes. AIDS 1991; 5:137-144.

13. Larder BA, Coates KE, Kemp SD. Zidovudine-resistant human immunodeficiency virus selected by passage in cell culture. J Virol 1991 65:5232-5236.

14. Favalli C, Jezzi T, Mastino A, Rinaldi-Garaci C, Riccardi C, and Garaci E. Modulation of natural killer activity by thymosin alpha 1 and interferon. Cancer Immunol Immunother 1985; 20:189-192

15. Favalli C, Mastino A, Jezzi T, Grelli S, Goldstein AL, and Garaci E . Synergic effect of thymosin alpha 1 and alpha- beta interferon on NK activity in tumor-bearing mice. Int J Immunopharmac 1989; 11: 443-450

16. Garaci E, Mastino A, Pica F, Favalli C. Combination treatment using Thymosin α 1 and interferon after cyclophosphamide is able to cure Lewis lung carcinoma in mice. Cancer Immunol Immunother 1990; 32:154-160

17. Garaci E, Mastino A, Favalli C . Enhanced immune response and antitumor immunity with combinations of biological response modifiers. Bull N Y Acad Med 1989; 65:111-119

18. Garaci E, Pica F, Mastino A, Palamara AT, Belardelli F, and Favalli C. Antitumor effect of thymosin α1/interleukin-2 or thymosin α1/interferon α,β following cyclophosphamide in mice injected with highly metastatic friend erythroleukemia cells. J Immunother 1992.

19. Favalli C, Mastino A, Grelli S, Pica F, Rasi G, and Garaci E. Rationale for therapeutic approaches with thymosin α 1, interleukin 2 and interferon in combination with chemotherapy. In: Goldstein AL and Garaci E, ed. Combination Therapies. New York: Plenum Press, 1992: 275-281.

THE PROBLEM OF INTERFERON SPECIES APPEARING IN PATIENTS WITH AUTOIMMUNE DISEASES

Ladislav Borecky[1], Vladimír Lackovic[1], Peter Kontsek[1], Norbert Fuchsberger[1] , Miroslav Kubes[1] and Jozef Rovensky[2]

[1]Institute of Virology, Slovak Academy of Sciences, Bratislava and
[2]Research Institute of Rheumatic Diseases, Piestany, Czechoslovakia

The appearance of interferon (IFN) in the serum of patients with AIDS, SLE, Argentinian hemorrhagic fever, bacterial meningitis etc. usually signalizes the beginning of an adverse phase of disease (see De Maeyer and De Maeyer-Guignard, 1988 etc). This led us to studies attempting to clarify whether the reported IFN activities in such cases were mediated by a structurally deviating ("pathological") or, "normal" IFN-species (Borecky et al., 1989). The diseases where such IFNs were found were often autoimmune (SLE, etc) or chronic with autoimmune components (AIDS, Down syndrome etc), and, the reported IFN activities were marked by thermo- and acid-lability (Preble et al., 1982; Eyster et al., 1983; Funa et al., 1984 etc).

In collaboration with the Institute of Rheumatic Diseases in Piestany, we studied cohorts of patients with systemic lupus erythematosus (SLE). SLE is a disease with growing incidence and chronic undulating course with alternating exacerbations and remissions (Ferrel and Tan, 1985). In our cohort of SLE patients, the presence of IFN was detected in about 15% of tested sera (Table 1). The average level (titer) of IFN was in general low, seldom exceeding 35 units per ml. In accordance with other studies (Abb, 1985, etc), the presence of IFN-activity in the sera coincided more or less with the clinical grade of disease.

The detected IFN activity usually reacted with the polyclonal anti-IFN alpha serum, however, the end-point of neutralization was seldom clear-cut. Also, the presence of IFN-like activity in the sera of patients was not persistent (Table 2).

Combination Therapies 2, Edited by A.L. Goldstein
and E. Garaci Plenum Press, New York, 1993

Table 1. Presence of IFN or Anti-IFN in sera of SLE patients.

	Healthy controls	SLE patients
Number of examinees	25	70
IFN positive	0	10
in %	0	14,3
Geometric mean of units/ml	8	36,5
Anti-IFN positive	0	13
in %	0	15,7

The antiviral test was used for IFN detection.

Table 2. Appearance and disappearance of IFN-alpha and Anti-IFN-alpha in sera of 4 SLE patients.

Test No.	Patients							
	G. A.		M. E.		M. M.		A. R.	
	IFN	A-IFN	IFN	A-IFN	IFN	A-IFN	IFN	A-IFN
1.	16	-	‹8	+	‹8	-	‹8	+
2.	‹8	+	‹8	-	16	-	‹8	-
3.	‹8	-	16	-	‹8	+	16	-
4.	32	-			16	-	‹8	+

A-IFN +: Neutralizing activity present.

In approximately the same percentage of patients that were found previously IFN positive, an IFN-neutralizing factor (named Anti-interferon) could be found during the period of IFN absence. In contradistinction to IFN, the anti-IFN activity was thermostable. We speculated that it might participate on the removal of IFN activity from the serum of IFN-negative patients. However, except of polypetide character, its biochemical properties remain at present unknown.

Next, the question was asked whether the SLE-IFN might exert some modulating effect on other reactive systems present in the organism. When compared with NK-cells in healthy controls or in the blood of IFN-negative patients, the activity of NK-cells in IFN-positive patients was depressed. The defect of SLE-NK cells seems to lay in inability to produce and release an unknown cytolytic factor that normally mediates the effect of NK-cells on target cells (Fig. 1).

In accordance with other studies, the SLE patients have also a depressed IL-1 and IL-2 system (Sibbit et al., 1983; etc) (Table 3).

In view of the problems encountered in isolation of IFN from sera of SLE patients in purified and sufficient amounts, in further studies a thermo- and acid-labile IFN fraction found by Chadha (1985) in normal human leukocyte IFN preparations was used. Such fractions (AL-IFN) can be obtained from the "A" peak of supernates of virus-stimulated

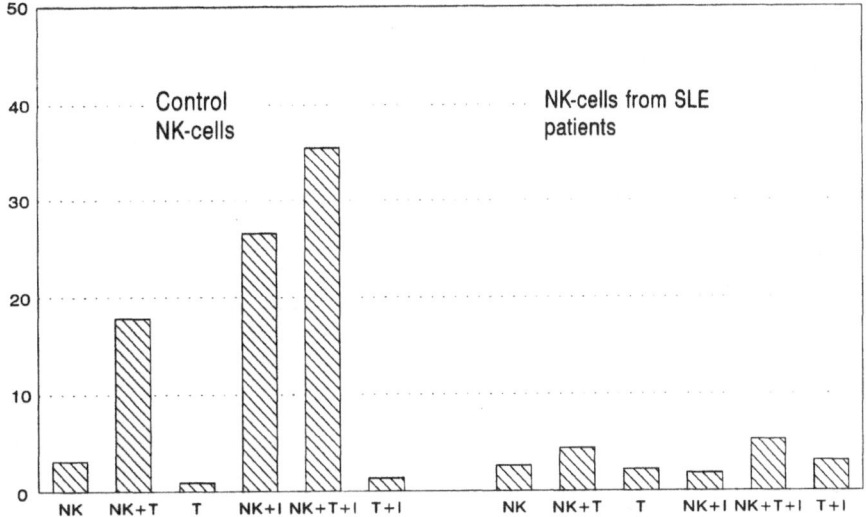

Fig.1. Inability of NK-cells from SLE patients to produce a cytotoxic factor after contact with K562 cells. The ratio of effector to target cells 20:1. After 18 hrs/36°C incubation, the cell-free supernate was added to target cells (K562) and the cytotoxocity was determined by 51 Cr release; T : K562 ; I : Interferon alpha (500 U per ml).

Table 3. NK-cell activity, IL-2 and IL-1 production in SLE patients.

Cohort	NK-cells (basal)	NK-cells after[1] IFN stimulation	Production (U/ml) IL-2[2]	IL-1[3]
Healthy control	59,3+17,4 (n=30)	67,7+15,2 (1,1) (n=30)	3,9+1,8 (n=7)	31,9+7,9 (n=8)
SLE - all	33,5+17,4 (n=50)	35,8+18,7 (1,1) (n=50)	1,5+1,0 (n=13)	5,6+8,6 (n=8)
SLE - IFN positive	25,5+11,3 (n=8)	24,8+7,5 (1,0) (n=8)	1,0+1,1 (n=6)	<1,0 (n=4)

[1] 500 U/IFN/ml. [2] PMBC (5.10^6 per ml) were stimulated with 25 ug/ml Con A for 24 hrs. [3] Adherent cells (10^6 per ml) were stimulated with 10 ug/ml LPS (E. coli OIII:B4) for 24 hrs.

human donor-cells after Sephadex chromatography, provided that the routine acidification of the IFN preparation was

omitted (Borecky et al., 1989) (Fig. 2). We succeded in
obtaining monoclonal antibodies with high specificity for
this fraction (AL-IFN).

The high specificity (selectivity) of monoclonal
antibodies against AL-IFN offered a partial explanation for
various interpretations concerning the type of SLE- and other
acid- and thermolabile interferons. As shown in Table 4, in
contradistinction to the specific monoclonal antibody against
AL-IFN, the polyclonal antisera may show a partial crossreaction between the specific (IFN-alpha or IFN-gamma)
antigens and AL-IFN. This may happen when they contained in
immunizing preparations, in addition to the "main" antigens
also "minor", non-removed IFN-antigens such as AL-IFN. This
raised the possibility that the "atypical" AL-IFN may
represent a new subtype of IFN family or, a new cytokine with
antiviral activity.

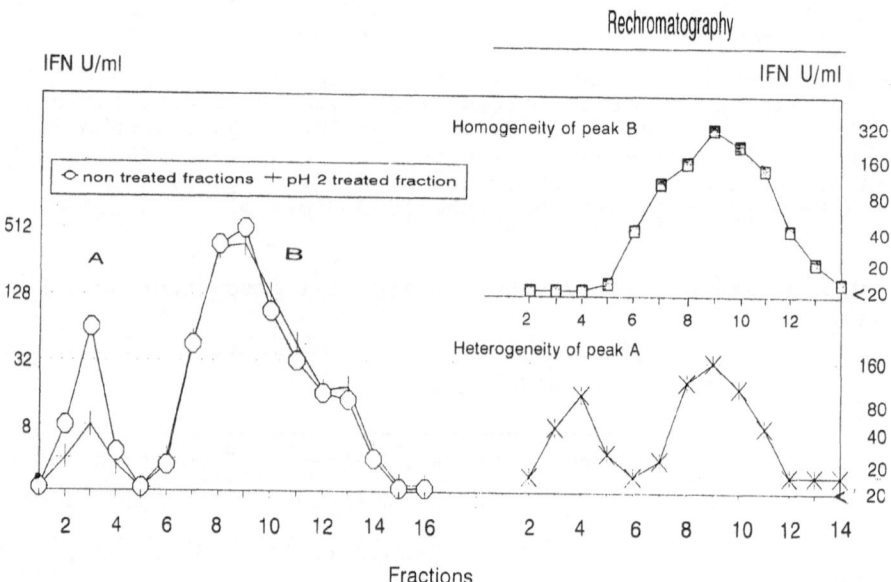

Fig.2. Complexity of peak A obtained after gel filtration of
human leukocyte IFN alpha

However, by courtesy of Dr. G. Bodo from Boehringer Co.
in Vienna, we recently included in our control tests a sample
of recombinant human IFN-omega 1, together with its specific
monoclonal antibody (Adolf, 1990). The employment of this
"new" IFN antigen has influenced the interpretation of the
AL-IFN problem.

As shown on Fig. 3, IFN-omega 1 and AL-IFN were cross-
neutralized by the two types of specific monoclonal
antibodies in a dose dependent manner. Since the monoclonal
antibody against AL-IFN showed also a partial neutralization
of the non-purified HIV-induced IFN (produced by CEM cells)
and/or serum with the SLE-IFN, these results suggest their

relatedness to IFN-omega 1. However, these results need further confirmation. Also, the acid- and thermolability of IFNs tested proved a rather non-reliable marker.

Table 4. Neutralization of antiproliferative activity ofvarious interferons in HL-60 cells with various anti-IFN antibodies

IFN species 100 U/ml	Neutralization[1] by:							
	Monoclonal antibodies to (ug per ml)				Polyclonal antibodies to (Dilutions)			
	AL-IFN alpha	IFN alpha	IFN beta	IFN gamma	AL-IFN alpha	IFN alpha	IFN beta	IFN gamma
AL-IFN	0,15	>10	>10	>10	10^{-4}	$>10^{-1}$	$>10^{-1}$	2.10^{-2}
IFN alpha	>10	0,2	>10	>10	10^{-3}	10^{-4}	$>10^{-1}$	$>10^{-1}$
IFN beta	>10	>10	0,3	>10	$>10^{-1}$	$>10^{-1}$	10^{-4}	$>10^{-1}$
IFN gamma[2]	>10	>10	>10	0,1	$>10^{-1}$	$>10^{-1}$	$>10^{-1}$	10^{-4}

[1]Amount (of Ig), or, dilution (of sera) which neutralizes 50% of antiproliferative activity of tested IFN. [2]10 units per ml of IFN-gamma were used in test.

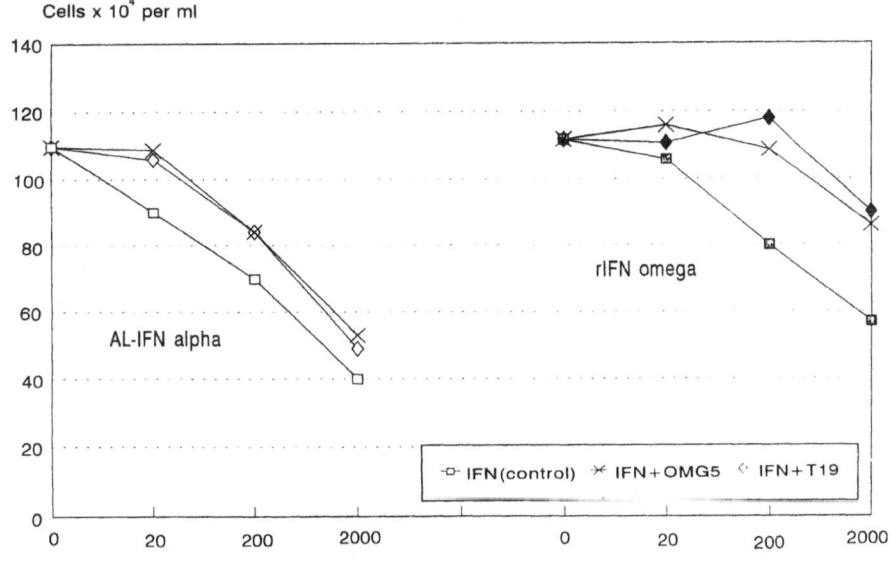

Fig.3. Crossreaction between Al-IFN and IFN-omega 1 in antiproliferative test

CONCLUSION

This studies support the view that, when produced in excess and acting outside of their normal cellular environment, IFNs and other cytokines may exert a deleterious effects in the organism (Gresser, 1982; Bocci, 1987; etc). They suggest that the SLE- and other AL-IFNs do not necessarily represent a deviating (atypical, "pathological") IFN alpha species but may be related to IFN-omega which is a less studied subtype of IFN-alpha family (Roberts et al., 1989; Adolf, 1990; etc). This view finds support a) in earlier reports that the pathological "TRI" inclusions can be reproduced also in vitro in Raji cells exposed to "normal" interferon beta (Rich, 1981); b) several reports found normal exogenous IFN accelerating the lupus-like disease of NZB/W mice (Engleman et al., 1981; etc); c) so far, no significant curative effect of IFN treatment was reported in autoimmune patients; and, finally, d) the acid and thermolability does not seem to be a reliable marker for differentiating "normal" and "pathological" IFNs.

REFERENCES

Abb, J.: Serum interferon and clinical manifestations of infection with human T-lymphotropic virus type III. Med. Microbiol. Immunol. 174/4, 205-210, 1985.

Adolf, G.R.: Monoclonal antibodies and enzyme immunoassays specific for human interferon (IFN) omega 1: Evidence that IFN-omega 1 is a component of human leukocyte IFN. Virology 175, 410-417, 1990.

Bocci, V.: Metabolism of protein anticancer agents. Pharmac. Ther. 34, 1-19, 1987.

Borecky, L., Kontsek, P., Novak, M., and Lackovic, V.: Human acid- and thermolabile interferon-like substance: selective reactivity with a monoclonal antibody. Antivir. Res.12, 195-204, 1989.

Chadha, K. C.: Acid labile human leukocyte interferon. In F. Dianzani and G.B. Rossi (Eds.): The Interferon System, Raven Press, New York, 1985, pp. 35-41.

De Maeyer, E., and De Maeyer-Guignard, J.: In Interferons and Other Regulatory Cytokines, J. Wiley Interscience, New York, 1988.

Engleman, E.G., Sonnefeld, G., Dauphinee, M., Greenspan, J.S.,Tala, N., McDevitt, H.O., and Merigan, T.C.: Treatment of NZB/NZW F1 hybrid mice with Mycobacterium bovis strain BCG or type II interferon preparations accelerates autoimmune disease. Arthritis Rheum. 24, 1396-1402, 1981.

Eyster, .E., Goedert, J.J., Poon, M.Ch., and Preble, O.T.: Acid-labile alpha interferon: A possible preclinical marker for the acquired immunodeficiency syndrome in hemophilia. New Engl. J. Med. 309/10, 583-590, 1983.

Ferrel, P.B., and Tan, E.M.: Systematic Lupus Erythematosus. In Rose, N.R. and Mackay, J.R. (Eds.): The Autoimmune Diseases, Acad. Press, London, 1985, pp. 29-57.

Funa, K., Anneren, G., Alm, G.V., and Bjoksten, B.: Abnormal

interferon production and NK cell responses to
interferon in children with Down syndrome. Clin. Exp.
Immunol. 56/3, 493-500, 1984.

Gresser, I.: Can interferon induce disease? In I. Gresser
(Ed.):Interferon 4, Acad. Press, London, 1982, pp.95-127

Preble, O., Black, R.J., Friedman, R.M., Klippel, J.H., and
Vilcek, J.: Systemic lupus erythematosus: Presence in
human serum of an unusual acid labile leukocyte
interferon. Science 216, 429-431, 1982.

Rich, S.A.: Human lupus inclusions and interferon. Science
213, 772-775, 1981.

Roberts, H.M., Imakawa, K., Niwano, Y., Kazemi, M., Malathy,
P.V., Hansen, T.R., Glass, A.A., and Kronenberg, L.H.:
Interferon production by preimplantation sheep embryo.
J.Interferon Res. 9, 175-187, 1989.

Sibbitt, W.L., Mathews, P.M., and Bankhurst, A.D.: Natural
killer cell in Systemic lupus erythematosus. Defects in
effector lytic activity and response to interferon and
interferon inducers. J. Clin. Invest. 71, 1230-1239,
1983.

INDEX